# Ballantyne's Deafness

## Sixth edition

Edited by

JOHN GRAHAM, FRCS,

Royal National Throat, Nose and Ear Hospital, London

and

MIKE MARTIN, OBE,

The Mike Martin Consultancy, Sussex

W

WHURR PUBLISHERS

LONDON AND PHILADELPHIA

© 2001 Whurr Publishers

First published 2001 by
Whurr Publishers Ltd
19b Compton Terrace, London N1 2UN, England and
325 Chestnut Street, Philadelphia PA 19106, USA

Reprinted 2002

**British Library Cataloguing in Publication Data**
A catalogue record for this book is available from the
British Library.

ISBN: 1 86156 170 9

Printed and bound in the UK by Athenaeum Press Ltd,
Gateshead, Tyne & Wear

# Contents

## Chapter 16                                                          258

Psychological aspects of acquired hearing loss
*Laurence McKenna*

## Chapter 17                                                          272

Deafness and mental health
*Peter Hindley and Nick Kitson*

## Chapter 18                                                          288

Hearing aids
*Mike Martin*

## Chapter 19                                                          311

Cochlear implants
*Huw Cooper*

## Chapter 20                                                          232

Implantable hearing aids
*Anders Tjellström*

# Preface to the Sixth Edition

It is a common observation that with the retirement of a pioneer in any field, that individual will need to be replaced by a team of people. John Ballantyne wrote the first edition of this book more than 40 years ago – in 1960 – as a monograph, with a single author. This, the sixth edition, is written by 18 authors and with the encouragement of two editors.

This is the first edition of *Deafness* without the direct involvement of John Ballantyne himself, although the Ballantyne family continues to be represented by Deborah, John's daughter, who is among the list of authors. With this edition we have changed the title to *Ballantyne's Deafness* in acknowledgement of John Ballantyne's authorship and editorship over the past 40 years and with the intention of firmly identifying this and future editions as a continuation of his work.

From an otologist's point of view, the past 40 years have produced many changes. At the time of the first edition, Rosen's stapes mobilization procedure was the new treatment for otosclerosis, superseding fenestration. Myringoplasty involved skin grafting and it was five years since Zollner had published his observations on types of hearing conduction following tympanoplasty. For the audiologist, the pilot studies which eventually led to universal screening of the hearing of infants and young children in the UK had recently been published, but no objective electrophysiological tests of hearing were available. Trials of radiotherapy to shrink the adenoids had taken place and been discredited and grommets had not yet been suggested to treat middle-ear effusion. The first edition predicted immunization for rubella, advances in treatment for rhesus haemolytic disease of the newborn, further discussion between those advocating 'oralism' and signing in the education of deaf children, and the need for further work in determining aetiology in the congenitally deaf.

The first edition was intended to be read by those interested in deafness, those working in the field of deafness and those experiencing deafness and its consequences. It was a truly interdisciplinary book, intended to allow, for example, otologists, teachers of the deaf, public health audiologists and paediatricians to find out more about each others' activities in the field of deafness. It was also intended to be an introduction to the subject of deafness for non-professionals, for the families and friends of people with hearing loss, for members of professions not involved in deafness and for general medical practitioners.

The book's popularity was reflected in the need for four further editions: in 1970, 1977, 1984 and 1993. This sixth edition has consolidated some chapters, expanded others to keep up with fields such as cochlear, bone-conduction and middle-ear implants, and has brought in some new authors, with fresh insights into existing topics.

The preface to the fifth edition stated that the book was not intended to be a textbook of audiology, but rather 'a general introduction to this complex subject'. The aim of this edition is still to occupy the middle ground between that of the newcomer to the field of deafness and that of the established expert; it is also intended to bridge the widening gap between each of the diverging paths by which current research continues to advance. We also recognize that hearing and deafness are part of the wider field of human communication and that this field has expanded well beyond the horizons that were visible 40, or even 14, years ago,

The editors are most grateful to a distinguished panel of authors for providing contributions of a uniformly high standard. We are confident that this sixth edition of *Ballantyne's Deafness* will successfully continue the aims set out by John Ballantyne when his book first appeared.

*John Graham*
*Mike Martin*
*May 2001*

# Contributors

**Patrick Axon**
Manchester Royal Infirmary
Manchester

**Deborah Ballantyne**
Istituto di Clinica ORL
Rome

**Martin Burton**
Oxford Hearing and Balance Centre
Radcliffe Infirmary
Oxford

**Ross Coles**
MRC Institute of Hearing Research
Nottingham

**Huw Cooper**
The Midlands Cochlear Implant Programme
Selly Oak Hospital
Birmingham

**Anne Duffy**
Hamilton Lodge School for the Deaf
Brighton

**Adrian Davis**
MRC Institute of Hearing Research
Nottingham

**John Graham**
Cochlear Implant Unit
Royal National Throat, Nose and Ear Hospital
London

**Valerie Hazan**
Department of Phonetics and Linguistics
University College London
London

**Jonathan Hazell**
The Tinnitus and Hyperacusis Centre
London

**Peter Hindley**
Deaf Child and Family Team
Springfield Hospital
London

**Nick Kitson**
Deaf Child and Family Team
Springfield Hospital
London

**Mike Martin**
The Mike Martin Consultancy
Loxwood
West Sussex

**Laurence McKenna**
Royal National Throat Nose and Ear Hospital
London

**Richard Ramsden**
Manchester Royal Infirmary
Manchester

**James Robinson**
Gloucester Royal Hospital
Gloucester

**Anders Tjellström**
Department of Otolaryngology
Sahlgren's Hospital
Göteborg

**Peter Watkin**
Audiology Department
Whipps Cross Hospital
London

**Tony Wright**
Institute of Laryngology and Otology
London

# List of abbreviations

| | |
|---|---|
| AABR | automated auditory brainstem response |
| AAOHNS | American Academy of Otolaryngology – Head & Neck Surgery |
| ABI | auditory brainstem implant |
| ABLB | alternate binaural loudness balance |
| ABR | auditory brainstem response |
| ACE | advanced combination encoder |
| AGC | automatic gain control |
| AIP | Adult Implant Profile |
| ALD | assistive listening device |
| AP | action potential |
| APR | auropalpebral reflex |
| ARHL | age-related hearing loss |
| BAHA | bone-anchored hearing aid |
| BDA | British Deaf Association |
| BEA | better ear average |
| BOA | behavioural observation audiometry |
| BSA | British Society of Audiology |
| BSER | brainstem-evoked response |
| BSL | British sign language |
| BTE | behind the ear (hearing aid) |
| BW | body worn (hearing aid) |
| CAP | compound action potential |
| CERA | cortical-evoked response audiometry |
| cf | critical frequency |
| ChIP | Children's Implant Profile |
| CI | confidence interval |
| CIC | completely in the canal (hearing aid) |
| CIS | continuous interleaved sampling |
| CM | coclear microphonic |
| CMV | cytomegalovirus |

| CNS | central nervous system |
|------|------------------------|
| CNV | contingent negative variation |
| COA | cervico-oculo-acoustic |
| CROS | Contralateral Routing of Signals |
| CSF | cerebrospinal fluid |
| CT | computerized tomography |
| dB | decibel |
| DC | direct current |
| DHA | District Health Authority |
| DPOAE | distortion product otoacoustic emission |
| EABR | electrically evoked auditory brainstem response |
| ECNL | equivalent continuous 8-hour noise level |
| ECochG | electrocochleography |
| ENT | ear, nose and throat |
| ERA | electric response audiometry |
| ESR | erythrocyte sedimentation rate |
| FM | frequency modulation |
| HIE | hypoxic ischaemic encephalopathy |
| HL | hearing level |
| HOH | hard of hearing |
| HPD | hearing protective device |
| HVDT | health visitors' distraction test |
| Hz | Hertz |
| IEC | International Electrotechnical Commission |
| IHC | inner hair cell |
| ISO | International Standardization Organization |
| ITC | in the canal (hearing aid) |
| ITE | in the ear (hearing aid) |
| LEA | local education authority |
| LDL | loudness discomfort level |
| LTASS | long-term average speech spectrum |
| MMR | measles, mumps and rubella |
| MRC | Medical Research Council |
| MRI | magnetic resonance imaging |
| NDCS | National Deaf Children's Society |
| NF1 | neurofibromatosis type 1 |
| NF2 | neurofibromatosis type 2 |
| NIHL | noise-induced hearing loss |
| NOHL | non-organic hearing loss |
| NSH | National Study of Hearing |
| OAE | otoacoustic emission |
| OAV | oculo-auriculo-vertebral |

| | |
|---|---|
| OHC | outer hair cell |
| OME | otitis media with effusion |
| OSPL | output sound pressure level |
| PAM | postauricular myogenic response |
| PCHI | permanent childhood hearing impairment |
| PET | positron emission tomography |
| PTS | permanent threshold shift |
| RCED | real ear-to-coupler difference |
| REAR | real ear-aided response |
| REIG | real ear-insertion gain |
| REIR | real ear-insertion response |
| RETSPL | reference equivalent threshold sound pressure level |
| REUR | real ear-unaided response |
| RNID | Royal National Institute for Deaf People |
| SAS | simultaneous analogue stimulation |
| SFOAE | stimulus frequency otoacoustic emission |
| SP | summating potential |
| SPL | sound pressure level |
| SR | stapedius reflex |
| SRT | speech recognition threshold/ stapedius reflex threshold |
| SVR | slow vertex response |
| TEOAE | transient evoked otoacoustic emission |
| TRT | tinnitus retraining therapy |
| TTS | temporary threshold shift |
| UCL | uncomfortable loudness level |
| UNS | universal neonatal screening |
| VRA | visual reinforcement audiometry |
| WHO | World Health Organization |

# Chapter 1
# Deaf and hard of hearing people

## Mike Martin

The dictionary defines 'deaf' and 'deafness' as 'wholly or partly without hearing', and for most people who have no direct connection with deaf people that is a full enough description. However, that definition does not indicate the problems that arise from deafness.

To understand the problems caused by deafness it is important to view the effects of deafness on what Peter Denes (Denes and Pinson 1993) calls the 'Speech Chain' (Figure 1.1). This emphasizes the fact that deafness has an overall effect on human communication in all aspects of life. Helen Keller (1910), probably the most famous deaf blind woman and the subject of the play and film *The Miracle Worker*, wrote that:

> I am just as deaf as I am blind. The problems of deafness are deeper and more complex, if not more important, than those of blindness. Deafness is a much worse misfortune. For it means the loss of the most vital stimulus – the sound of the voice that brings language, sets thoughts astir and keeps us in the intellectual company of man.

This statement reinforces the dramatic effects of deafness on the Speech Chain and hence human communication.

Figure 1.1 shows the Speech Chain and provides a basis for understanding why deafness affects the development of speech and language and the reason why oral and, in some cases, written communication is affected. The importance of this concept is that, as with all chains, it is only as strong as the weakest link. Consequently, in the case of deafness, the weak link is the ear (the auditory system), which, if damaged, has a knock-on effect on the whole communication process.

Communication must also be seen as going beyond speech and must include the awareness and use of sound for determining all aspects of the environment we live in.

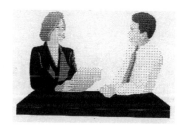

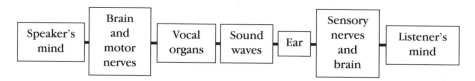

| Speaker's mind | Brain and motor nerves | Vocal organs | Sound waves | Ear | Sensory nerves and brain | Listener's mind |

**Figure 1.1:** The Speech Chain.

# Terminology

A considerable number of different terms are used to describe people who have a hearing loss. Indeed, in this and other chapters, words such as deaf, hearing impaired, hard of hearing, etc., may be used in a range of different ways. The terms are not always exclusive to a particular group and often there is a need to be careful as to whether a word is used in a technical or a general sense. Some words used in a technical sense actually give offence to deaf individuals.

We can start at a very general level and, as this book is entitled *Deafness*, consider what we mean by the term 'deaf'. When you ask many people if they have a hearing loss the first thing they will tell you is that they are not 'deaf'. The question is: if they are not deaf what are they?

First of all, there is a functional distinction that many people make between the descriptions 'deaf' and 'hard of hearing'. The term 'deaf', for many people, implies a total loss of hearing, whereas the term 'hard of hearing' means that they have a loss of hearing that is not at all total. The situation starts to become confusing, particularly as we have already used the term 'hearing loss'. The following are terms that are commonly used to describe deafness and deaf people as well as a description of what is normally meant by their use.

### Hearing loss

The ability of an individual to hear is measured clinically in terms of a comparison with a standardized set of data e.g. (ISO 389-1 1998), derived from groups of people who are deemed to be 'otologically normal' and therefore have 'normal hearing'. An otologically normal person is defined as someone who 'is in a normal state of health who is free from all signs or symptoms of ear disease and from obstructing wax in the ear canal, and who has no history of undue exposure to noise'. This definition is further refined by limiting the age range of otologically normal subjects to 18 to 30 years, in order to remove changes in hearing due to age.

Any deviation from that norm, measured in decibels (dB), is called a 'hearing level' (HL). If that hearing level is such that it is worse than the norm then it is termed a 'hearing loss', which is the non-technical term most people use to describe the level of their hearing.

However, people will often use words to describe the various degrees of hearing loss. It is possible to come to a broad agreement on what the words mean based on the results of pure-tone audiometry and the pure-tone audiogram, which are described in Chapter 5.

Table 1.1 indicates the terms that have been given to average values of hearing level by the British Society of Audiology (BSA 1988) to provide a basis for comparing the level of people's hearing in general terms. While there are many variations in the values quoted, they are indicative of the levels of hearing loss associated with widely used terms.

**Table 1.1:** Audiometric descriptors based on the average of pure-tone hearing threshold levels at 250, 500, 1000, 2000 and 4000 Hz

| Audiometric descriptor | dB HL |
| --- | --- |
| Mild hearing loss | 20–40 |
| Moderate hearing loss | 41–70 |
| Severe hearing loss | 71–95 |
| Profound hearing loss | > 95 |

Averages do not imply any particular configuration of hearing loss and do not prevent additional terms, such as 'profound high-frequency hearing loss', being used.

Given that people may classify themselves, or others may classify them, in terms of their degree of hearing loss, e.g. having a mild, moderate, etc., loss, they are also likely to classify themselves into one of the following groups. How people describe themselves in the following groups will depend on a number of factors, including: their degree of loss, its onset, their preferred mode of communication and their wish to have a cultural identity.

This hearing loss is also technically a 'hearing impairment', which then causes a 'hearing disability' and consequently a 'hearing handicap'. The formal definitions of the terms impairment, disability and handicap are given by the World Health Organization (WHO 1980) and are as follows:

- Impairment: any loss or abnormality of psychological, physiological or anatomical function leading to a disability and possible handicap.
- Disability: any restriction or lack (resulting from an impairment) of ability to perform an activity in the manner or within the range considered normal for a human being.
- Handicap: a disadvantage for a given individual, resulting from an impairment or disability, that limits or prevents the fulfilment of a role that is normal (depending on age, sex and social or cultural factors) for the individual.

In the context of deafness, the impairment is the damage to the auditory system, which is commonly physiological in nature, and the disability that this creates is a loss of function (hearing), which in turn prevents a person from hearing sounds. When a person cannot hear sounds that are important at a particular time and in a particular environment, this creates a handicap in that situation. While the impairment and the disability are there all the time, the handicap will only become apparent when there is a need to detect or recognize sound patterns. Consequently the handicap of deafness is very situation-specific, which tends to make understanding the needs of deaf people complex.

## Hard of hearing (HOH)

Most people who have mild to severe degrees of hearing loss and who benefit from amplification, will call themselves 'hard of hearing'. In fact, many will tell you very positively that they are not 'deaf' but have some problem with their hearing. Hard-of-hearing people form the majority of those with a hearing loss and are predominantly over the age of 60. Chapter 2 gives details of the distribution of hearing loss with age and severity.

Because hard-of-hearing people have developed a hearing loss after they have acquired speech and language, usually in later life, they will communicate by speech and hearing. They will rely on lip-reading (speech-reading) to a varying degree, and the use of hearing aids to support their communication. The effects of a poor acoustic and visual environment and poor communication skills on the part of people speaking to them will significantly affect their ability to communicate. It is worth pointing out that hearing-impaired people's ability to lip-read varies enormously and cannot be taken for granted.

## Deaf

The term 'deaf' may be used in a number of ways and is mainly, but by no means exclusively, used to describe people who are severely or profoundly deaf. Their hearing loss is such that hearing aids will not allow them to understand speech without lip-reading, although they may provide information on sounds around them, called environmental sounds, and support lip-reading. Consequently many deaf people do not use hearing aids because their benefit is so limited.

However, the main use of the term 'deaf' is related to those people who were born deaf or who went deaf before they acquired normal speech and language, i.e. they are prelingually deaf. A consequence of such deafness is that it can have a profound effect on their development. Hence the need for early diagnosis and treatment. For many such people their preferred mode of communication is by the use of sign language. While sign language is recognized as a minority language in its own right, it is not widely used in the general community. The effect of this is to produce a cultural grouping of deaf people who often refer to themselves as the 'deaf community'.

## Deafened

The term 'deafened' includes those people who can be described as deaf, due to their degree of hearing loss, but who became deaf in later life, after acquiring speech, language and literacy skills within what is accepted as the normal range for any individual. Such people will communicate by using speech and lip-reading. Their speech may lose some of its intelligibility due to the inability to monitor speech production, but does not present a significant communication problem to most people. If a person is a good lip-reader it may be difficult to know that that person has a profound hearing loss. In general, most of these people will not wish to use sign language.

## Deaf blind

A small group of people are born, or acquire, both a severe or profound hearing loss and a similar degree of visual impairment. Which impairment came first is important. A person who is born deaf and then acquires a severe visual problem will have more serious communication problems than a person whose primary impairment is visual and who then acquires a hearing impairment.

Communication with deaf blind people is mainly restricted to tactile means. However, it is very important in all cases of hearing impairment to take note of the visual acuity of the individual. Equally, it is very important with visually impaired people to take note of any hearing problems. Very few deaf blind people are able to read Braille and the majority will rely on finger-spelling and signing on the hand. Spartan is the simplest means of communication, whereby block capitals are drawn on the palm of the hand and can be undertaken, albeit slowly, by anyone.

# Consequences of deafness

The ability to communicate freely with other people is taken for granted until something, such as a hearing loss, impedes this natural process. The problems caused by deafness may, if taken as only relating to the ear, appear simply troublesome. However, deafness can have a devastating effect on the quality of everyday life. One of the problems in bringing this fact home to both lay and professional people is that the effects of deafness are very situation-specific. A hearing-impaired person who is a good lip-reader may appear to follow every word in a one-to-one, face-to-face conversation in a good light when they know what is being talked about. However, they may be quite unable to cope if the conversation is with a small group of people who are talking freely among themselves, or when the speakers are in a bad light or a bad position. A deaf person can only attend to one person at a time and cannot hear interjections or the nuances of what is said. The effect of hearing loss does depend on the age of onset of the loss, the type of loss and its consequent effect on speech perception, and on the attitudes and abilities of the individual, as well as the support they receive from family, friends and professionals.

Deafness often leads to a loss of confidence on the part of a deaf or hard-of-hearing person. The person may find it difficult to know when the subject under discussion has changed or when to enter the conversation, as they may not be aware when someone else is speaking. This problem is made worse if the person is unable to lip-read or has a visual handicap as well and cannot see clearly who is speaking.

When asked to list problems that they consider important, hard-of-hearing people appear at first to produce a list that contains somewhat trivial items. Barcham and Stephens (1980) asked some 200 hearing-aid users to list the problems they face as a result of their hearing loss that they considered important. Table 1.2 lists those items considered to be a major problem by those who completed the questionnaire.

**Table 1.2:** Problems faced and considered major by hard-of-hearing people as a result of their hearing loss

| Problem | % of responses |
| --- | --- |
| Listening to TV/radio | 48 |
| General conversation | 34 |
| Doorbell | 24 |
| Group conversation | 23 |
| Speech in noise | 23 |
| Telephone bell | 20 |

The results in Table 1.2 were obtained some 20 years ago but they are still very representative of the everyday problems that hearing-impaired people face today. While failing to hear the door bell or telephone bell may appear trivial, it is an example of something that becomes a limiting factor for elderly people wanting to live on their own.

## Professionals associated with deafness

Deafness requires a multidisciplinary approach and involves a wide range of professionals. The following section attempts to clarify the roles and functions of these professionals and is based on the *Careers in Audiology* booklet compiled by the BSA (1998), which provides full details of each profession.

*Audiological physician*

A physician concerned with disorders of hearing and balance, who has a postgraduate degree in audiological medicine.

*Audiological scientist*

A scientist with a postgraduate degree in audiology concerned with the identification and diagnosis of hearing impairment and the rehabilitation of hearing-impaired adult and child patients.

*Community doctor in audiology*

Predominantly a paediatrician, often with a postgraduate degree in audiology, who provides audiological services for children and their families.

*Educational audiologist*

A teacher of the deaf who has undertaken additional approved training leading to a recognized qualification in paediatric and educational audiology. Undertakes assessment of hearing-impaired children, audiological habilitation, the fitting and evaluation of hearing aid systems, and advising parents and professionals on audiological matters.

*Hearing aid audiologist (hearing aid dispenser)*

Dispenses hearing aids in the private sector and is registered with the Hearing Aid Council in accordance with the Hearing Aid Council Act 1968.

*Hearing therapist*

Assesses the rehabilitative needs of those with acquired deafness and provides help with communication using hearing aids, environmental aids, and the skills of speech-reading and auditory training.

*Industrial audiometrician*

Undertakes the assessment of the hearing of people working in noisy industry and the categorization of the results. May also select and provide hearing protectors and recommend appropriate action to prevent hearing damage.

*Lip-reading teacher*

Helps people with acquired deafness to develop their lip-reading and observational skills and to maximize the use of their residual hearing.

*Medical technical officer (audiology), also known as an audiology technician*

Their work includes the assessment of hearing and the fitting of hearing aids, and advising on their use within the NHS.

*Otolaryngologist (ENT surgeon)*

Responsible for the diagnosis and medical, surgical and rehabilitation management of disorders and injuries of the ear, nose and throat, including head and neck cancer and speciality facial plastic surgery. When particularly specializing in diseases of the ear is called an otologist.

*Social worker with deaf people*

Undertakes a wide range of services to deaf, deafened and hard-of-hearing people and their families dealing with situations relating to deafness and a broad range of social problems.

*Speech and language therapist*

Undertakes the assessment and treatment of all types of communication disorders in children and adults. Therapists working with deaf people have a higher qualification in a speciality concerned with deafness and its effects on communication.

*Teacher of the deaf*

A qualified teacher who has undertaken additional training leading to a qualification to teach children with impaired hearing.

## Conclusion

When faced with a person who has a hearing loss, it is essential to take into account the whole person, not just his or her hearing loss. The effect of deafness is complex and far-reaching. Each professional involved in the management of that person is important in the care of the patient. But as the patient progresses through the management system the relative importance of the professionals changes, as do the needs of the deaf person. Consequently an awareness of the differing needs of the patient and of the professional who will contribute best to their wellbeing is important. Above all it is important to listen to the individual's problems. Due to the varying nature of the effects of deafness, care has to be taken not to place a patient in any category without careful consideration, backed up by as much objective and subjective information as it is possible to get. This requires time, which often is not provided for, to make a proper assessment of the hearing-impaired person.

# Chapter 2
# The prevalence of deafness and hearing impairment

ADRIAN DAVIS

Deafness and hearing impairment should be one of the most important public health issues in the UK for the coming decades of the new millennium. Not only will there be a premium on communication in the coming years, but people will live longer and healthier lives. Those longer lives need sound communication as a basis for a high quality of life and the independence that is a right of all. However, the extent to which commissioners of healthcare will allocate deafness and hearing impairment an appropriately high priority for provision will depend on a number of interacting factors: public opinion, lobbying by pressure groups, local and national politics, as well as financial limitations. But the major influence on the prioritization of provision should be an informed knowledge of:

- the number of people affected by deafness
- the limitations imposed on deaf people by society and the disability and handicap experienced by particular groups of individuals related to their degree of deafness, age and expectations
- the predominant aetiologies of deafness
- the quality and overall efficiency of service provision for deafness.

We need to consider the statement 'Do those that need a service, get it; and do those that get it (a) benefit and (b) get a good-quality service?'

This chapter attempts to look at these four potential (essentially epidemiological) inputs to the prioritization of services for deafness, with the greatest attention being given here to the first – the prevalence of deafness. The two terms 'prevalence' and 'deafness' give potential for confusion. The term 'prevalence' is used here to refer to the number of people in a defined population with a stated characteristic at a particular time (e.g. the number of people who had a hearing problem in 2000).

10

Sometimes the prevalence is stated as a percentage of the population. A term related to prevalence is 'incidence', which is defined as the number of new cases in a defined population with a stated characteristic over a particular time period (e.g. the number of people with a new hearing problem arising between 1 January 2000 and 31 December 2000).

The term 'deafness' has many dimensions, some of which are explored elsewhere in this book. Unfortunately, 'deaf' or 'deafness' has a number of unwanted connotations. From a practical point of view, it is often difficult to decide how and where to draw the line between who is 'deaf' and who isn't, particularly when carrying out a survey to determine the prevalence of 'deafness'. To overcome this terminological problem, in the rest of this chapter the more easily quantifiable term 'hearing impairment' is used.

The prevalence of hearing impairments and their change over the demographic variables of gender, socioeconomic group and, most importantly, age, are essential ingredients in the planning of audiological and ear, nose and throat (ENT) services. At the broadest level the purchasers of healthcare can estimate the needs of the population from the prevalence of hearing impairment. In the system in use in the UK, the commissioning may become devolved to the local level, e.g. primary care group, where the prevalence is sufficient; other methods of purchasing hearing healthcare might be seen in a similar mode, e.g. with managed healthcare in the US. Even within these systems there is a role of wider policy decisions to be made, e.g. in negotiating contracts for hearing aids. At the extreme, of course, individuals can pay for their own healthcare. Obviously these needs will vary according to the age groups and severity (and type, as explained in other chapters in this book) of hearing impairment. The audiological healthcare providers share this interest in the overall marginal levels of need. They also have an interest in:

- the extent to which the public seek out their services
- whether the mix of services is appropriate for the population served (both now and in the future)
- the extent to which the services supplied meet the demand
- the quality of the service offered (and how it is perceived by consumers of healthcare).

Knowledge of the extent to which external factors influence the prevalence of hearing impairment (e.g. meningitis in children, noise exposure in adults, genetic susceptibility to noise and ageing) at particular ages may help in defining what scope there is for primary prevention of hearing pathology. However, as external factors seem to play a small (but sometimes critical) part in the population prevalence of hearing impairment, the main public health emphasis should be on early intervention to limit the long-standing forms of hearing disability that can have severe handicapping effects on individuals.

Information concerning the prevalence of hearing impairment has been used by a wide variety of professional bodies and individuals for a variety of purposes, e.g. educators in planning educational opportunities for the hearing-impaired child and adult; social workers and nurses who have responsibility for the elderly; physicians planning their practice approach and targets; and market researchers ascertaining the number of potential clients for new products.

Another large set of individuals who asked for prevalence information are those who are either hearing impaired themselves, are closely related to someone with a hearing disability or working for a hearing-related organization (e.g. RNID, NDCS, Hearing Concern, BDA; see List of abbreviations pp. xv–xvii). Knowledge of the extent to which the prevalence of hearing impairments changes with age, the natural history of hearing impairments and the relative contribution of aetiological factors, such as noise exposure, can be important factors in the counselling of many hearing-impaired people. In addition it could help to determine priorities within an organization.

The prevalence of hearing impairment as an indicator of population need for hearing services should not be estimated by performance indicators, such as the number of hearing aids fitted last year or the size of the waiting list for hearing aids, because of the hidden nature of hearing impairments and the substantial size of the existing unmet need. This estimate can only be ascertained at present by population measures, usually through surveying of the appropriate population. For prevalences in excess of 2%, this is feasible, although a large study would be required for an accurate assessment of prevalences in the region of 2–5%. Evaluation of the approximate prevalences for rare conditions (e.g. the number of people who might benefit from a cochlear implant) requires other survey techniques.

The following section discusses, in a minimal way, some pertinent aspects of method. The chapter will then concentrate on:

- the prevalence of hearing impairment in adults, and its variation with age
- the prevalence of hearing impairment in children
- the adequacy of the services for hearing-impaired people.

## Methods for the National Study of Hearing

The data on hearing impairment in adults are taken predominantly from the National Study of Hearing (NSH), which was conducted by the MRC

Institute of Hearing Research (Davis 1989, 1995). The fieldwork for the four individual studies comprising the NSH was conducted between 1980 and 1986. Three of the four main samples taken for the survey (in excess of 50 000 people were contacted by a postal questionnaire) were concentrated in Cardiff, Glasgow, Nottingham and Southampton; the fourth sample was taken from the UK, balancing the sample over health regions. These surveys gave self-reported information on the population's hearing, tinnitus and use of the public health system. However, there is a severe limitation on using just this information for planning purposes, due to the extent to which the young have a tendency to overrate their disability for a given level of hearing impairment and the old consistently to underrate their disability. As a result of this and for other scientific reasons, over 3000 people representative of the adult population received extensive audiological investigation. The data on hearing impairment originate from the 2708 people aged 18–80 years who underwent audiological investigation.

## The prevalence of hearing impairment in adults

There are a large number of measures of hearing impairment, the most general being the hearing threshold levels obtained for pure tones at different frequencies. To simplify the information available from the pattern of these thresholds over frequency (the audiogram), an index of impairment has been used for the average hearing threshold level over the frequencies 0.5, 1, 2 and 4 kHz, in the better ear. This measure (better ear average, BEA) tends to underrate the problems that a person with asymmetrical hearing might have, but is probably one of the better predictors of overall hearing disability, which includes the ability to hear speech in a background of noise and the ability to use environmental sound cues appropriately.

The prevalence of hearing impairment is shown in Figure 2.1. About 30% of the adult population has an impairment in at least one ear, with two thirds of these having an impairment in the better ear at 25 dB hearing level (HL) or greater. Between 20 and 30% of adults also have great difficulty hearing speech in a background of noise. This is not surprising, as most people find this task difficult. However, Davis (1995) showed that this degree of reported difficulty was associated with a hearing threshold that was considerably raised compared with those who did not complain. Tinnitus, which is highly associated with hearing impairment, is reported in about 10% of people to occur spontaneously (i.e. not only after loud sounds) and to last for more than five minutes.

The prevalence for a range of severity of hearing impairment is presented in Table 2.1, showing that 16.1% of the adult population in the UK, aged 18–80, have BEAs of 25 dB HL and greater. The statistical bounds

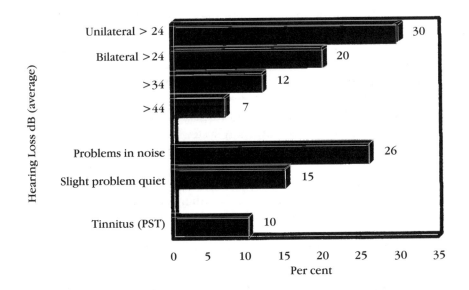

**Figure 2.1:** The overall prevalence of impairment and reported disability in those aged 18 years and over in Great Britain.

of this estimate are also shown in Table 2.1: at BEAs of 25 dB HL and greater, the prevalence estimate lies between 15.0 and 17.3%, with a high degree of confidence (95%). As the severity of hearing impairment increases the prevalence decreases. Beyond levels of 45 dB HL, which has a prevalence of about 4%, the prevalence estimates may be subject to systematic biases rather than to random error from sampling. However, they are the best available in the UK for bilateral severe and profound hearing impairments. Thus at a severity of 65 dB HL and greater the best estimate is about 11 people per 1000, at 95 dB HL and greater about 2 per 1000 and at 105 dB HL and greater about 1 per 1000. On the worse ear, however, there were about 6 per 1000 at 105 dB HL and greater.

Generally, at degrees of severity of 45 dB HL and greater there are no substantial differences between men and women in the percentage having hearing impairments. Below that men have a substantially higher chance of having a mild-to-moderate hearing impairment. At 25 dB HL and greater the prevalence estimate is 18.1% (confidence interval (CI) 16.4–19.7%) for men and 14.4% (CI 12.8–16.0%) for women. This difference is almost certainly due to the greater degree and duration of noise exposure experienced by men aged 40 years and older compared with women. As noise affects thresholds in the 4 kHz region more than at lower frequencies, this difference, which is slight for BEA, is greatly increased at high frequencies (3–8 kHz).

**Table 2.1:** Estimate of the prevalence of hearing impairment as a percentage of people in the UK, aged 18–80 years, with different degrees of severity of hearing impairment in the better ear*

| Severity of hearing impairment (dB HL) | Prevalence estimate | Low CI | High CI |
|---|---|---|---|
| 25+ | 16.1 | 15.0 | 17.3 |
| 35+ | 8.2 | 7.4 | 9.1 |
| 45+ | 3.9 | 3.4 | 4.4 |
| 55+ | 2.1 | 1.7 | 2.5 |
| 65+ | 1.1 | 0.8 | 1.4 |
| 75+ | 0.7 | 0.5 | 1.0 |
| 85+ | 0.4 | 0.2 | 0.7 |
| 95+ | 0.2 | < 0.1 | 0.5 |
| 105+ | 0.1 | < 0.1 | 0.4 |

*The thresholds have been averaged over the frequencies 0.5, 1, 2 and 4 kHz to obtain an average level of hearing impairment. The low and high 95% CIs are also shown n = 2662 (people with acceptable audiograms).

The majority, 87%, of the hearing impairments at 25 dB HL and greater are of a sensorineural type rather than having a substantial conductive component. (See Chapters 8–10 for an explanation of the difference between the types of hearing impairment. The criterion used here to qualify for a conductive component was an average difference of 15 dB between the air- and bone-conduction thresholds.) The proportion with no conductive component on the worse ear is less than on the better ear, at 69%. At a greater severity than 25 dB the proportion of people with no conductive component on the better ear decreases to 82% at 35 dB HL and greater, and to 69% at 45 dB HL and greater.

The prevalence of hearing impairment at all severities in the population is highly dependent on age. This is the case even for profound hearing impairments, indicating that most hearing impairments are acquired. At 95 dB HL and greater, the estimate in terms of numbers is about 100 000 people in the UK, of whom probably about 15 000 were impaired prelingually. For young age groups the proportions of prelingually impaired are much higher than the average figures suggest. The proportion of the profoundly impaired individuals who could be candidates for cochlear implants obviously depends on the actual audiometric and other selection criteria used by different centres, but might be as low as a few per cent or as high as 50%.

The proportion of hearing-impaired people with visual impairments is high, as ageing is a common factor in the increasing prevalence of both these sensory impairments. However, the number of people with substantial visual disability and severe hearing impairment or worse is not currently known with any degree of statistical precision, but is unlikely to be more than 1 in 10 000.

In terms of prevalence of hearing impairment as a function of age (at 25 dB HL and greater), Figure 2.2 gives some indication of the change with age, when equally pooled over gender. Until the age of about 45 years, mild hearing problems are rare, so that the prevalence estimates (triangles, read off the left-hand axis) are small and in the margins of reliability. Beyond the age of 50 the prevalence estimates are well over 10%, approaching 50% by 70–74 years of age. The median BEA (50% of the sample having better hearing and 50% having worse) as a function of age is also shown in Figure 2.2 (this is pooled over men and women for simplicity and is shown by the filled circles, read off the right-hand axis). The median is a better indicator than the prevalences of the gradual way in which thresholds change with age, even below 50 years. The median BEA increases at about 2.5 dB per decade in people aged 20–40 years, but at up to 10 dB per decade in those aged 60–80. Figure 2.2 shows the close way in which the prevalence and the median are related in the population.

The number of people in the UK with hearing impairments of different degrees of severity, taking gender into account, can be deduced from the prevalence of hearing impairment and the demographic profile. Table 2.2 shows the estimated number of hearing-impaired people using the

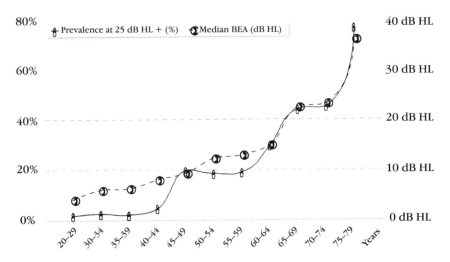

**Figure 2.2:** The prevalence of hearing impairments at a BEA of 25 dB HL and greater and of median BEA as a function of age, pooled over women and men.

mid-1990s estimates for the age and gender profile of Great Britain. There are about 8.58 million people with BEA hearing impairments of 25 dB HL and greater. This decreases to about 2.94 million with moderate degrees of impairment. There are substantially more women than men with hearing impairments, despite roughly equal prevalences, because more women survive into the seventh, eighth and ninth decades of life. Indeed at 45 dB HL and above, Table 2.2 shows that about a quarter of those disabled by this level of impairment are women of 80 years or older.

Over the next two decades, due to increasing survival, the number of hearing-impaired people will probably rise by 20%, in line with other chronic disabilities. Thus by the year 2016 there may be 700 000 people with severe hearing impairments (65 dB HL and greater) compared with an estimated 580 000 in 1988. The number of people with profound hearing impairment is of interest, because on the one hand they have very special needs, but on the other hand they are possible candidates for cochlear implantation. The data presented in Table 2.2 suggest that in the age range 18 years and above, there are under 200 000 people in Great Britain who are profoundly deaf. The estimates are open to much speculation because of the rarity of this degree of deafness. The prevalence of 150 000 people includes those with deafness that has been

**Table 2.2:** Estimates of the number of people (in thousands) in Great Britain with hearing impairments, as a function of age group, gender and severity of impairment for the better ear at 25, 35, 45, 65 and 95 dB HL averaged over the mid-frequencies (0.5, 1, 2 and 4 kHz). The estimates for the 18–80 age group are less subject to bias than those for the 81+ age group

| Gender | Severity | 18–60 | 61–80 | 81+ | Total |
|--------|----------|-------|-------|-----|-------|
| Female | 25+      | 911   | 2184  | 1377 | 4472 |
| Male   |          | 1220  | 2302  | 586  | 4108 |
| Total  |          | 2131  | 4486  | 1864 | 8580 |
| Female | 35+      | 373   | 1314  | 1216 | 2903 |
| Male   |          | 544   | 1209  | 484  | 2237 |
| Total  |          | 917   | 2523  | 1700 | 5140 |
| Female | 45+      | 183   | 618   | 923  | 1724 |
| Male   |          | 288   | 514   | 414  | 1215 |
| Total  |          | 471   | 1132  | 1337 | 2940 |
| Female | 65+      | 48    | 169   | 322  | 539  |
| Male   |          | 87    | 125   | 146  | 359  |
| Total  |          | 136   | 294   | 469  | 898  |
| Female | 95+      | 5     | 21    | 59   | 85   |
| Male   |          | 33    | 13    | 19   | 65   |
| Total  |          | 38    | 34    | 78   | 150  |

acquired in the adult years as well as those adults who were either born with that degree of impairment, e.g. because of rubella or inheritance, or who acquired it during childhood, e.g. because of meningitis. If we accept that there are probably 20 000–30 000 people with profound deafness from childhood (see below), this means that a substantial proportion, about 80%, of profound deafness is acquired. The distribution with age shows that it is not only more common in the over-80 age group, but the absolute numbers are greatest in this age range. This represents a great challenge to reduce the dependency that is brought about by this deafness, which it is unlikely to be reduced by cochlear implantation at this age. However, there is much scope for the role of cochlear implantation in the younger age groups, if it is acceptable to the individual and society and meets agreed standards of quality and cost-effectiveness.

Tinnitus, i.e. noises in the ears or in the head, correlates highly with the individual's hearing impairment. The best predictor of tinnitus is the severity of hearing impairment in the worse ear at high frequencies. Over one in three adults reports some tinnitus, mainly transient, but this section concentrates on the 10% who report tinnitus that lasts for more than five minutes and is present not only after very loud sounds. About half of this tinnitus group report that their tinnitus is moderately or severely annoying. Bilateral tinnitus is reported in about 3% of those with better hearing thresholds than 25 dB HL in the worse ear at high frequencies, with unilateral tinnitus reported in about 2%. These tinnitus prevalences increase in line with severity of impairment to 10% (bilateral) and 15% (unilateral) for those with 85 dB HL or more in the worse ear averaged over the high frequencies (5% of the population).

The prevalence of tinnitus is very susceptible to small changes in the protocol that defines the precise condition of concern, and in any tinnitus study this has to be well controlled. However, the results of two UK studies (Coles, Davis and Smith, 1990; Sancho-Aldridge and Davis 1993) show that there is no doubt that the quality of life for 2% of the population may be moderately affected by tinnitus, and that for perhaps as many as 5 per 1000, or about 0.3 million people in the UK, quality of life is greatly affected by their tinnitus.

Nearly 7% of the population have consulted a doctor about tinnitus. The main statistical factors predicting consultation are the severity of the tinnitus, annoyance and the degree of hearing impairment. However, socioeconomic group and age are the best predictors of the third who were seen by the family doctor and who were subsequently referred to a hospital department.

# The prevalence of hearing impairments in children

The NSH did not gather much information on the prevalence of hearing impairment among children. The European Communities report *Childhood Deafness in the European Community* (Martin et al. 1981) puts the lower bound on hearing impairment prevalence at around 1 per 1000 in children with a BEA of 50 dB HL born during 1969 and ascertained by 1977 (i.e. 8 years of age). This is a good benchmark to take for the birth cohorts in the 1980s and 1990s. While the part played by rubella in the UK has decreased, there has been a large increase in the number of pre-term babies with hearing impairments who survive. This group may account for up to 40% of the hearing-impaired children in some districts.

Haggard and Hughes (1991) have reported in detail on the problems of otitis media with effusion (OME or glue ear). This does not concern us here, because its individual consequences are not as severe as for those with 'permanent' impairments. However, Davis and Wood (1992) report a small-scale study in the Nottingham Health District on the 1983–86 birth cohort, and Fortnum and Davis (1997) report a much larger study on the Trent Region 1985–1993 birth cohort, which is further elaborated in a policy context by Davis et al. (1997). Both these studies have some validity in the context of planning screening, diagnostic and rehabilitative facilities for hearing-impaired children.

In the Nottingham DHA 1983–86 birth cohort we estimated that 1.8 (CI 1.4–2.3) per 1000 children in this birth cohort were fitted with a hearing aid – this is 1 in every 566 children – by the age of about 3 years. This covers all degrees of hearing impairment, including unilateral impairments. For bilateral hearing impairments 50 dB HL and greater, the estimate was that there were 1.3 (CI 0.9–1.8) children per 1000. Of the 1.3 per 1000, 1.0 was diagnosed as having hearing impairment present from birth, and with a significant sensorineural component.

The Trent Ascertainment Study (Fortnum and Davis 1997) gave estimates over a wider geographical area. It showed that there were considerable variations over time and place in Trent, as we might expect from such a rare condition. In some districts in some years there might be no children with permanent childhood hearing impairment and in other years there may be two or three times the mean number of children. This makes planning and commissioning services for children a very difficult task at an average district level with perhaps 4000–6000 births per year. We estimated that there were 1.33 (CI 1.22–1.45) children per 1000 live births with permanent hearing impairments (PCHI) in the better ear of 40 dB HL or greater across the mid-frequencies (0.5, 1, 2 and 4 kHz) by the age of 5 years. The estimate for congenital PCHI was 1.12 (CI 1.01–1.23) per 1000 live births, of which 0.24 (CI 0.20–0.30) per 1000 were profoundly hearing impaired at 95 dB HL or greater. This suggests that congenital profound deafness accounts for about a quarter of all hearing-impaired children.

As the severity criterion increases the prevalence decreases. Thus at 50+, 70+ and 95+ dB HL the estimates were 1.10, 0.59 and 0.31 per 1000 children with PCHI by the age of about 5 years. Of the profoundly hearing-impaired children, about 1 in 3225 at the age of 5 years, about one fifth had acquired pathologies, predominantly meningitis. If these data are representative of other UK districts this suggests that about 250 children per birth cohort (about 800 000 per annum) have a profound hearing impairment. Probably between 40 and 60 of these profoundly impaired children may have had meningitis as a primary aetiological factor, so it is essential that all children surviving meningitis are given a formal hearing assessment.

Over the next decade, substantial inroads may be made in understanding the nature and causes of PCHI. About 30% of the children with PCHI have been in neonatal intensive care for 48 hours or longer. This history raises the likelihood that they have a hearing impairment by about eightfold. The precise reasons for this are unclear. There are no doubt a combination of factors, including the use of ototoxic drugs, hyperbilirubinaemia, anoxia and other events such as intra-cranial haemorrhage. It may be that no one factor is responsible but that it is a combination of factors that are important. Included in those factors could be the increased susceptibility to noise that early birth may add to other problems. Genetic factors are probably responsible for a greater proportion of the severe and profound hearing impairments. In a population study of the Trent Region, Connexin-26 mutations have recently been shown to be associated with quite a high proportion of profound hearing impairments (Dr Mick Parker, personal communication) – maybe as many as a third of congenital impairments. Many other genes are being identified as associated with congenital and progressive deafness (see www.ihr.mrc.ac.uk for updates on progress and links to other sites that have information on genes associated with deafness).

## Services for hearing-impaired people

Detailed information and evidence about services for hearing-impaired people are only slowly becoming available in terms of:

- the coverage, timeliness and effectiveness of prevention programmes (e.g. paediatric/neonatal screening, vaccination, noise conservation, pre-retirement screening)

- the extent to which those who might benefit from advice or a hearing aid have their needs met
- the extent to which the quality of the service provided meets the needs of the individual (e.g. failure rate of hearing aids, non-use rate, waiting times for initial consultation, quality of ear moulds, availability of rehabilitative support).

There is some recent information available concerning hearing screening for children. Fortnum and Davis (1997) show that the median age of amplification, as shown by the age at which a first hearing aid was fitted, was 26 months for all children with PCHI of 40 dB HL or greater. For children with profound impairments this was younger (12 months) and for the large numbers with impairments between 40 and 69 dB HL it was older (43 months). The infant distraction test that has been used routinely throughout the UK has done a reasonably good job in detecting those with severe and profound deafness by the age of 12 months, but is failing quite substantially those children with moderate impairments.

Recent work on neonatal hearing screening in the UK and in the US is summarized in Davis et al. (1997). This recommends that the UK moves towards a universal neonatal hearing screen as the most preferred practice rather than the infant distraction test. This should enable a better screening coverage overall and a high yield of children with congenital PCHI at an affordable cost. However, it needs to have good health and education services in place so that parents and hearing-impaired children are given a good-quality service. This is an extremely important issue, because early identification gives us a potential to work with parents and hearing-impaired children to limit the impact of hearing impairment. However, if handled inappropriately there is a greater potential for long-lasting damage to families and their children. The target should be to detect all hearing-impaired children with at least moderate impairments by the age of 3 months and to begin habilitation, with or without amplification, by 6 months of age.

Consumer satisfaction and the image of hearing services are both very important. Hearing services do not necessarily have a good image with other professionals and members of the public. Even for fairly selected groups the level of 'consumer dissatisfaction' with the hearing aid is quite high. This work needs to be extended on a representative sample, but levels of 34% dissatisfaction were shown. Population studies that we have carried out show that these dissatisfaction rates may be a slight overestimate. In terms of parents' dissatisfaction with hearing services, it is difficult to take the initial report as indicative of the real satisfaction or dissatisfaction because of the highly emotive timing of services and adaptation to the news of hearing impairment. However, qualitative evidence shows that there are a substantial number of families who are greatly worried by the way they and their children have been treated. This perception does not always meet with professional acceptance, but should be seriously considered, because how the service is perceived is important for outcomes and should drive the need to continuously refine and improve services. For adults the dissatisfaction is a product of a number of issues, which can be summed up as accessibility of services, availability of good-quality hearing aids, provision of good rehabilitation services, appropriate repair and advice services, and the timing of the services.

The proportion of people who have ever had a hearing aid is shown in Table 2.3, using data available from the NSH, a study carried out by the Independent Television Commission (ITC) (Sancho-Aldridge and Davis 1993) and a more recent study carried out as part of the MRC National Study of Ear, Nose and Throat Symptoms. The prevalence estimate from the NSH is about 4%, with approximately 3% of the adult population now using an aid. The smaller NSH household study and ITC study, which have wider-ranging samples, show slightly lower prevalences at 3.2% and 3.6%. The most recent study, carried out in 1998, shows a small but significant increase in hearing-aid possession since the mid-1980s, particularly in the over-70 age group.

**Table 2.3:** Estimates for the prevalence of hearing aid possession among adults

| Age group (years) | NSH (1) | NSH (2) | NSH (3) | NSH (4) | ITC (5) | MRC (6) |
|---|---|---|---|---|---|---|
| 18–30 | 0.5 | 0.5 | 0.3 | 0.3 | 1.3 | 0.6 |
| 31–40 | 0.8 | 0.7 | 0.4 | 0.5 | 1.0 | 0.8 |
| 41–50 | 2.0 | 2.0 | 1.2 | 1.0 | 1.0 | 1.4 |
| 51–60 | 3.1 | 2.7 | 2.1 | 2.8 | 4.6 | 3.5 |
| 61–70 | 6.7 | 6.4 | 4.9 | 6.3 | 6.5 | 7.9 |
| 71–80 | 13.9 | 13.6 | 11.6 | 12.7 | 15.6 | 17.8 |
| 81–90 | 26.1 | 26.1 | 19.3 | 30.3 | 28.3 | 30.7 |
| 18–90 | 4.0 | 3.9 | 3.0 | 3.2 | 3.6 | 4.2 |
| N = | 35 841 | 18 682 | 18 682 | 10 777 | 4636 | 32 734 |
| Year | 1980–86 | 1984–96 | 1984–86 | 1982 | 1991 | 1998 |
| Population | Four cities in GB | Four cities in GB | Four cities in GB | GB | GB | GB |

(1) the NSH overall, (2) the NSH phase 3 (possession of aid), (3) the NSH phase 3 (current use of aid), (4) the NSH household survey (5) the Independent Television Commission (ITC) survey and (6) a recent household survey as part of the MRC National Study of Ear, Nose and Throat Symptoms.

At ages below 50 years the studies do not have sufficiently high numbers to make statistically meaningful comparisons. At ages over 50 there is a surprising degree of agreement among the studies, indicating that provision has probably not changed substantially (as a proportion of the age-stratified population) over a few decades. This is disappointing, because there has been a considerable interest in providing hearing aids as early as possible to the adult population. Also there has been a substantial change in the technology that is available. However, it is not clear to what extent this new technology is available to the NHS hearing services.

Eighteen per cent of the 71- to 80-year-old group may have a hearing aid in 1998, but 3% do not use it and 6.6% do not use it most of the time. As can be seen from Figure 2.2, hearing impairment changes rapidly in this age group, and it is probable that at least 50% of this group would benefit from an aid. There is obviously scope for better quality services and the first step in providing those services needs to be a more aggressive approach to providing better and more appropriate services at an earlier age. Even for those aged 50–60 years, unmet need is substantially greater than provision. To prevent severe hearing disability and handicap developing in old age it is important to begin educating the pre-retirement groups, because 10–15% or more of those aged 50–65 years would benefit from hearing-aid provision and rehabilitation (Davis 1991; Stephens et al. 1991). This education can only be successful if the image of hearing services and hearing aids is substantially improved, accessibility is improved and long-term audit of the services is conducted routinely.

The main factor influencing take-up of hearing-aid services in the NSH sample was the severity of the hearing impairment. In addition to this type of impairment, the socioeconomic group of the patient and whether the patient reported tinnitus also contributed to the pattern of take-up. Thus people with conductive impairments and/or tinnitus and those from non-manual socioeconomic groups were more likely to possess a hearing aid for a stated level of hearing impairment (Davis 1991).

For people who receive a service, Table 2.3, taken at face value, suggests that about a quarter of those who have had an aid no longer use it (some for valid reasons, e.g. hearing considerably improved). Reasons for complete non-use were investigated in the NSH (Fortnum and Haggard 1984). The four main categories distinguishing non-users from users, being that aids were:

1   too loud
2   too noticeable
3   made whistling noises
4   were fitted with little or no explanation of how to use them.

Among those using their aid for less than 4 hours per day, the three main distinguishing complaints were:

1   high background noise levels
2   difficulty manipulating controls
3   battery accessibility.

## Summary

- There are about 8.6, 5.1, 2.9 and 0.15 million adults in the UK with bilateral hearing impairments of at least 25, 35, 45 and 95 dB HL respectively over the frequencies 0.5, 1, 2 and 4 kHz.
- Prevalence of all severities of hearing impairment increases rapidly with age after 50 years, and up to one in three of the hearing impaired is over 80 years of age.
- There is substantial unmet need in terms of people who would benefit from a hearing aid and/or advice on hearing tactics (Field and Haggard 1989). Only 19, 33 and 55% of people with a bilateral impairment of at least 25, 35 and 45 dB HL respectively have tried a hearing aid.
- There is substantial dissatisfaction among those who do receive a hearing aid. There is a great need to monitor outcomes and audit routine satisfaction as well as technological problems in hearing-aid services.
- Some aspects of dissatisfaction could be overcome if appropriate access to services was available from an early age (e.g. 50–60 years of age) and if counselling had been made available (e.g. hearing therapists).
- The introduction of more appropriate technology (e.g. non-linear processing hearing aids or other more sophisticated digital hearing aids) and management procedures into the NHS audiology service would no doubt both improve the image of the service and increase benefit to those with hearing impairment, if targeted at those who would most benefit.
- Congenital hearing impairment is a substantial public health problem affecting more than 1 in 1000 people. Present services do not identify these children at an appropriate age. Neither do they overwhelmingly give a service that is of the highest quality, particularly in terms of the coordination of services. This suggests that the phased introduction of universal neonatal hearing screening is an urgent requirement that should be linked to substantial service improvement over the coming decade
- By the age of 3 years, it is possible that 2 in 1000 children may benefit from a hearing aid. Only one in eight of these aided children has a

profound hearing impairment. Cochlear implants should be investigated as a possible intervention for all such children. However, there should also be a substantial investment in the habilitation and education of those with moderate impairments as there has been considerable under-investment in this area.

* Acquired profound hearing impairment, usually as a result of meningitis, contributes 10–20% of the profoundly impaired children. Advances in vaccination may help prevent some of the consequences of meningitis in the next decade. We also expect considerably greater understanding of the genetic bases of congenital and acquired hearing impairments.

## Conclusions

Consideration of the prevalence of several aspects of deafness has shown that hearing pathologies, impairments and disability represent a substantial public health problem, both in terms of numbers (for adults) and severity of handicapping consequences (for children and adults). As yet, the public health goals and targets have not been clearly stated in the UK, and thus there is no model based on a coherent, consistent consensus for local audiological services to adopt. Better levels of provision within current service arrangements are required, together with some quality assurance procedures to ensure the same quality of service to the consumer. However, there is clear evidence that new forms of provision are needed to give benefit to the sizeable numbers whose needs are not met within the current framework of audiological services.

## Acknowledgements

I would like to thank all the staff who have helped in the design, execution and management of the NSH. Thanks also to Dai Stephens and Heather Fortnum who made comments on the earlier edition.

# Chapter 3
# Structure and function of the ear: its anatomy and how we hear

TONY WRIGHT

The ear is probably the most remarkable and certainly the most unlikely structure in the body. This chapter describes and depicts the structure of the ear and explains, to the best of present knowledge, how it all works. Structure and function are so closely tied together that it is almost impossible to describe one without the other.

Convention and convenience have divided the structure of the ear into three separate parts – the outer, middle and inner ear (Figure 3.1). Each has a separate function but each function has to work perfectly for hearing to be normal. No attempt will be made here to describe the various diseases or disorders that can affect hearing – this will be left to later chapters in the book; what this chapter sets out to achieve is to describe the normal.

## The outer ear: structure

In the adult, the outer ear consists of the external pinna or auricle (Figure 3.2) and the external ear canal, which extends about 25 mm inwards. The external ear canal ends at the tympanic membrane (eardrum), which is a thin, almost circular, membrane stretched across the depths of the ear canal. The pinna consists of a springy, elastic cartilage with a complex shape and an extension about one third of the way down the ear canal. This extension is not a complete tube, being open at its anterior superior portion between the tragus and the superior rim of the helix (Figure 3.2). (This notch allows the surgeon one route of access to the depths of the ear canal and middle ear without cutting the cartilage. Such an incision is called an endaural incision.) The cartilage of the pinna and the canal is covered on both sides by a tough membrane called the perichondrium. The cartilage itself has no blood supply and all the nutrients needed to keep it intact are derived from the perichondrium. Between the

26

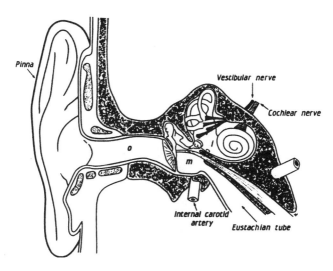

**Figure 3.1:** Schematic diagram of outer (o), middle (m) and inner (i) ears. The light shading represents the cartilage of the pinna and ear canal while the heavier shading is the temporal bone.

perichondrium and the skin that covers the pinna and lines the ear canal, there is only a very thin layer of fibrous tissue. However, behind the ear in the postaural or postauricular region there are several small muscles in this subcutaneous layer. These postauricular muscles run between the cartilage of the pinna and the skull and, in humans, have very little function except in those who can move their ears and thereby amuse children at parties. In many other animals, however, these muscles have an important role in moving the ears, both to collect more sound and to help in locating the source of sound. The postauricular muscles are supplied by small branches of the facial (VII) nerve, and contract slightly, but detectably, in response to sound, thereby forming part of the postauricular myogenic response (PAM).

The external ear canal is formed by the cartilaginous portion, which accounts for the outer one third, and a bony portion, which comprises the rest. There is really very little soft tissue between the skin and the perichondrium or periosteum (which covers the bony portion). However, in the outer cartilaginous portion there are lots of small hairs with their associated oil-secreting glands (sebaceous glands), and also a number of modified sweat glands (ceruminous glands), that together produce a mixture of proteins, mucopolysaccharides and lipids. The whole ear canal as well as the external surface of the tympanic membrane is covered with skin. A fundamental property of skin is to grow. Everywhere else in the body the skin grows upwards towards the surface where the dead layers of

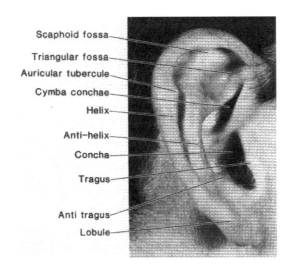

Scaphoid fossa

Triangular fossa

Auricular tubercule

Cymba conchae

Helix

Anti-helix

Concha

Tragus

Anti tragus

Lobule

**Figure 3.2:** The external ear of the author. The presence of tragal hairs indicates the passing of youth.

skin flake off and show themselves, for example, as dandruff on the scalp. If this were to happen in the ear canal, then the canal would very quickly become completely filled by layers of dead skin (keratin). What in fact happens, however, is that the skin of the ear canal migrates from the depths outwards, at about the same rate as fingernails grow. At the cartilaginous portion the layers of skin become mixed with the secretions of the sebaceous and sweat glands, the resultant concoction being called wax. As well as being water resistant, wax also has the important properties of being antibacterial and antifungal which helps preserve the integrity of the ear canal and reduce the chance of infection. Wax production is under the control of several factors and various skin conditions, fevers, local irritations and the psyche all alter the amount and quality of the wax produced, thereby altering the resistance of the ear canal to infection.

The nerves that carry sensation from the external ear and ear canal are derived from a number of sources and this diversity accounts for the ear commonly being affected by referred pain, i.e. disease at one site causing pain in another. The nerves involved in supplying the ear are listed in Table 3.1.

## The outer ear: function

Before sound reaches the tympanic membrane it is collected by the auricle and then passes along the ear canal. The auricle in humans

**Table 3.1:** Sensory nerves of the auricle and ear canal

| Nerve | Derivation |
| --- | --- |
| Greater auricular | Cervical root C2 and C3 |
| Lesser occipital | Cervical roots – C2 |
| Auricular | Vagus (X) nerve |
| Auriculotemporal | Mandibular branch of trigeminal (V) nerve |
| Facial | Facial (VII) |

makes only a small contribution to enhancing the amount of sound entering the ear canal, by reflecting it from its curved surfaces towards the exernal opening of the canal. This effect can be further improved by cupping the hand behind the ear and it was used in some primitive types of acoustic hearing aid.

The ear canal also has features that enhance the amount of sound reaching the tympanic membrane. When sound enters an appropriately sized tube, which is closed at one end, there is resonance in that tube so that the pressure at the open end is low while that at the closed end is high. Resonance enhancement at the tympanic membrane occurs in the human ear, so that over the frequency range 2–7 kHz, i.e. over the frequencies used mainly for hearing and distinguishing speech, there is about a 30-fold gain in the sound pressure (i.e. 15 dB) at the tympanic membrane (Figure 3.3).

Thus there has been some enhancement of the airborne sound reaching the tympanic membrane. The problem is how to transmit this sound and convert it into a form that is suitable for passage through the fluids of the inner ear. This task is achieved by several different features in the anatomy of the tympanic membrane and middle ear, which, together, permit most of the sound reaching the membrane to get into the inner ear.

## The middle ear: structure

The middle-ear space consists of the tympanic cavity (the tympanum), which connects not only with the posterior parts of the nose – the nasopharynx, by way of the eustachian tube – but also with air-filled spaces in the mastoid bone behind the ear canal and the middle ear.

The boundary between the ear canal and the middle ear is the tympanic membrane. This is also frequently called the eardrum, which is a misnomer because a drum consists not only of the membrane but also of the supporting walls and the air inside. Nevertheless, the tympanic membrane is a thin, almost oval disc, slightly broader above than below,

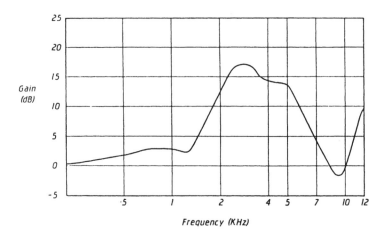

**Figure 3.3:** A graph showing the enhancement of sound at the level of the eardrum. The gain for different frequencies, shown along the base of the graph, is increased by different amounts with the maximal gain in the mid-range of frequencies.

forming an angle of about 55° with the floor of the ear canal (Figure 3.4). The largest diameter is 9–10 mm, measured diagonally from posterosuperior to anteroinferior (Figure 3.5). Most of the edge of the membrane is thickened to form a rim of fibrous tissue and cartilage called the annulus. It is inserted into a groove or sulcus in the bony ear canal and thereby holds the membrane tautly in place. The sulcus does not extend all the way around the ear canal because, at the top, both anteriorly and posteriorly, the thickened annulus turns to run centrally in the membrane and reach the malleus handle as the anterior and posterior malleolar folds. This means that there is a small portion of tympanic membrane without an annulus at its rim. This is the uppermost portion of the membrane and is called the pars flaccida. The much larger portion of the membrane, below the malleolar folds, is called the pars tensa. Both the pars flaccida and the pars tensa have a similar structure: there is an outer layer of skin, a middle layer of fibrous tissue and an inner mucosal layer, which is continuous with the lining of the tympanic cavity.

The skin layer is very thin and consists of cells that migrate outwards from the centre of the membrane. The middle layer has numerous fibrous strands which, in the pars tensa, are arranged both radially, like the spokes of a wheel, and circumferentially. These fibres give the membrane its tautness and allow it to keep its curved shape. The fibres in the pars flaccida are much fewer and are not organized into any such arrangement.

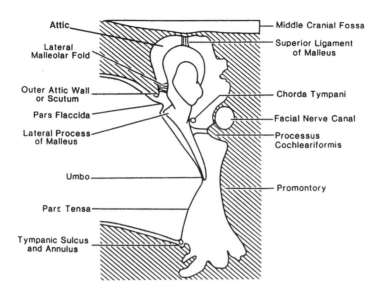

**Figure 3.4:** Diagram of cross-section of ear canal and middle ear. The section has passed through the joint between the malleus and the incus, the former being viewed from behind (posteriorly).

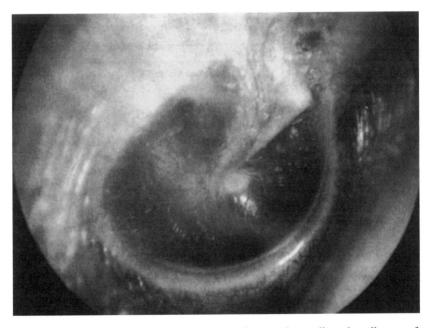

**Figure 3.5:** Photograph of right tympanic membrane: the malleus handle runs from the centre of the membrane (the umbo) upwards and forwards to the lateral process, a prominent white swelling which forms a good landmark.

The middle ear itself can be thought of as a room with four walls, a floor and a ceiling. The outside wall is mainly taken up by the tympanic membrane and the bony rim that supports it. The front wall holds the trumpet-shaped opening of the eustachian tube and above that a small bony canal holding a muscle called the tensor tympani. The back wall separates the middle ear from the mastoid cavity, although there is an opening called the aditus to the mastoid antrum in the top corner (Figure 3.6). The inside wall separates the middle ear from the inner ear and has two small openings in it. The oval window, which is the upper of the two, carries the stapes, while the round window is closed by a thin membrane, which is obscured from view by a bony overhang. Beneath the floor of the middle ear, and at the front, is the internal carotid artery as it ascends and then turns forwards to run medial to the eustachian tube before entering the skull to supply the brain. Blood returning from inside the skull leaves via the sigmoid sinus, and the top of one of the curves lies at the back part of the floor of the middle ear, where it is called the jugular bulb because it represents the beginning of the jugular vein in the neck. The roof of the middle ear is thin bone, which separates it from the inside of the skull and the middle cranial fossa containing the temporal lobes (Figure 3.6).

## The contents of the middle ear

The middle ear contains: air, bones (ossicles), muscles and nerves and, with the exception of the air, these will be described in turn.

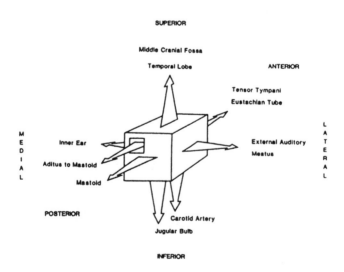

**Figure 3.6:** Schematic diagram of the relationships of the right middle ear.

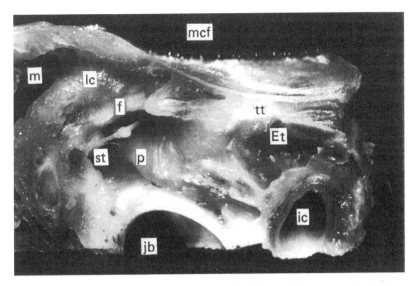

**Figure 3.7:** Photograph of the inner, medial wall of the middle ear. mcf: middle cranial fossa; m: mastoid; lc: lateral semicircular canal; f: facial nerve; st: stapedius tendon running to stapes; p: promontory; jb: jugular bulb; tt: tensor tympani; Et: eustachian tube; ic: internal carotid artery.

## The ossicles

A chain of three small bones connects the tympanic membrane with the inner ear via the oval window. The malleus (hammer) consists of a handle and a head. The handle is attached to the tympanic membrane and can be seen from the outside when the tympanic membrane is inspected with an otoscope. The head of the malleus is surrounded by air and lies in the upper parts of the middle-ear space called the epitympanum or attic (Figure 3.4). The malleus is attached to the body of the incus (anvil) by a joint and, descending from the body back into the middle ear, is the long process of the incus, which makes contact with the head of the stapes (stirrup) (Figure 3.8). The stapes has an arch and a footplate, and it is the footplate that lies in the oval window attached to the bony window frame by a thin elastic membrane (the annular ligament). The whole ossicular chain is suspended by membranes and ligaments so that it transmits sounds very efficiently.

## The muscles

Two muscles can be found in the middle ear. The tensor tympani lies in a bony canal in the top of the eustachian tube and the muscle runs backwards across the upper part of the inner wall of the middle ear. The

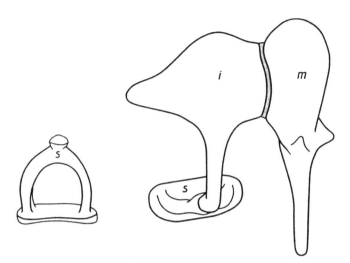

**Figure 3.8:** Diagram of malleus (m), incus (i) and stapes (s).

tendon of the muscle then runs round a small pulley called the processus cochleariformis to cross the middle ear and insert into the back of the malleus handle. This muscle is supplied by a branch of the trigeminal (V) nerve. The stapedius muscle arises from the back wall of the middle ear and its tendon passes through a small tube-like projection of bone – the pyramid – to insert into the head of the stapes. The stapedius is supplied by the facial (VII) nerve (see Figure 3.7)

The action of both these muscles is to stiffen up the ossicular chain, thereby reducing the transmission of some sounds but, interestingly, at least the stapedius also contracts just before the owner speaks, although the function of this is unclear.

**The nerves**

The largest nerve to run through the middle ear is the facial (VII) nerve on its way from the brainstem to supply the muscles of the face and control virtually all aspects of facial movement. The nerve passes out from the brainstem and crosses the so-called cerebellopontine angle, a small space filled with cerebrospinal fluid, to enter the internal auditory meatus along with the acoustic and vestibular nerves on their way to the inner ear. The facial nerve passes between the cochlea in front and the balance portions of the inner ear behind to reach the inner wall of the middle ear (Figure 3.9). It then turns backwards at the geniculate (knee-like) ganglion and runs in a bony canal (the fallopian canal) above the oval window and the stapes. When the nerve reaches the back wall of the middle ear, it turns down to run in the bone between the mastoid and the middle ear until it escapes from the base of the skull through the opening called the stylo-mastoid foramen. The nerve then turns forwards to pass through the parotid gland, where it breaks up into five branches to supply the muscles of facial expression.

The other major nerve that runs through the ear is the chorda tympani. This nerve carries the sensation of taste from the anterior two thirds of the tongue and travels up to enter the front wall of the middle ear just above the eustachian tube opening and near the attachment of the tympanic membrane. The nerve then runs in the middle layer of the tympanic membrane itself, behind the malleus handle to cross the membrane and reach the back wall of the middle ear where it joins the facial nerve and accompanies it to the brain.

The facial nerve and the chorda tympani both take rather irregular routes to pass through the ear. This strange situation has arisen from the way the middle ear has evolved as an out-pouching of nose and pharynx, inserting itself between the inner ear and the skin outside.

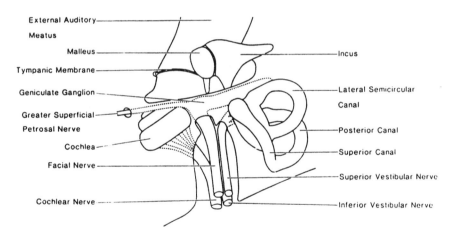

**Figure 3.9:** Diagram of the path of the facial nerve through the temporal bone. In this view you are looking down on to the base of the skull in the region of the inner ear. Technically this is the floor of the middle cranial fossa. The facial nerve is passing out between the cochlea in front and the semicircular canals behind to reach the genicu-late ganglion.

## The eustachian tube

The middle ear needs to be filled with air at more or less normal atmos-pheric pressure in order to be able to work. It is generally felt that the correct functioning of the eustachian tube is the most important factor in maintaining normal ventilation of the middle ear.

The eustachian tube runs from the middle ear to the nasopharynx in a forward, slightly inward and slightly downward direction. It is about 36 mm long and, like the ear canal, has a bony and a cartilaginous portion. The bony portion is effectively an extension of the bony walls of the middle ear and starts as a wide opening which over its 12 mm length narrows down to the isthmus, which is the narrowest part of the eustachian tube with a diameter 2 mm.

The cartilaginous portion of the tube is 24 mm long, although the cartilage does not form a complete circle. There is a solid back wall and curved roof, which continues to form part of the front wall (Figure 3.10). The rest of the front wall consists of a fibrous membrane completing the tube. One of the muscles of the palate – the tensor palati – arises, in part, from the edge of the curved cartilage forming the roof and front wall of the eustachian tube. The other end of the muscle runs into the soft palate, spreads out like a fan, and meets and joins the same muscle from the other eustachian tube. When the muscle contracts the soft palate becomes firm, but the eustachian tube is also opened a little.

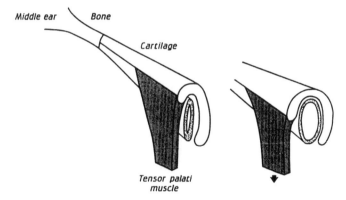

**Figure 3.10:** Diagram of the action of the eustachian tube. The cartilage walls of the inner portion of tube have the tensor palati muscle attached. When this contracts the cartilage buckles and the tube opens a little.

The nasal end of the tube opens in the side wall of the nasopharynx and the cartilaginous walls form a bump beneath the mucosa lining the nose. The tube is lined at the nasal end by nasal mucosa which, like respiratory mucosa anywhere in the body, has the following:

* single cells producing mucus, the so-called goblet cells
* mucous glands

- cells carrying hair-like cilia, which beat and move the mucus towards the nasopharynx.

Getting closer to the ear, the concentration of these three features reduces but, nevertheless, the eustachian tube still has all the features of respiratory mucosa (Figure 3.11).

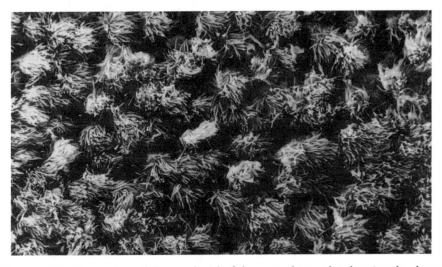

**Figure 3.11:** The surface of the nasal end of the eustachian tube showing the dense carpet of cilia. In life, these beat in unison to move mucus from the middle ear to the nose.

## The mastoid air cells

The mastoid bone is a rounded mass of bone at the base of the skull, part of which can be felt behind the ear. One of the large muscles controlling movement (the sternomastoid) is attached to its lower end, and running within it is the sigmoid sinus on its way to becoming the jugular bulb in the floor of the middle ear. The air-filled spaces of the middle ear connect with a small air-filled space in the mastoid bone called the mastoid antrum. Everyone has a mastoid antrum and most people have, arising from the antrum, a large number of air-filled spaces separated by thin sheets of bone so that the whole thing resembles a honeycomb. In this situation, the mastoid is called a cellular or aerated mastoid. In a smaller group of people, and frequently in people with (or who have had) long-standing middle-ear disease, there is a very restricted development of air cells so that the mastoid is mainly bone – this is called sclerotic. Whether the lack of air cells causes or is caused by the middle-ear disease is not firmly established.

# The middle ear: function

All animals that hear, whether they live under water or on land, have some form of inner ear with the auditory sensory cells (hair cells) bathed in fluid. For animals that live under water (excluding mammals), the transfer of sound waves from the surrounding water to the fluid in the inner ear is relatively efficient and all there is between the outside water and the inner-ear fluids is a thin membrane. However, when life adapted itself to living on land a mechanism evolved for the transfer of airborne sounds to the fluids of the inner ear. This mechanism is the middle ear, which has the same basic arrangement in all land mammals. There is a taut tympanic membrane, an air-filled middle ear and a collection of bones connecting the membrane to the inner ear. There has been considerable diversity in the evolution of the middle ear, e.g. birds have a single bone, the columella, while in humans there are three, and in many rodents the malleus and incus are fused together. In mammals, as well as the middle ear there is also the external ear, which has features that assist the transfer of airborne sound to the middle ear.

Why is this rather complex arrangement necessary? When sound is projected at the surface of a body of water, virtually all of it is reflected back and perhaps only 0.5% gets into the fluid. This is why echoes are so good in areas where mountains surround lakes. The technical explanation for this effect is that the impedance of air, i.e. the resistance of air to the passage of sound, is very different from the impedance of a liquid. (The impedance of air is 415 N s/m$^3$ and that of the cochlear fluids is 150 000, i.e. 1.5 ($10^5$ N s/m$^3$.) Where the impedance of two adjoining substances is quite different, then the transfer of sound from one to the other is poor. What the middle ear does, to about a 60% level of efficiency, is to overcome the mismatch of the impedances of air and the cochlear fluids. The middle-ear mechanism has thus been called the middle-ear transformer or impedance matcher.

The impedance of air is 415 newton seconds per cubic metre or Ns/m$^3$ and that of cochlear fluids is 150 000 i.e. $1.5 \times 105$ N sm$^3$)

**Middle-ear transformer mechanism (Figure 3.12)**

1  There is a large area of tympanic membrane to absorb the incoming sound, which is then transferred to the very much smaller area of the stapes footplate. Thus a large amount of sound pressure is concentrated on to a small area.
2  The tympanic membrane, although taut, is not rigid. If it were rigid then a considerable amount of sound would be reflected from it. Instead the membrane buckles or gives a little with the incoming sound

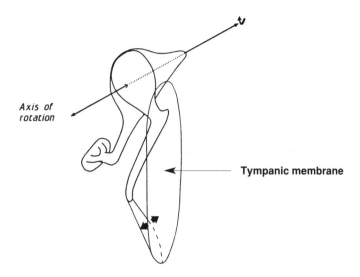

*Axis of rotation*

**Tympanic membrane**

**Figure 3.12:** Diagram of the middle-ear transformer mechanism: there is a large area of tympanic membrane to collect sound, which is transferred to the smaller area of the stapes footplate. The tympanic membrane also buckles, which increases its absorptive powers and there is a small lever effect due to the different lengths of the malleus and incus.

and these forces are transmitted to the malleus handle, which is firmly attached to the very centre of the membrane.

3  The arrangement of the malleus and incus creates a lever-like effect so that the rather low-pressure, wide-ranging movement caused by airborne sound at the tympanic membrane is converted to smaller but higher pressure waves at the stapes.

Overall, therefore, the action of the middle ear is to convert the rather low-pressure, large-displacement, airborne sound waves reaching the tympanic membrane into high-pressure, small-displacement waveforms, which are more suited for transmission through the fluids of the middle ear.

*Prerequisites for the transformer mechanism*

For the middle-ear transformer to be optimal, certain conditions need to be fulfilled.

1  The tympanic membrane must be intact and flexible. Perforation reduces the effectiveness of sound collection to a certain degree – although the hearing effects of a tiny hole are not measurable by standard techniques. A tympanic membrane made rigid by scarring and thickening (tympanosclerosis) also loses its effectiveness in absorbing sound.

2  The ossicles must be intact and mobile. Any dislocation or discontinuity stops the transfer of the collected sound from the tympanic
   membrane and causes a considerable hearing loss. Similarly, any condition that restricts the mobility of the malleus, incus and stapes impairs
   sound conduction to the inner ear and causes a hearing loss.
3  There needs to be air on both sides of the tympanic membrane at about
   the same pressure for hearing to be optimal. A middle ear full of fluid
   causes the tympanic membrane to lose its mobility so that, instead of
   buckling, sound is reflected back into the ear canal. The mobility of the
   ossicles will also be reduced and add to the problems. However, even
   with a middle ear full of the thickest, stickiest fluid, sound can get
   through and, providing the cochlea and auditory nerve are intact, the
   individual will not be profoundly deaf.

If the air pressure in the middle ear is low (as can happen during
aeroplane descents), the tympanic membrane becomes pushed inwards
by the relatively high pressure in the external ear canal. This prevents
normal sound absorption and, again, reduces the hearing although not to
the degree of having a middle ear full of fluid.

## Maintenance of middle-ear ventilation and drainage

The middle ear and mastoid are lined by a tissue that absorbs oxygen from
the air in contact with it and, at the same time, releases small amounts of
carbon dioxide, produced by the body's metabolism, in much the same
way as the lungs do, although on a far smaller scale.

The classic theory of how the middle ear is ventilated suggests that
overall there is a predominance of absorption of gas by the lining mucosa
so that the gas pressures in the middle ear drop slowly. Every few minutes
the individual swallows or, less frequently, yawns, and the eustachian tube
is pulled open a little so that a small amount of air ascends the tube to
replenish that which has been absorbed. Over a prolonged time, and with
normal eustachian tube function the middle-ear pressures remain stable
and at about the level of the external air pressure. Various experimental
work in humans has suggested that about only 1 mm$^3$ of air per ear per day
is needed to maintain equilibrium. Any condition that impairs the function
of the eustachian tube results in a failure of middle-ear ventilation and
reduces middle-ear pressure. If this pressure is low enough, indrawing or
retraction of the tympanic membrane occurs.

The lining of the middle ear is a form of respiratory mucosa and so may
respond in the way that respiratory mucosa elsewhere in the body does to
infection (bacterial or viral), allergy, irritation and so on, by producing
mucus. This mucus is normally moved by the motile cilia (quite different

from the stereocilia of cochlear hair cells), which line the eustachian tube, towards the opening of the tube in the back of the nose, and the mucus is then swallowed.

Any condition that alters the effectiveness of the cilia in moving the mucus causes a build-up of mucus in the middle ear.

# The inner ear: structure

The inner ear contains the sensory structures – the hair cells – which act as microphones to convert incoming sound into electricity for transmission to the brain via the acoustic nerve. The arrangement of these cells is, at first sight, rather complicated because in mammals they are housed in a coiled-up tube resembling a snail's shell, called the cochlea. In an attempt to make the anatomy easier to understand the coil is unrolled to form a straight tube as shown in Figure 3.13. In fact, birds have an inner ear formed in this way, which is called the lagena rather than the cochlea.

This single tube is filled with fluid and is split in half along its length by a partition, which does not quite extend to the apex. The small gap at the end is called the helicotreme and allows communication between the space above the partition, called the scala vestibuli, and the space below, called the scala tympani. The bony opening at the basal end of the scala tympani, next to the middle ear, is the round window and this is closed over in life by the round-window membrane. The opening of the scala vestibuli is the oval window, which is filled by the footplate of the stapes

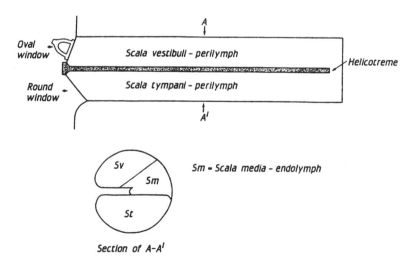

**Figure 3.13:** Diagram of the uncoiled cochlea with a cross-section shown below.

attached to the rim of the window by the annular ligament. The scala vestibuli also connects with those parts of the inner ear that deal with balance and this relationship can be seen in Figure 3.14. The fluid filling the two scalae is called perilymph and has a similar composition to the cerebrospinal fluid, which bathes the brain and with which it is in contact through a small bony tunnel called the cochlear aqueduct. This opens in the scala tympani near the round window.

If the tube is cut across from A to A1 in the diagram and the cut end of the tube looked at, then some additional structures become visible (Figure 3.13). The partition separating the scala vestibuli from the scala tympani is half bone and half a thin membrane, known as the basilar membrane. Arising from the bony partition is a second thin membrane, which extends to the side wall and forms a sloping roof to a third compartment, called the scala media or cochlear duct. This thin membrane is called Reissner's membrane. The scala media is therefore a triangular tube that is closed at the apex but communicates at the base with the series of canals and ducts forming the balance portion of the inner ear. In humans, the scala media is coiled through two and a half turns, this whole collection of canals and ducts being called the membranous labyrinth. It is filled with endolymph, an unusual fluid that has high potassium levels, low sodium levels and an electric potential of 80 mV. The constituents of the endolymph in the

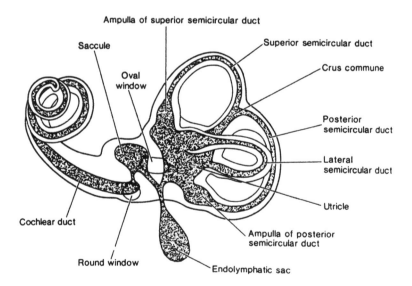

**Figure 3.14:** Diagram of the complete inner ear: the scala media is also called the cochlear duct and is shown shaded. It connects with the balance portions of the inner ear – the saccule, utricle and semicircular canals – by way of the ductus reuniens.

cochlea are maintained by the stria vascularis, which lies on the side wall of the scala media. This structure has a very rich blood supply and under the microscope looks very similar to some of the tissues of the kidney.

### The contents of the scala media (Figure 3.15)

The floor of the scala media is flat and consists of an inner bony portion and an outer membranous part. On the membranous portion there is a small ridge called the organ of Corti, which contains the auditory sensory cells (Figure 3.16). These cells consist of a long body containing the nucleus, with nerve fibres attached to one end and a thickened plate called the cuticular plate at the other. Projecting from the surface of the cuticular plate is a cluster of hair-like structures called stereocilia (Figure 3.17). These are fine, rigid rods, made of actin packed to form a crystalline structure, and linked together by small interconnections to form a stereociliary bundle. There are two separate types of hair cell. The inner hair cell (IHC) has a short, rounded, cell body and many nerve fibres attached to its base. The outer hair cell (OHC) has a long tubular body and fewer nerve fibres, which, when stimulated, can change the tension within its walls. The IHCs form a single row extending along the length of the scala media, while the OHCs are arranged in three or four irregular rows. A scanning electron micrograph of part of the human organ of Corti shows

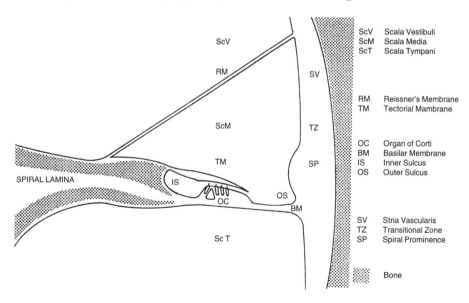

| | |
|---|---|
| ScV | Scala Vestibuli |
| ScM | Scala Media |
| ScT | Scala Tympani |
| | |
| RM | Reissner's Membrane |
| TM | Tectorial Mambrane |
| | |
| OC | Organ of Corti |
| BM | Basilar Membrane |
| IS | Inner Sulcus |
| OS | Outer Sulcus |
| | |
| SV | Stria Vascularis |
| TZ | Transitional Zone |
| SP | Spiral Prominence |
| | |
| | Bone |

**Figure 3.15:** The scala media or cochlear duct shown diagrammatically in cross-section.

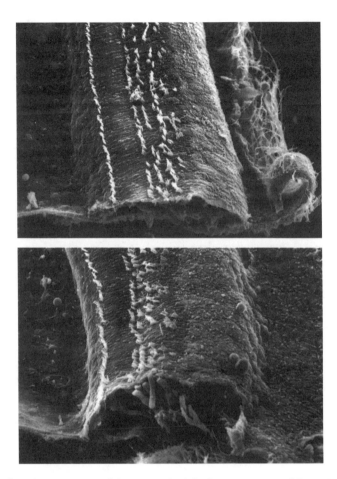

**Figure 3.16:** A short portion of the cut end of the human organ of Corti. In the upper picture, the cut edge of the basilar membrane is also seen and its fibrous nature can be appreciated. Projecting from the surface of the organ of Corti are the hair cell bundles, and these are seen to be arranged into a single row of inner hair cells and several rows of outer hair cells. In the lower, more oblique micrograph, the cut edge of the organ of Corti can be seen. A few of the sausage-shaped bodies of the outer hair cells are visible.

the arrangement of hair cells (Figure 3.18). In life, the organ of Corti is covered by a soft, gelatinous membrane called the tectorial membrane, which arises from the bony portion of the floor of the scala media and stretches over the sensory cells to attach to the outer parts of the organ of Corti. The tips of the stereocilia of the OHCs are attached to the underside of the tectorial membrane but those of the IHCs stand free in the endolymph. A cross-section of the organ of Corti shows the relationship to the tectorial membrane (Figure 3.19).

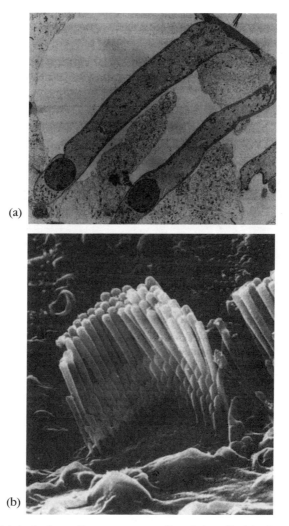

(a)

(b)

**Figure 3.17:** (a) A single auditory sensory cell or hair cell: this electron micrograph shows the cell running diagonally across the illustration. At the upper (right) end can be seen some short hairs projecting from a thickened surface plate. At the base of the cell body is a darkly staining nucleus. (b) The surface view of the top end of a single human outer hair cell. Projecting from the surface plate is a cluster of stereocilia. Although they look flexible, in life these are rigid structures that pivot about their bases when deflected.

A closer view of the surface of the organ of Corti shows that in humans there is a rather irregular arrangement of the hair cells with missing OHCs and often extra IHCs (Figure 3.18). This is quite different from the arrangement in many experimental animals, which is remarkably regular.

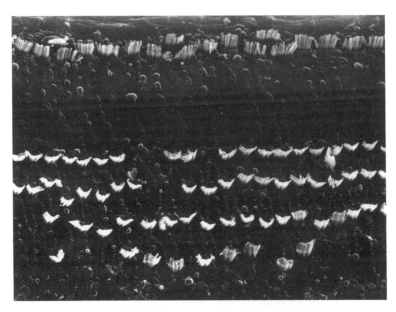

**Figure 3.18:** A surface view of a segment of the human organ of Corti. This section is one fifth of a millimetre across. There is a single row of inner hair cells with occasional extra cells, and a variable number of rows of outer hair cells with frequent missing cells and quite remarkable irregularity.

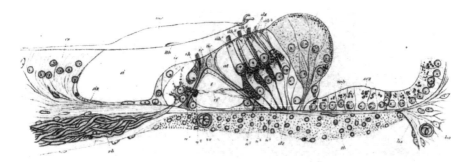

**Figure 3.19:** A cross-section of the organ of Corti. This picture is taken from the works of Retzius, completed in 1884. The tectorial membrane has retracted a little from the organ of Corti during preparation and would in life attach to the organ of Corti outside the outer hair cells.

Overall there are about 3000 IHCs and 12 000 OHCs in each cochlea of a young person. As the years pass these numbers decline at a regular rate. Surprisingly, most of the nerves carrying information to the brain arise from the IHCs and each IHC has about 10 fibres attached to it. These fibres run inwards towards the centre of the cochlea to join with fibres from the rest of the organ of Corti and form the acoustic nerve. This then runs inwards with the vestibular (balance) nerve and facial nerve through a bony canal called the internal auditory meatus to reach the brainstem (Figure 3.19). From here, and by complex pathways, the nerve fibres ascend through the brain to reach the central auditory cortex where the perception of sound occurs. There is no space here to describe these pathways in any depth but a block diagram of some of the names will help with some of the terminology in the chapters on objective hearing tests (Figure 3.20).

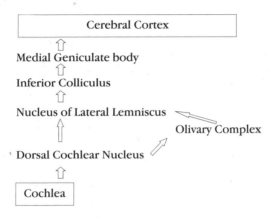

**Figure 3.20:** Block diagram of the main ascending auditory pathways.

# The inner ear: function

As mentioned earlier, the auditory sensory cell or hair cell is the focal point of the hearing mechanism. External sound converges on the hair cells, which are thereby stimulated and correspondingly produce electrical signals, which are then carried by the acoustic nerve fibres to the brain.

### Hair cell function

The mechanism by which the hair cell converts sound to electrical energy is incompletely understood but relies on the following features (Figure 3.21):

- The endolymph which bathes the surface of the stereocilia has a high potassium content and a +80 mV electrical potential.
- The inside of the IHC has a relatively low potassium content and a potential of −45 mV.
- There is, therefore, a steep gradient of both potassium concentration and electrical potential across the upper surface of the IHC and its stereocilia.

- Distortion of the stereocilia opens up spaces in the surface membranes (ion channels) and through these, potassium ions flow down their concentration gradient.
- This causes the voltage of the inside of the cell to alter, becoming less negative, and the cell is then said to have depolarized.
- If the degree of depolarization is large enough, little packets of chemical transmitters (neurotransmitters) are released in large numbers from the base of the cell and cross the narrow space to be absorbed by the nerve fibres, which are closely attached to this basal region of the cell.
- These neurotransmitters in turn cause the nerve fibres to depolarize, in much the same way that the hair cell body depolarized, except in this case a chemical rather than a mechanical stimulus was the initiating feature.
- The nerve fibre then carries this electrical signal along its length and at the other end releases further neurotransmitters to stimulate the nerve to which it is in turn connected. There are a whole range of neurotransmitters in the nervous system, many of which are only just being discovered.

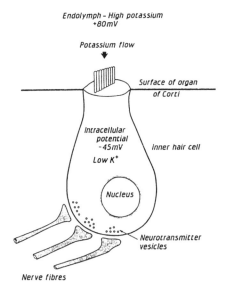

**Figure 3.21:** Schematic diagram of an inner hair cell: the endolymph bathing the upper surface of the hair cell and stereocilia has high potassium ($K^+$) levels and a positive electrical potential. The inside of the hair cell has a low potassium level and a negative potential so that there is a steep gradient across the hair cell membrane. This gradient probably provides the basis for the remarkable sensitivity of the hair cell to stimulation.

**Sound transmission within the cochlea**

The previous section has shown how sound stimulates individual hair cells. The problem for discussion in this section is how sound is carried through the cochlea from its arrival at the oval window by way of the stapes, and how all the different pitches present in complex noise are distinguished. From the section on structure, it will have become apparent that along the length of the cochlear duct there are progressive changes in the dimensions of various structures. In going from base to apex the basilar membrane becomes wider and more flexible, the hair cell bodies and the stereocilia of the OHC and IHCs increase in length, and the size of the scala media increases. With other changes, this gradient creates conditions within the cochlea that result in specific regions of the scala media being responsive to particular pitches or frequencies of sound.

As sound pressure enters the cochlear fluids at the oval window, waves are set up in this fluid. You can imagine this as resembling the waves that result when a stone is thrown into a pond, except that instead of spreading out as they would in the pond the waves are channelled along the cochlea. These pressure changes are transmitted across the basilar membrane, with the round window membrane, which is in contact with the air of the middle ear, acting as the compensatory membrane to the movements of the stapes footplate (Figure 3.22). This second window is necessary because of the incompressibility of fluid, and if the round window is totally obstructed then a significant hearing loss results.

What happens to create this wave in the cochlea is that near the base of the cochlea the stiffness of the basilar membrane limits vibration, whereas near the apex the basilar membrane is more lax and it is the mass of the membrane, together with the organ of Corti, that limits vibration. Where vibration is stiffness-limited, there is little delay in the vibrations actually occurring, whereas if vibration is mass-limited there is some delay as the applied pressure has to overcome the inherent inertia. Thus, when a single pitch or frequency is applied to the stapes, the basilar membrane starts to move first at the base and progressively further along the cochlear duct. There is thus the appearance of a travelling wave moving up the cochlea and this was first observed by Georg von Békésy in the 1940s (von Békésy 1980). For each individual frequency there is a combination of the conditions of stiffness and mass which results in maximal movement of the basilar membrane. Thus the wave grows in size as it passes along the cochlea until it reaches maximum amplitude, and then fairly suddenly the increasing mass component damps down further vibration and the wave dies out.

It has been found that high-frequency sound has the peak of its travelling wave near the base, while low frequency sound peaks near the apex.

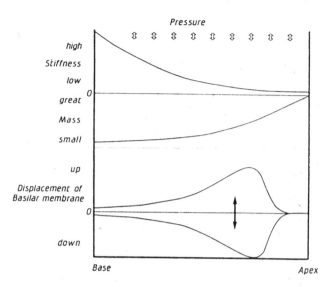

**Figure 3.22:** Schematic diagram of the generation of the travelling wave within the cochlea. The base of the cochlea is represented at the left of the graph with the apex at the right. The top curve represents the stiffness of the basilar membrane, which decreases on going from base to apex, while in the graph below the mass of the organ of basilar membrane and the organ of Corti is seen to increase. The resulting displacement of the basilar membrane following the application of sound pressure is seen in the lower compartment, the solid lines representing the overall wave envelope. This is von Békésy's travelling wave.

Thus for a single frequency of sound there is a point of maximum resonance of the basilar membrane. What probably happens in this region is that the basilar membrane, along with the organ of Corti, is moved relative to the tectorial membrane which is fixed to the bony floor of the scala media at the spiral limbus (Figure 3.23). As this movement occurs there is fluid displacement in the space (the inner sulcus) between the spiral limbus, tectorial membrane and organ of Corti, and this causes bending of the IHC's stereocilia with their subsequent depolarization. Close to the threshold of hearing at one pitch, perhaps only a few IHCs are stimulated. As the sound becomes more intense the travelling wave increases in size so that more than just a few IHCs are stimulated by the fluid movement in the inner sulcus. More nerve fibres are then stimulated and the sound appears louder.

Thus, built into the anatomy of the cochlea is a system that analyses the frequency of the sound applied to it and also gives a measure of its intensity. When von Békésy first described his travelling wave he realized that the peak of the wave (see Figure 3.22) was much too broad to be able to account for the ear's ability to distinguish pitches that were very close together. For example, a trained ear can distinguish frequencies that differ

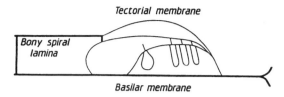

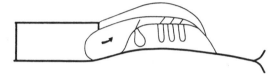

**Figure** 3.23: Diagram representing the changes that occur with basilar membrane movement. As the membrane rises, the organ of Corti moves relative to the more rigid tectorial membrane and the stereocilia of the outer hair cells are deflected, while fluid movement under the tectorial membrane causes displacement of the inner hair cell stereocilia.

by only 1 Hz or less in the range of speech frequencies, whereas it took a change of tens of hertz to shift the peak of the travelling wave sufficiently to stimulate adjoining IHCs. von Békésy thought that further analysis of frequency took place in the brain, but in the 1950s, and with the advent of microelectrode technology, various workers – notably Evans (1975) and Kiang et al. (1970) – were able to insert electrodes into single fibres of the acoustic nerve. They could thus test the response of single fibres coming from the IHCs to applied sound (Figure 3.24).

With the appropriate sound reaching the ear the nerve fibre fires off volleys of nerve impulses and this can be recorded as a response. The experiment performed held the intensity of the sound constant and swept across a range of frequencies. At low-level sounds a fibre coming from a single IHC was only responsive at a single critical frequency. As the sound intensity was increased a little, it was found that the fibre became responsive to a slightly wider range of frequencies and this band of response increased still further as the intensity was raised (Figure 3.25). The shape of the outline of this band of responsiveness is called the frequency tuning curve. The tip of the curve is very sharp in healthy animals and the nerve fibre is 'sharply tuned'. If the electrode were placed in another fibre, a similar frequency tuning curve could be obtained but with a slightly shifted critical frequency. Thus whole families of overlapping tuning

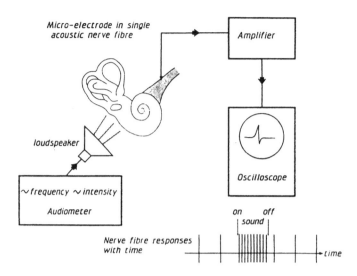

**Figure 3.24:** Highly schematic diagram of the experimental set up to test the responses of a single fibre of the acoustic nerve.

curves could be built up from the different fibres of an acoustic nerve. If the OHCs were missing or the animal became depleted of oxygen the sharpness of these tuning curves was lost.

It thus became apparent that von Békésy's idea that the analysis of frequency was performed in the brain was wrong because the nerve fibres leaving a healthy cochlea had already been 'tuned' to specific frequencies.

It was also realized that the cochlea had to be healthy with intact OHCs for this tuning to work and in fact von Békésy had had to use the ears of dead animals and humans to perform his research. He had also had to use extremely intense sound to be able to see the movement within the cochlea and this sound level was well above the natural range of the inner ear. As technology improved it became possible to measure movement of the basilar membrane in live, healthy animals at more reasonable sound pressures. Sellick and others in 1982 were able to show that instead of the rather flat top to von Békésy's wave there was, in fact, a very sharp, 'finely tuned' peak of basilar membrane movement (Figure 3.26). This enhanced peak required a healthy cochlea, normal intact OHCs and was easily lost by minute pressure changes within the cochlea.

Nevertheless, however the calculations were performed and whatever values were given to the stiffness and the mass of the cochlear structures, it has not been possible to match the predicted movements of the basilar membrane as a passive responder to incoming sound with those actually observed in experiments. It is now strongly felt that there is, within the

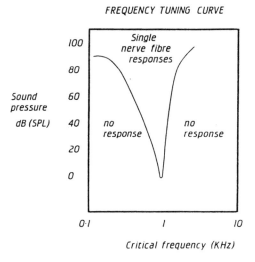

**Figure 3.25:** Graph of the responses of a single fibre of the acoustic nerve. Across the base of the graph are shown the different frequencies applied to the ear and at the side the pressure of that sound in decibels. The area within the solid line indicates where the nerve fibre is responding. So, for this particular fibre the critical frequency (cf), i.e. the frequency at which the stimulation is minimal to obtain a response, is 1 kHz. The whole graph is called a frequency tuning curve and the sharp point indicates that the fibre is 'finely tuned'.

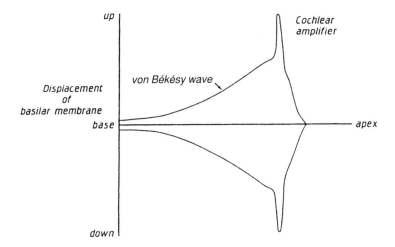

**Figure 3.26:** Revised view of von Békésy's travelling wave. At or near the peak of von Békésy's wave there is a small area of active movement that sets the basilar membrane into an enhanced displacement. This cochlear amplifier requires energy and the presence of healthy outer hair cells.

cochlea, an active process, or cochlear amplifier, which results in the fine-tuning of von Békésy's wave, and which requires the OHCs for its function. The precise mechanism of this 'amplifier' is yet to be established but the system is mechanically active and relies on the OHCs that have the ability to alter their length and tension, acting, perhaps, like coiled springs within the organ of Corti. It is possible that when they are appropriately stimulated a small segment of the basilar membrane, organ of Corti, stereocilia and perhaps tectorial membrane goes into an enhanced resonance powered by the OHCs.

This released energy enhances the sensitivity of the cochlea and results in only a few inner cells being stimulated at a low threshold at one frequency. More recently it has been possible, using fine electrodes, to record from the IHCs themselves. Cody and Russell (1987) have shown quite conclusively that depolarization of the IHCs is also finely tuned so that the stimulus reaching the stereocilia of the IHCs must itself be finely tuned, thereby confirming Sellick's finding that the movements of the basilar membrane are critical factors in the ear's ability to discriminate pitch.

### Cochlear echoes

In 1978, Kemp found that after a short burst of sound there was, after a short delay, an output of sound from the inner ear. If this sound coming out of the ear was analysed, it was found to be very similar to the sound that had been put in and so was named the cochlear echo, or more formally the otoacoustic emission (OAE). After initial scepticism from some of the scientific community, it became apparent that this was a real effect and when the calculations were performed it was realized that more sound could be got out of the cochlea than was put in. For the echoes to be heard, the animals had to be healthy and there had to be functioning OHCs. The Kemp effect was therefore a mechanically active, energy-requiring amplifier and its discovery predated the realization of the need for such an amplifier to be present within the cochlea to account for the ear's ability to discriminate pitch. What is probably happening is that some of the energy generated by the internal cochlear amplifier, which sets the basilar membrane into enhanced resonance, leaks back out of the cochlea to be detected as an echo. As soon as the OHCs start to malfunction, this echo is reduced and then lost.

Thus, OAEs not only have a role in the theory of hearing but also have the potential, now being realized, of providing a very sensitive indicator of hearing loss, or even of a developing hearing loss, because loss of the emissions can precede a loss of hearing as recorded on pure-tone audiograms (see also Chapter 6 for audiometry based on inner ear physiology).

# Chapter 4
# Introduction to acoustics and speech perception

Valerie Hazan

To understand the communicative difficulties faced in everyday life by deaf listeners who use aural–oral communication, it is important to have some basic knowledge of how speech is produced and perceived by listeners with normal hearing. The aim of this chapter is therefore to provide a basic introduction to the processes involved in the production of speech, the transmission of speech in the form of sound waves and the decoding of these sound waves by the listener in order to achieve understanding of the message.

## Speech production

### The Source-filter model

The production of speech sounds involves the interaction between a source of sound and a 'filter', which will shape the source to produce a wide range of different sounds. This process is described by a simple model known as the Source-filter model.

### Sound source

Speech sounds can be produced with one of two sound sources. The most common is the sound source produced by the vibration of the vocal folds in the larynx. The vocal folds can be set in motion by the flow of air from the lungs passing between them once they have been brought together. A fall in air pressure caused by the rapid flow of air between the vocal folds causes them to snap shut; once this has occurred, air pressure builds up beneath the vocal folds and the vocal folds open again. The rate of vibration of the vocal folds is, to a certain extent, physiologically determined, as it is related to the size of the larynx and of the vocal folds. This process of regular opening and closing of the vocal folds occurs, on average, 125 times a second in adult male speakers and 225 to 250 times a second in adult female speakers. However, the rate of vocal-fold vibration is also under the speaker's control and can be altered during an utterance to produce changes in the perceived intonation of an utterance. Vocal-fold vibration produces a sound that very much resembles a 'buzz'; the acoustic composition of this 'buzz' will be described on page 61. A speech sound is said to be voiced if its production involves vocal-fold vibration. All sounds in the word 'manually', for example, are voiced and the vocal-fold vibrations can be felt by placing a finger on the throat while uttering this word.

A second source of sound is noise (or turbulence) produced by forcing air through a narrow constriction somewhere in the mouth. This noise source sounds more like a 'hiss' and is used in the production of consonants such as the ones in the words 'sash' or 'fish', for example.

*Filter*

The shaping that is applied to the sound source is determined by the phenomenon of 'resonance'. A resonator is an object that has a 'preferred' rate or frequency at which it likes to vibrate, which is determined by its volume or length. Examples of resonators include a pendulum, a swing, a tuning fork and a cavity filled with air. If a resonator is set in free motion, it will naturally vibrate at its preferred frequency, known as the *resonant frequency*. Large resonators (e.g. a pendulum on a long string or an empty milk bottle) have a low resonant frequency while small resonators (e.g. a pendulum on a short string or a milk bottle almost filled with water) have a high resonant frequency.

In speech production, the whole of the vocal tract, which is the airway that includes the throat, the mouth and nasal cavity, constitutes the filter. The vocal tract can be thought of as a series of connected, air-filled chambers or cavities. By changing the position of *articulators*, such as the tongue, the jaw and the lips, during the production of speech sounds, the speaker will be changing the size of various cavities within the vocal tract. Each of these cavities is acting as a resonator and will have a 'preferred' frequency or small range of frequencies at which it will vibrate. As the sizes of the various cavities change, so do their resonant frequencies. As resonant frequencies change, so does the *timbre* or quality of the speech sound produced. Moving the tongue from the back of the mouth to the front of the mouth, for example, will change the vowel quality from /u/ as in 'booed' to /i/ as in 'bead'. As resonant frequencies are determined by cavity size, male speakers, who generally have larger vocal tracts than female speakers, will generally produce sounds that contain resonances at lower frequencies. In fact, as no two speakers have identical vocal tract configurations and sizes, no two speakers will produce identical sound patterns.

In speech production, a distinction is made between vowel sounds, which are produced with an open vocal tract, and consonant sounds for which there is a constriction or even complete occlusion in the vocal tract.

## Vowel production

In the production of vowels, the vocal folds are vibrating (unless the vowel is whispered), the vocal tract is open and a change in vowel quality is achieved by a smooth movement of articulators, such as the jaw, tongue or lips. In phonetics, vowels are described and classified in terms of the position of the tongue during their production: whether high or low, whether front or back. In vowels such as /ɑ/in 'dart', the articulators are relatively steady throughout the sound, whereas in diphthongs such as /ɛi/ as in 'date', the articulators move smoothly during the production of the vowel from positions appropriate for the production of /ɛ/ as in 'bet' to those appropriate for /ɪ/ as in 'bit'.

## Consonant production

A number of different descriptors are used to classify the consonants of a language. First, consonants are described in terms of their *manner of production*. For example, consonants known as plosives (e.g. the initial consonants in 'bowl' or 'till') are produced with a complete closure at some position within the vocal tract, followed by a rapid release once the air pressure has forced the occlusion open. Fricatives (such as the initial consonants in 'fill', 'sill', 'vile') are produced with a constriction within the vocal tract through which air is forced. Nasals (such as the initial consonants in 'mile', 'nil') involve a lowering of the soft palate, which allows air to exit through the nasal cavity while there is an occlusion at some point within the oral cavity.

Another descriptor is the consonants' *place of articulation*. This is determined by the place within the oral tract where an occlusion or constriction occurs. For example, the initial consonant in 'bile' is called a bilabial, as closure occurs at the lips.

Finally, consonants are described in terms of their *voicing*, i.e. whether or not their 'source' involves vocal-fold vibration. The initial consonants in 'mile' and 'nil', for example, are described as voiced, whereas the initial consonant in 'pile' is described as voiceless, as it is produced without vocal-fold vibration.

A full phonetic description of speech sounds used by the languages of the world can be found in the International Phonetic Alphabet chart, which contains symbols for around 70 main consonant types and 30 vowels. Of course, each language will only use a subset of vowel and consonant sounds. British English (Received Pronunciation accent) is particularly rich in vowels (20 as opposed to five in Italian, for example) and also includes around 24 consonant categories. The size of the vowel and consonant inventories of a language are an important consideration when considering speech perception and production by people with a hearing impairment as they do to a certain extent determine the inherent 'difficulty' of a language, at the phonetic level at least.

## Acoustics of sound waves

### Basic concepts

Once they exit the vocal tract, speech sounds are propagated as pressure disturbances in the atmosphere, i.e. as a series of compressions and rarefactions of air molecules. The air molecules themselves make only very small movements but the pressure disturbance propagates outwards from the sound source. This results in changes in air pressure above and below atmospheric pressure. These pressure variations that constitute sound are often represented on a 'waveform', which is a plot of pressure variations over time. It may be helpful to first describe the waveform of the purest sound that exists: the sinewave (or 'pure tone'), which is the sound that is produced by a tuning fork. A pure tone has a very smooth and regular waveform and a single cycle of this waveform (see Figure 4.1) represents a single cycle of compression and rarefaction of air molecules. Pure tones are widely used in the measurement of hearing.

The two parameters that are plotted on the axes of a waveform display are time (x-axis) and amplitude (y-axis). On the time axis, we can see that the

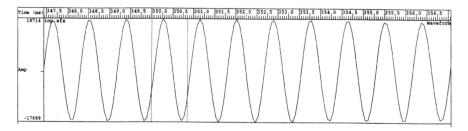

**Figure 4.1:** Waveform of a sinewave (or 'pure tone'). Time is represented on the x-axis and amplitude on the y-axis. Two vertical lines show the period of a single cycle of the sinewave (around 0.8 milliseconds).

waveform forms a certain pattern that repeats after a certain lapse of time. The time taken to complete a cycle is called the *period* and the term *frequency* is used to describe how many cycles are completed in a specific timespan. The standard measure used to measure frequency is the Hertz (1 Hz = 1 cycle per second): a pure tone that has a frequency of 200 Hz therefore has 200 complete cycles of vibration per second. The human ear is sensitive to a wide range of frequencies: healthy young listeners can normally hear sounds with frequencies ranging from about 20 Hz to 20000 Hz. The auditory sensation of frequency is the *pitch* of the sound. Pitch is defined as 'the attribute of auditory sensation in terms of which sounds may be ordered on a musical scale'. A doubling in frequency is perceived roughly as a doubling in pitch, i.e. a 400 Hz tone is heard as 'twice as high' as a 200 Hz tone, and an 800 Hz tone is heard as 'twice as high' as a 400 Hz tone. Two tones that vary with such an interval are said to be an octave apart.

The y-axis displays the *amplitude* of the sound, which is related to pressure variation. Human listeners are normally sensitive to an extremely wide range of air pressure differences: the ratio between the pressure of the loudest sound which can cause pain and the softest sound we can perceive is about 10 000 000:1. The unit most commonly used to measure sound levels, the decibel (dB), measures not absolute amplitude but the pressure ratio between a sound and some reference sound. The decibel scale is a convenient one of representing the very large pressure ratios that we are sensitive to in a concise way. Indeed the decibel is calculated as 20 times the logarithm of the pressure ratio between two sounds. Let us take as an example a measured sound which is 10 000 (or $10^4$) times more intense than the reference sound: the logarithm of this ratio $10^4$ is 4 and the decibel value is consequently $20 \times 4 = 80$ dB. There are a number of different reference sound levels used but a common one is the sound level corresponding to a pressure of 20 micropascals (considered to be the pressure of a just audible sound at frequencies around 1000 Hz); this scale is called dB sound pressure level (SPL) and is the one used in sound level meters. Another common decibel scale used in audiology is the dB hearing level (HL) scale. This uses as a reference sound level the pressure corresponding to the average threshold of hearing for a given frequency, as measured by international standards organizations on a large number of healthy young listeners (ISO 389-1).

The auditory sensation of amplitude is the *loudness* of a sound. Loudness is therefore a subjective attribute that is measured indirectly by getting a listener's impressions of the relation between sounds of different intensities. We are not equally sensitive to the loudness of sounds at different frequencies. For example, a 1000 Hz tone at 20 dB SPL will sound louder than an 8000 Hz tone at 20 dB SPL.

## Complex periodic sounds

A sinewave or 'pure tone' is described as a 'periodic' sound because the same cycle repeats over time. Most sounds have a much more complex pattern of vibration than the sinewave but may still be considered periodic, as their cycles repeat over time: these are called complex periodic sounds. An example of such a complex periodic waveform is that of the vowel /ɑ/ as in 'bard' in Figure 4.2; this can be compared with that of a simple periodic waveform in Figure 4.1.

A major breakthrough in the description of waveforms was made by a mathematician called Fourier in the early part of the 19th century. Fourier was able to show that all complex periodic waveforms were in fact made up of a set of pure tones. Within a complex periodic sound, these component pure tones are all multiples of the frequency at which the waveform repeats (called the *repetition* frequency). If this repetition frequency is 100 Hz for example, other component tones present in the complex periodic sound will have a frequency that will be some multiple of 100. Such component tones are called *harmonics* and the repetition frequency is also called the *fundamental frequency*.

The waveform is not a very useful display if one is interested in the frequency composition of sounds, as it does not display harmonics and their relative intensity. Such information can be obtained by analysing sounds using a bank of electronic filters and displaying the output as a *spectrum*, which plots frequency against amplitude. It goes beyond the scope of this chapter to give a technical account of signal analysis, but an important point to remember is that the spectrum of a sound obtained from such an analysis is affected by the type of filters used and is not an exact representation of the signal.

On such a display, each component pure tone or harmonic is represented by a vertical line. If we look at a schematic representation of the

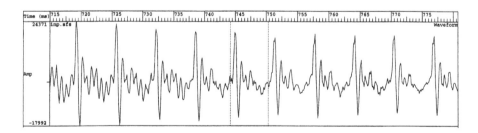

**Figure 4.2:** Waveform of vowel /ɑ/ (as in 'bard'). Time is shown on the x-axis and amplitude on the y-axis. The vertical lines show the duration of a single cycle of the vowel.

spectrum of the sound produced by vocal-fold vibration (*glottal pulse*) (see Figure 4.3a), we see that it is made up of a large number of harmonics, which are equally spaced in terms of their frequency, and that the higher harmonics are of lower intensity than the lower harmonics. If we look at the spectrum of the vowel /ɜ/, as in 'bird', we can see that it is made up of the same harmonics as the glottal pulse, which was the source of the sound. However, instead of seeing the intensity of the harmonics decreasing from left to right along the frequency axis, we now see a number of peaks in the spectrum: some harmonics are much more intense than others. These peaks result from the process of the 'filter', i.e. the action of the vocal tract. As was described above, cavities within the vocal tract have certain resonant frequencies, i.e. frequencies at which they like to vibrate. If there are harmonics in the sound source that are at or close to these resonant frequencies, they will be amplified as the result of the action of the resonator, hence the peaks in the spectrum. The frequency response (Figure 4.3) displays the resonant frequencies for the configuration of the vocal tract during the production of the vowel /ɜ/.

When describing speech sounds, we call each of these resonance peaks a *formant*. Formants are labelled as follows: the formant which is lowest in frequency for a given sound is called the first formant (abbreviated as F1), the next lowest is the second formant (F2), etc. Vowels are characterized by the position and distance between their formants (e.g. /i/ as in 'bead'

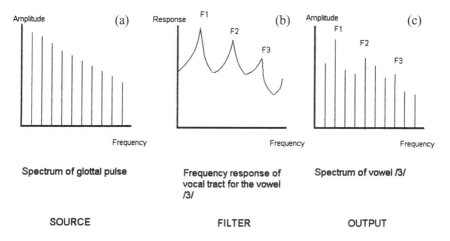

**Figure 4.3:** Schematic representations of the spectrum of a glottal pulse (sound source), of the frequency response of the vocal tract, and of the spectrum for the vowel /ɜ/. The resonant frequencies or formants are labelled as F1, F2 and F3. The amplitudes of individual harmonics change as a result of the action of the filter but their spacing is not affected.

has a low-frequency first formant and a high frequency (>2000 Hz) second formant while /ɑ/ as in 'bard' has a high first formant and low second formant). The patterning of the first two formants is usually sufficient to distinguish all vowels.

In Figure 4.3c, we therefore see that the *spacing of harmonics* in the spectrum of the vowel is determined by characteristics of the sound source (rate of vocal-fold vibration), but that the peaks in the spectrum or formants are determined by characteristics of the filter. Perceptually, harmonic spacing will be perceived as determining the pitch of the sound, while resonant peaks are perceived as determining the timbre or quality of the sound (e.g. whether the vowel heard was /i/ or /ɑ/). These two aspects of the sound can be altered independently: when uttering 'ah?' or 'ah!', we are changing the rate of vocal-fold vibration hence changing the perceived intonation pattern of these words, but the vocal tract configuration does not alter and therefore the perceived vowel is the same. If we utter 'ah' and 'eh' on a monotone pitch, the rate of vocal vibration remains the same but the vocal tract configuration changes, hence a chance in perceived timbre.

**Aperiodic sounds**

Certain speech sounds are not periodic, i.e. they have waveforms that do not show any regularity in time. Such sounds are those for which the sound source is turbulent noise. Turbulent noise sounds contain a large number of pure tones that are not equally spaced. The spectrum of aperiodic sounds is therefore continuous: there are so many component pure tones within it that one no longer sees lines representing individual harmonics. In aperiodic sounds, the overall shape and peaks of the spectrum is still determined by characteristics of the filter: articulators will be in different positions for sounds such as the initial consonant in 'sin' or 'fin' and the overall shape of the spectrum will reflect the presence of resonant peaks.

**Spectrographic representations of speech sounds**

The spectrum is a useful representation of the frequency (or 'spectral') composition of speech sounds but, as it represents a 'snapshot' of a sound at a given moment, it does not give any indication of how a signal changes with time. A picture of both the spectral composition of sounds and of how they change in time can be obtained using a third type of display known as the *spectrogram*. This plots time on the x-axis against frequency on the y-axis, with amplitude shown as the darkness of the trace. The spectrogram is particularly meaningful for speech perception research, as the signal analysis done to produce it is known to be quite similar to the analysis carried out within the cochlea which breaks down a complex signal into its components. The acoustic patterns that we see on spectrograms therefore resemble, to a certain extent, patterns of excitation along the basilar membrane within the cochlea.

Even a basic knowledge of the frequency compositions of different speech sounds can lead to a better understanding of which sounds are likely to be particularly difficult to discriminate by listeners with a hearing loss. A spectrogram of the word 'mats' is shown in Figure 4.4. This word includes a variety of speech sounds: a nasal consonant, a vowel, a plosive consonant and a fricative consonant. The approximate times at which each sound begins and ends are indicated in the legend to Figure 4.4, although speech scientists will argue that speech cannot really be segmented in such a linear manner. Dark areas represent frequencies at which there is energy in the signal.

It can be seen that different vowels and consonant categories have quite different acoustic patterns. Vowels are very characteristic as they contain a series of dark horizontal bands. Each of these bands represents a formant, hence a resonant peak in the signal. Consonants produced with different manners of articulations show quite different and characteristic patterns on spectrographic displays. Plosives (see 't' in Figure 4.4) are characterized by a strong burst or pulse (vertical line on display) which

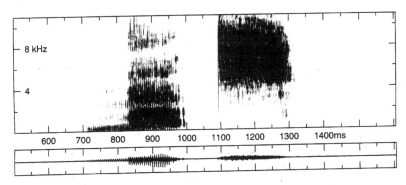

**Figure 4.4:** Spectrogram and waveform of word 'mats'. On the spectrogram, time (in milliseconds) is indicated on the x-axis and frequency (in kilohertz) on the y-axis. The sound 'm' starts at about 700 ms, the vowel around 820 ms; the release of the consonant /t/ can be seen as a vertical pulse at around 1100 ms and the final /s/ immediately follows it. The first two formants of the vowel are seen as two dark bands around 600 Hz and 1500 Hz. The energy in the first two sounds 'ma' is mostly in the low-frequency region below 3000 Hz, while the energy in the final two sounds 'ts' is mainly above 4000 Hz. It can be seen from the waveform that the vowel is the most intense sound in the word.

corresponds to the release of the occlusion. Fricatives (see 's' in Figure 4.4) are seen as large bands of random marks that represent friction or noise. Nasals (see 'm' on display) have similar formants to vowels, although of lower intensity, and again have most of their energy in the low-frequency region of the spectrum. Consonants produced with the same manner of articulation but which differ in their place of articulation will have similar patterning but will have their main energy in different frequency ranges. For example, for alveolar consonants such as the initial consonants in 'tin' and 'sin', the energy in the burst is concentrated in the high-frequency region (> 5000 Hz), while for labial consonants such as the initial consonant in 'pin', it will typically be below 1000 Hz. Consonant sounds will vary not only in their frequency composition but also in their relative intensity.

**Issue of variability**

Speech is characterized by a great deal of variability. We have already seen that the dimensions of individuals' vocal tracts will, to a certain extent, determine the resonant frequencies of certain speech sounds. A certain degree of variability is therefore due to the difference in these dimensions linked to the sex, age and size of the speaker.

However, the acoustic patterns of any given individual will also vary from utterance to utterance as a result of a wide range of factors. These factors include the following.

- Speaking style: vowels produced in casual or sloppy speech will not be as clearly articulated as vowels produced during careful or formal speech. Vowel formant frequencies will consequently not be as distinct from each other.
- Speaking rate: sound patterns produced at a fast speaking rate will differ in terms of their frequency and duration to those produced in slow speech.
- Physical state: sound patterns produced when an individual is highly stressed or ill will be different from those produced in a normal state.
- Coarticulation: the consonant/vowel environment in which a sound is produced will affect its frequency and duration.

# Speech perception

A final link in the speech chain is the process of decoding the speech signal in order to understand a message. This phase includes a stage known as auditory processing, in which the speech signal reaching the ear is broken down into different patterns of excitation along the basilar membrane. This process is reviewed in Chapter 3. In this section, we are concerned with the next stage, which is the process by which these patterns of excitation are interpreted as particular sounds, words and sentences. This process is, of course, complicated by the fact that speech is inherently so variable, as discussed above. A listener somehow needs to be able to recognize the similarity between, say, the vowel in the word 'bad' produced by a young child and a tall adult, even though the acoustic patterns in both cases will be quite different in fundamental and formant frequencies, duration and intensity. The process by which this is done (known as *normalization*) is still not totally understood and the fact that a young child can fairly effortlessly learn to recognize speech sounds despite all this variability is also a source of wonder.

## Sources of information used in speech perception

To understand a message, the listener makes use of a number of different sources of information. Clearly, it is important to be able to decode acoustic patterns, but there are many situations in which much of the signal is quite inaudible due to the presence of loud background noise, for example, or the presence of a significant hearing impairment. Yet, a listener can often understand the gist of the message in these poor listening conditions. The three main sources of speech perception information will be described in turn.

### Acoustic cues

A listener needs to a certain extent to be able to identify which vowels and consonants have been produced before accessing lexical information to recognize words. We have seen that acoustic patterns for individual speech sounds are quite characteristic but also quite complex. Do we need to decode all aspects of the signal in order to recognize a speech sound, or are certain elements of the speech signal strong markers to the identity of the sound?

Numerous speech perception experiments have been carried out in the past 40 years to answer these questions. The turning point in speech perception research was the invention of the sound spectrograph, which for the first time made acoustic patterns 'visible', and of the early speech synthesizers, which enabled researchers to construct artificial speech and manipulate acoustic patterns. Using synthetic speech, it is possible to construct sounds in which only one acoustic pattern (say, the frequency of a plosive burst) differs between two consonants. If a change in the characteristics of a single acoustic pattern leads to a change in the consonant perceived, it is clear that this pattern is somehow a 'marker' to the difference between these two sounds. By doing exhaustive research of this kind, *acoustic cues* were identified: sound patterns that are markers of specific features of a sound (e.g. voicing, place and manner of articulation). As each speech sound in the language is a unique combination of these features, the recognition of a combination of acoustic cues that mark such features can lead to the correct recognition of a sound.

Speech is designed to be 'robust', i.e. resistant to interference by background noise. Part of this robustness is due to the fact that each phonetic feature is marked by more than one acoustic cue. For example, the feature of place of articulation in plosives is marked by the frequency of the burst but also by the direction and extent of movement in the second and third formants at the beginning of the vowel. Perception of either of these cues alone can be sufficient to perceive the correct place of articulation of the sound.

Information about speech sounds can also be gleaned from much less detailed cues, such as the amplitude envelope of the speech signal and the duration of different segments. This can be shown by the fact that it is possible to understand a signal which consists of noise shaped to have the same amplitude envelope and duration characteristics as real speech even though all detailed acoustic patterns are missing.

## Contextual information

A lot of emphasis in speech perception research has been on the identification of acoustic cues. However, there has also been a realization that a speech message can be understood even when a great majority of acoustic cues cannot be heard. This may happen, for example, when listening to speech masked by noise or passed through a channel which filters out many of its component frequencies (e.g. speech heard through a telephone). Listeners must therefore rely also on other sources of information. The term *contextual information* is used to describe all the cognitive information that listeners use, i.e. vocabulary knowledge, knowledge of the world, of the grammatical structure of the language, of the person uttering the message, etc. Most messages that we perceive are presented in some kind of context, and are fairly or even highly predictable from the previous information perceived. For example, if we hear 'For your birthday, I baked a', grammatical knowledge tells us the last word is likely to be a noun, 'cultural' knowledge tells us about traditions used to celebrate birthdays and lexical knowledge will enable us to retrieve the word 'cake'. We therefore use predictability to narrow down what we expect to hear. Perception of only a few gross acoustic cues is then sufficient to confirm expectations. It has been suggested that we adapt our speech to the degree of predictability of the message: we can afford to speak quite sloppily when, say, chatting to a partner about domestic matters, as the message will be highly predictable from the context. However, when the information communicated is new and unpredictable, we use more careful and clearly articulated speech, as the listener will make more use of acoustic information.

Studies have shown that listeners differ in the degree to which they are able to use these cognitive sources of information. Some listeners may, for example, be able to disguise a certain degree of hearing loss by making very efficient use of contextual information, while others will be less efficient at compensating for the loss of acoustic cues.

### Visual cues

A third important source of speech perception information is the visual information gleaned from looking at the speaker. This effect can be quite striking and easily experienced if one first just listens to speech in a noisy environment with eyes closed and then looks at the speaker. The feeling is often that of going from total lack of comprehension to understanding. One reason that visual cues are so helpful is that they provide information about who is speaking, when and where. This allows the listener to tune in to the speaker, to more easily pick out the speech from the background noise thanks to timing information, and to localize the speech in relation to the noise. Recently, the term 'speech-reading' has been used in preference to lip-reading, as visual information consists of much more than just reading the lip movements of the speaker. Speech-reading also provides segmental information, i.e. information about features of the individual sounds produced. It provides, to a certain extent, information about the place of articulation of the sounds. Sounds articulated at the front of the mouth such as the initial consonants in 'pin', 'bin' and 'mitt' are clearly recognized but consonants produced further back in the vocal tract are difficult to distinguish from each other. Visual cues may indirectly give information about the manner of articulation, although this relies on quite subtle timing differences that many speech-readers do not grasp. However, they provide no information about whether a sound is voiced or voiceless as vocal-fold vibration is 'invisible': the initial consonants in 'sue' and 'zoo', for example, which differ solely in whether they are voiced or voiceless, cannot be discriminated using speech-reading alone. Speech perception via speech-reading alone is therefore a difficult task as a language such as English, for example, has so many pairs of consonants that have the same manner and place of articulation but different voicing. Again, individual listeners seem to vary quite widely in their ability to speech-read.

## Speech perception in the presence of a hearing impairment

The aim of this chapter is ultimately to give a better understanding of the problems that listeners with a hearing impairment may encounter in understanding speech. We must therefore consider the way in which hearing impairment can affect the use of the sources of information described above.

### Raised audibility thresholds

Deafness will affect auditory processing in many ways. The most obvious manifestation is that audibility thresholds are raised. This may be compensated by amplification provided via a hearing aid. But in the case of profound deafness, even strong amplification may not make some parts of the speech audible as a listener may, for example, have no measurable hearing for frequencies above 2000 Hz. As a result, the acoustic cues contained in certain frequency bands may be totally lost to the listener. For many listeners with a hearing impairment, this loss will primarily affect sounds that have important acoustic cues in mid-to-high-frequency ranges. These are fricative consonants, such as the initial and final consonants in 'fizz' and 'sieve', and certain plosive consonants which have their main energy in the higher-frequency range, such as the initial and final consonants in 'date'. By looking again at the spectrogram in Figure 4.4 and masking out the frequency range over, say, 2000 Hz, one gets an idea of how many of the acoustic patterns are lost. A broad view of how speech sounds are mapped within the hearing range, in terms of their relative amplitude and frequency, can be obtained by looking at what is commonly known as the 'speech banana' superimposed on the pure-tone audiogram (Figure 4.5).

### Poor frequency resolution

A second very damaging effect of sensorineural deafness, which does not apply to purely conductive losses, is the way in which it affects frequency resolution, i.e. the ability, within the auditory system, to decode a complex waveform into its component patterns. It was argued above, that the spectrogram was a fair representation of the different patterns of excitation that occur along the basilar membrane. When frequency resolution is affected, the signal is analysed with much broader filters and, as a result, patterns that are close in frequency will merge and no longer be resolved

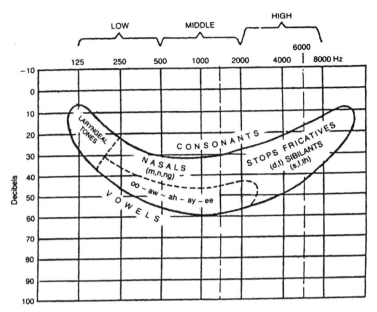

**Figure 4.5**: Figure giving a broad view of the main frequency and amplitude composition of different speech sound categories, superimposed on the pure tone audiogram. This diagram is sometimes called the 'speech banana'.

as separate patterns of excitation. In the presence of background noise, speech intelligibility will be further reduced because noise that is analysed through the same broad auditory filter as an acoustic pattern will have a strong masking effect on this part of the speech signal. Auditorily, this degraded frequency resolution has the effect of 'blurring' the signal, just as an imperfect visual resolution leads to a blurred image. Unfortunately, the difference between visual and auditory blurring is that whereas visual blurring can be corrected with lenses, auditory blurring cannot be corrected via the use of a conventional hearing aid. The degree of impairment in frequency resolution cannot be predicted from the pure-tone audiogram. 'Psychoacoustic' tests that evaluate frequency resolution do exist but are quite lengthy to administer and are not routinely used in the audiology clinic.

The degree to which a hearing loss will affect an individual's ability to perceive speech is therefore to a certain extent linked to the degree of the loss and to whether the loss is sensorineural or conductive. With today's powerful hearing aids, a moderate-to-severe loss that is not associated with too great an impairment to frequency resolution can be compensated for quite well. With severe-to-profound sensorineural losses, the effect is less predictable and individual variability in performance is much greater. As was mentioned earlier, this can be explained in part by factors such as frequency and temporal resolution, which are not routinely evaluated clinically. Ultimate attainment in speech perception is also highly dependent on a number of factors that are difficult to quantify, such as age at diagnosis, age at hearing aid fitting or type of aid. As mentioned above, individuals also vary in both their ability to make use of visual cues for speech-reading and their ability to use contextual information to aid in speech recognition. These factors will therefore also affect the ultimate attainment in terms of speech recognition of a person with a hearing loss and help explain why two people with identical audibility thresholds can vary so widely in their comprehension of speech.

**Effect of hearing loss on speech development**

In children with normal hearing, the development of speech is a slow and complex process that appears to begin soon after the cochlea is formed in the womb. Indeed, after birth, infants have been shown to 'recognize' sounds that they heard on a regular basis during the later part of the pregnancy (nursery rhyme read aloud daily, theme tunes of favourite 'soaps'). Although they do not hear fine details of speech sounds in the womb, they can hear high-amplitude, low-frequency components of the sounds that carry information about the intonation and rhythm of nursery rhymes or musical pitch of tunes.

Even by the age of four weeks, infants can hear fine distinctions between sounds; they increase their rate of sucking when the syllable 'pa', which they hear played out repeatedly from a loudspeaker, changes to the syllable 'ba'. At this stage, however, the discrimination is purely auditory and the infant has not learned to associate a sound with a specific 'label': they hear the difference between the two syllables but do not know which is 'pa' and which is 'ba'. Also, they seem able to discriminate sounds of all languages. It seems likely that during the first year, through repeated exposure to the sounds of their own language, infants become more attuned to the speech sounds that exist in their language and become desensitized to sounds which do not. At the same time, they gradually learn to associate speech sounds that they hear with the vowels and consonant labels that occur in their language.

Speech sounds are acquired in a fairly hierarchical way, with the ability to identify a sound usually preceding the ability to produce it. It seems that speech sounds which have their distinctive acoustic patterns in the low-frequency range (say, below 2000 Hz) are acquired earlier than speech sounds which have acoustic patterns in the higher-frequency range. As a result, intonation patterns and vowels are perceived early, and nasal and plosive consonants are usually acquired before fricatives, such as the initial and final consonants in 'sa<u>sh</u>' or '<u>fish</u>', or affricates such as the initial consonant in '<u>ch</u>eese'. The acquisition of speech perception and production is a slow process and children are not truly adult-like in their ability to perceive speech until the age of 12 or even older.

How does hearing impairment affect this process of development? As discussed above, much development occurs during the first year of life, long before there are any clear signs that the child can understand and produce words. If a hearing impairment remains undiagnosed during this period, a child is deprived of much of this early exposure to speech that is so crucial to further development. Once fitted with a hearing aid, a child receives some auditory input, but this may still be distorted due to poor frequency resolution and to the effects of the amplification. If the loss is severe to profound, certain sounds (such as 'f' and 's', which have patterns in the high-frequency range) may remain totally inaudible despite the amplification. Given early exposure to sound (through early fitting of aids for example), and an emphasis on the use of the auditory channel for perceiving speech, the prognosis for speech development may be good for many deaf children, but development is likely to be much delayed relative to children with normal hearing, and some speech sounds may never be acquired if the child cannot hear them. Especially in the case of profound losses, it is very difficult to predict how well a child may develop oral speech, as development will be affected by factors as diverse as their frequency resolution ability, the age of onset of deafness and age of fitting of hearing aids, their ability to use visual and contextual information, their educational background, frequency of use of hearing aids, type of hearing aid and amount of auditory training/stimulation. This difficulty in diagnosing how successful a child will be in his or her ability to understand and produce intelligible speech is one of the complicating factors in deciding whether to choose an education mode primarily based on aural/oral or manual approaches and in deciding if a child should be offered a cochlear implant.

# Chapter 5
# Subjective audiometry

Deborah Ballantyne and Mike Martin

Subjective audiometry is the starting point for measuring the hearing level of people with suspected hearing loss. It may be broadly defined as auditory tests that require an overt response from the person being tested. This is in contrast to objective audiometry, which requires no overt response from the individual and relies on the measurement of a physiological response to the test stimulus.

Subjective audiometry mainly uses pure tones as the test stimuli, except for the evaluation of speech recognition ability.

Pure-tone audiometry is the most widely used form of subjective testing. It provides basic information about a person's level of hearing and is relevant to the diagnosis and treatment of that loss as well as to the patient's rehabilitation and, in the case of children, their education.

## Diagnostic strategy

People presenting themselves to an ENT specialist may be surprised to find that they are not given a pure-tone audiometric test straight away. The reason for this is that some treatment, for example removal of wax, may be required first. There are a whole battery of tests that can be used to assess the severity of hearing loss and its cause: only relevant tests are undertaken to make the most efficient use of clinical time. Tests are selected with a view to making a diagnosis in the shortest possible time. Before ordering tests, the specialist will obtain a good history of the patient's problems and possibly perform a general medical examination.

### Tuning fork tests

In today's electronic world, it may be surprising that an instrument as old as a tuning fork may still be used. However, tuning fork tests can quickly tell a specialist whether a patient's hearing loss is conductive or sensorineural and which ear is affected. Figure 5.1 shows a typical tuning fork used for clinical purposes. These forks are of low frequency, e.g. 256 or 512 Hz, and are activated by gently striking the free end of the prongs while holding the fork at the stem. The fork is then either placed near the entrance to the ear canal, without touching the ear, for measuring air conduction, or the footplate is placed on the mastoid process or forehead for measuring bone conduction.

Three tuning fork tests are still widely used and are outlined below.

### Weber's test

This is a bone conduction test to distinguish a sensorineural from a conductive loss in unilateral deafness. The signal will be heard most easily in the ear with the conductive loss and the signal is said to be referred to that ear.

The test procedure is very simple: the tuning fork is placed on the forehead and the patient is asked in which ear they hear the tone. In a person with normal hearing, the tone will be heard centrally, in the middle of the head, or in both ears equally. With a unilateral sensorineural deafness the sounds will be heard in the ear opposite to the deaf one. However, in unilateral conductive deafness the sound will be heard louder in the deaf ear. This potentially ambiguous situation can usually be clarified using the Rinne test.

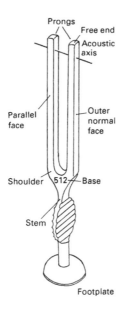

**Figure 5.1:** A 512 Hz tuning fork used in hearing tests.

*Rinne's test*

In this test, each ear is examined separately and the hearing by air conduction is compared with that by bone conduction to distinguish conductive from sensorineural losses.

The test procedure is to place the tuning fork close to the ear canal, but not touching the ear, with the tips of the prongs of the tuning fork level with the ear canal at a distance of about 2 cm and lined up with the ear canal. The patient is asked if they can hear the tone, then the footplate (heel) of the tuning fork is placed on the mastoid bone behind the same ear. The patient is asked which is louder: when the air-conducted sound is louder it is a Rinne positive response. If the bone-conducted signal is louder it is a Rinne negative response. In cases of severe sensorineural deafness, a false-negative Rinne response may be found. Here bone conduction in the deaf ear appears better than air conduction. This is because the vibration transmitted from the footplate of the tuning fork on to the mastoid bone is heard in the opposite ear, since it cannot be heard in the ear with the severe sensorineural deafness that is being tested. The true situation can be established by feeding a masking noise (for example from a mechanical noise generator called a Bárány Box) into the opposite ear. With this opposite ear masked the patient no longer hears any sound on that side when the footplate of the tuning fork is placed on the mastoid bone of the deaf ear. Rinne's test is then said to be falsely negative, i.e. it is really positive, indicating a sensorineural rather than a conductive deafness.

*Bing test*

The Bing test is a comparison of occluded and unoccluded bone conduction. The test is based on the occlusion effect whereby a bone-conducted sound is perceived to be louder when the ear canal of the test ear is blocked.

The test procedure is to apply the tuning fork to the mastoid process of the test ear and ensure that the patient can hear it. The tester then blocks the ear canal by pressing a finger into the entrance to the canal. The patient is then asked to say whether the sound is louder, softer or there is no change. An increase in loudness is known as a positive Bing and no change a negative Bing. No change implies a conductive loss and louder a sensorineural loss.

Table 5.1 is a summary of the relevance of the outcomes from the above tests.

**Table 5.1:** Examples of responses from diagnostic tuning fork tests

| Hearing loss | Weber | Rinne | | Bing | |
|---|---|---|---|---|---|
| | | Right | Left | Right | Left |
| No loss | Central | Positive | Positive | Positive | Positive |
| Bilateral sensorineural | Central | Positive | Positive | Positive | Positive |
| Unilateral sensorineural right | Left | Positive | Positive or false negative | Positive | Positive |
| Bilateral conductive | Central | Negative | Negative | Negative | Negative |
| Unilateral conductive left | Left | Positive | Negative | Positive | Negative |

# Pure-tone audiometry

Pure-tone audiometry is by far the most commonly used test procedure to measure hearing levels in routine clinical practice. It involves both threshold and supra threshold measurements of hearing based on overt responses from the subject to the test tones. A high degree of standardization for both procedures and equipment has led to a reliable form of testing. Figure 5.2 shows the factors that have to be taken into consideration in the performance of pure-tone audiometry.

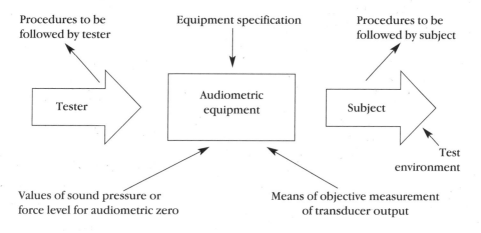

**Figure 5.2:** Factors affecting the measurement of hearing.

## The tester

The results from a subjective test will be dependent on how the test is performed. The tester must follow testing protocols that are laid down in a number of national and international standards (ISO 8253-1; ISO 6189).

## The equipment

A pure tone audiometer is an instrument that produces and controls the test signals. Figure 5.3 shows a typical clinical audiometer the performance of which is specified in national and international standards (IEC 60645-1). Figure 5.4(a) is a functional diagram of the audiometer where the signals to the patient may be presented via earphones, bone vibrator or with additional equipment through a loudspeaker for sound field measurements. Speech audiometry may also be undertaken using a pure-tone audiometer that has an external input for a tape recorder or CD player and a means of monitoring the signal level (Figure 5.4(b)).

The audiometer must be calibrated by measuring the acoustic output from the headphones using ear simulators (acoustic couplers or artificial ears). These are designed to measure the SPL from the earphone in a manner that relates to the use of the earphone on the ear (Figure 5.5). The output from bone vibrators is measured on a mechanical coupler (previously called an artificial mastoid). Figure 5.6 shows a typical device. All these devices are standardized (IEC 60318-1; IEC 60318-3; IEC 60318-6) as are the values of SPL required to obtain the threshold of hearing (ISO 389-1; ISO 389-3).

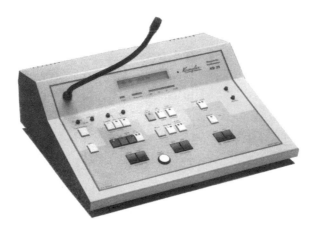

**Figure 5.3:** A typical diagnostic pure tone audiometer. Photograph courtesy PC Werth Ltd.

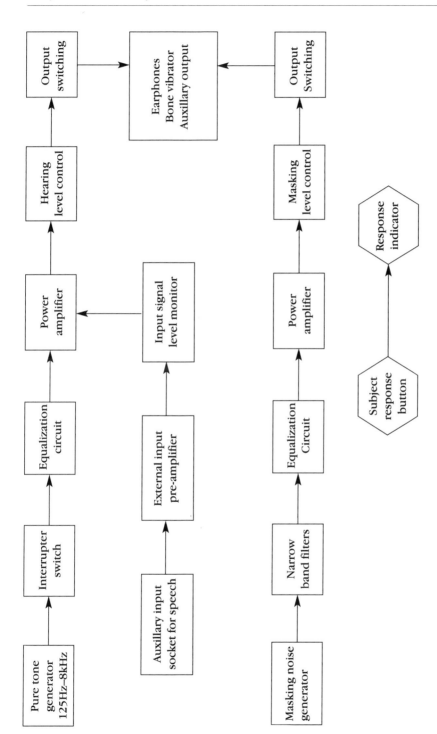

**Figure 5.4(a)**: Functional diagram of a diagnostic pure tone audiometer.

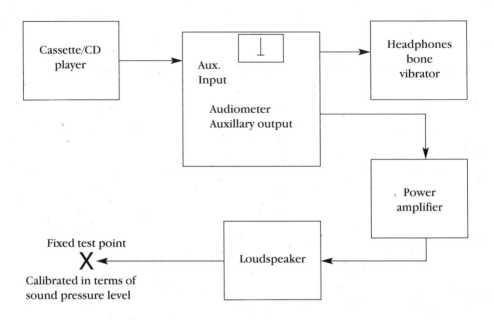

**Figure 5.4(b):** Functional diagram of the means to undertake speech audiometry using a pure tone audiometer.

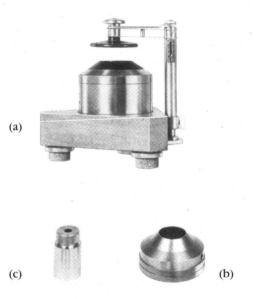

**Figure 5.5:** Ear simulators. (a) Wide-band artificial ear, (b) 6cc acoustic coupler, (c) 2cc acoustic coupler for the measurement of insert earphones. Photographs courtesy B&K Ltd.

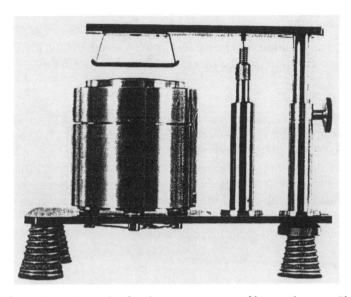

**Figure 5.6:** Mechanical coupler for the measurement of bone vibrators. Photograph courtesy B&K Ltd.

## The subject

It is important that subjects are properly instructed about what to do in the test and that they understand the task. People often do not realize how quiet the test signals that they have to respond to will be. It is also important that the manner in which they respond to the signal should be made clear. Again these requirements are specified in appropriate standards (ISO 8253-1; ISO 6189).

## The environment

To measure the threshold of hearing of a normally hearing person it is necessary to have very quiet listening conditions. The presence of ambient noise will mask the test signals and make the threshold of hearing seem worse than it really is. Consequently considerable care needs to be taken to ensure that audiometry is only undertaken in surroundings that have suitably low levels of background noise. Acceptable levels of background noise that have no effect on threshold measurements are set out in international standards (ISO 8253-1; ISO 6189).

The environment should also be visually quiet, with no people moving about and no distracting pictures, so that nothing distracts the subject's attention from the difficult task of detecting the presence of very quiet signals.

**The audiometer**

The pure-tone audiometer shown in Figure 5.4 is the basic instrument for all subjective audiometry. The functional parts are as follows.

*Pure-tone generator*

This produces pure tones over the frequency range 125 to 8000 Hz in fixed steps at the following standardized frequencies: 125, 250, 500, 750, 1000, 1500, 2000, 3000, 4000, 6000 and 8000 Hz. The tester selects the frequencies depending on the requirements of the test and the model of audiometer; not all frequencies are used or even present on all audio-meters. A small number of audiometers are available for high-frequency audiometry in the frequency range 8 to 16 kHz; these are mainly used for research and advanced clinical applications.

*Interrupter switch*

This switches the tone on and off and in some audiometers is capable of doing the reverse. It is normal practice in audiometry for the tone to be off and then switched on. The manner in which the interrupter switch works is closely specified to ensure that it does not produce spurious mechanical or electrical noise. An abrupt onset of the signal, or switching it off abruptly, can produce signals that the subjects hear even when they are not able to hear the test tone, thus producing a false level of threshold. Interrupter switches come in a variety of mechanical forms and some audiometers have automatic pulsing of the signal.

*Equalization circuit*

This part of the audiometer automatically compensates for the changes in the standardized values of SPL or force level required to obtain audiometric zero at different frequencies (see below under threshold of hearing).

*Power amplifier*

This provides amplification of the test signals and the power to drive the earphones and bone vibrator over the output range of the audiometer.

*Hearing level control/output attenuator*

This controls the level of the signal to the earphones and bone vibrator. It normally has 5 dB steps and covers a range from 10 dB below the threshold of hearing to at least 110 dB above threshold for most audiometers. This control is placed at the output of the audiometer to ensure that any electrical background noise in the instrument is kept to a minimum and does not influence the thresholds at normal hearing threshold levels.

## Output switching

Audiometers will normally have two earphones and the signal is switched by the tester from one phone to the other. The switching may also select the bone vibrator and route the signal to the auxiliary socket to drive an external amplifier and loudspeaker. The control will also determine where any masking signal, if used, is directed. For earphones this will normally be to the non-test ear.

## Earphones and bone vibrator

The earphones used on audiometers are chosen from a very small range of devices that have been the subject of international standardization. The earphones are an integral part of the audiometer and cannot be replaced or changed without altering the calibration of the whole equipment. The pressure of the headband that holds the earphones on the ear is also specified and if not correct can change the calibration. The bone vibrator is also specified in the same way.

## Subject response button

To provide a simple means for the subject to indicate the presence of the test signal, the availability of a hand-held push button is a distinct advantage. There is some form of visual indication, such as a light on the front of the audiometer, to indicate to the tester that the button has been pushed.

## Masking noise channel

This consists of a random noise generator whose output is filtered to produce narrow bands of noise centred on the frequency of the test tone being used. This has to be switched with the pure-tone generator and also requires an equalizing circuit to provide a stated SPL from the earphones. A separate output attenuator is required to control the level of masking. This control may be calibrated in terms of SPL or effective masking (see below). Where the audiometer can be used for speech audiometry broad band noise may be available.

An audiometer is a measuring instrument and therefore must be accurately calibrated if the results from using it are to be meaningful. Audiometers should be calibrated at least annually by a responsible test laboratory. However, checks should be undertaken daily by the tester before using the equipment. Requirements for calibration and checking are given in international standards (ISO 8253-1; IEC 60645-1).

## Threshold of hearing

One of the main tests undertaken in pure-tone audiometry is the measurement of the threshold of hearing of an individual and comparing this threshold with what is accepted as 'normal'. To do this it is necessary to have definitions of what is meant by 'threshold' and 'normal'. There then has to be a means of relating the subjective evaluation of threshold to the objective calibration of the audiometer. While this may appear to be a simple matter, it is extremely complex, as may be seen from the following.

The measurement of any subjective form of threshold relies on having criteria for threshold. In the case of hearing, the person being tested is asked to indicate when he or she thinks a sound is present; in other words when he or she can detect the presence of a sound. However, this detection may be affected by the instructions given to the subject. We may say 'only respond when you are really *sure* that you hear the sound' or 'only respond when you *think* you hear something'. These two sets of instructions will give different results, with the first giving a threshold which requires a louder sound than the second. Also the test signal could be presented only once, or it could be presented many times until a response has been achieved. The duration of the signal also has an effect: too short and it will not be heard until it is much louder, too long and it will create problems in administering the test and may even cause changes in threshold. Furthermore, different thresholds will be recorded if the test is started with the signal so that it is easily heard and then reduced until it is no longer heard, or the reverse.

Consequently, an agreed method for defining threshold has to be found. The compromise in pure-tone audiometry is that the number of times the test signal is presented is four and the subject is considered to have heard the signal if he or she responds to at least two of the four. The duration of the test signal should be around one second and not repeated in a rhythmic manner, which allows the subject to guess when the next tone will be presented. The test procedure is therefore one that starts with the signal being clearly heard by the patient. The signal is then reduced in level until it is no longer heard, then increased until the signal is heard again. The process is repeated to ensure a consistent response. The threshold that is normally recorded is the one found with the signal that starts below threshold and increases, i.e. an ascending threshold. These requirements are specified in international standards (ISO 8253-1; ISO 6189), which are adopted by most countries.

By taking the above factors into account it is possible to obtain very repeatable measurements of threshold.

The question then arises as to what is meant by a 'normal' person. The threshold of hearing changes with age and consequently, for conventional audiometry, the normal threshold of hearing is restricted to the age range 18 to 30 years. The state of health of the ear is important in defining normal subjects and the concept of an otologically normal person is used to define normal. The definition in ISO 389-1 of an otologically normal person is one 'in a normal state of health who is free from all signs and symptoms of ear disease and from obstructing wax in the ear canal, and who has no history of undue exposure to noise, to potentially ototoxic drugs, or of familial hearing loss'.

### Audiometric zero

Having defined what is meant by a normal person and the threshold of hearing, these concepts are used to provide the basis for defining the zero on the hearing level dial of the audiometer. This is called audiometric zero or zero dB hearing level and is the set of signal levels, for pure tones at different audiometric frequencies, with respect to which hearing threshold levels are measured.

The process for obtaining an objective measure of the subjective values for audiometric zero is as follows. The letters relate to Figure 5.7(a).

- First, a large group of otologically normal subjects have their threshold of hearing measured by an agreed procedure for a stated earphone or bone vibrator (A,B).
- The values of threshold are then statistically analysed for each audio-metric frequency. From these results an 'average' value is produced (C).
- The level of the electrical signal needed to produce that 'average' value for threshold from the earphone is then measured and noted (D).
- The earphone used to measure the thresholds is then placed on an appropriate ear simulator (E).
- The electrical signals from (D) are then applied to the earphone (F).
- The SPL generated in the ear simulator is then measured (G).

The result from this is that there is now a known value of SPL that is equivalent to the 'average' threshold level for that earphone and ear simulator combination.

The average value of SPL measured in the ear simulator is now called the *reference* value. It is not the value of sound pressure that is measured on the ears of real subject but is the *equivalent* to them. The measurement that is then used to calibrate the audiometer is the *reference equivalent threshold sound pressure level* or RETSPL.

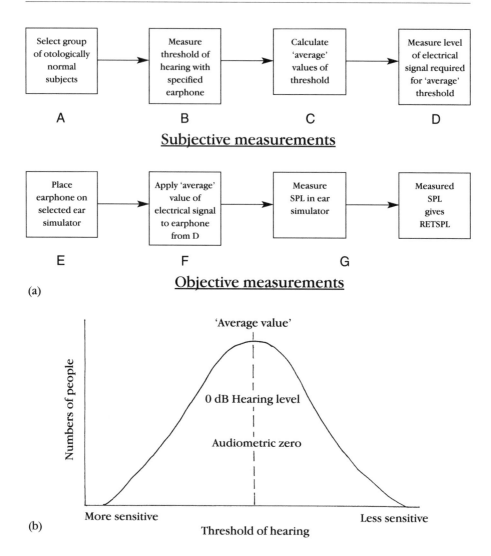

**Figure 5.7:** (a) Method for obtaining RETSPLs for earphone listening. (b) Distribution of normal hearing levels at one frequency. The 'average' value taken from the distribution becomes 0 dB on the HL dial of the audiometer and, in terms of SPL measured in an ear simulator, is also the RETSPL.

Figure 5.7(b) is an example of the results that might be obtained from a large group of normally hearing subjects whose results form an approximation to a normal distribution. This shows that there is no one value for the normal threshold of hearing and that normally hearing people can vary considerably in their hearing sensitivity. The importance of this is that it shows audiometric zero to be a statistical value and that because an individual does not have a threshold exactly on the central value it does not mean that they are not normal.

Ear simulators are devices that present an acoustic load to an earphone and contain a calibrated microphone to measure the SPL developed by the earphone under the earcap. The output from the calibrated microphone is fed into a measuring amplifier or a sound level meter, thus allowing the SPL generated in the ear simulator to be measured. Ear simulators may be divided into two groups: (a) those that are simple cavities that do not represent the acoustic properties of the external ear, called acoustic couplers; and (b) those that have an acoustic impedance representing that of the average adult ear, called artificial ears. Figure 5.5 shows typical ear simulators used for measuring the output from earphones used in audiometry. A device that approximates the mechanical properties of the mastoid process called a mechanical coupler, previously an artificial mastoid (Figure 5.6), is used to measure the vibratory output from bone vibrators.

Table 5.2 gives an example of RETSPLs for one type of earphone on two different ear simulators (ISO 389-1). It should first be noted that the SPL for threshold varies enormously, from 125 to 8000 Hz, and second, that different values of sound pressure occur in the different ear simulators for the same earphone.

The values in Table 5.2 are used to establish the output of the audiometer when its HL dial is set at 0 dB.

**Table 5.2:** Reference equivalent threshold SPLs (RETSPLs) for Telephonics TDH 39 earphone with MX41/AR ear cushion

| Frequency (Hz) | RETSPL – Artificial ear IEC 60318-1 dB | RETSPL – Acoustic coupler IEC 60318-3 dB |
| --- | --- | --- |
| 125 | 45 | 45 |
| 250 | 27 | 25.5 |
| 500 | 13.5 | 11.5 |
| 1000 | 7.5 | 7 |
| 2000 | 9 | 9 |
| 4000 | 12 | 9.5 |
| 6000 | 16 | 15.5 |
| 8000 | 15.5 | 13 |

### The audiogram

The results from a pure-tone audiometric test are recorded on a chart called an audiogram (Figure 5.8). The audiogram has 0 dB, normal hearing, at the top of the chart and increasing hearing levels towards the bottom of the chart. Therefore, the further down the chart the threshold is, the greater the hearing loss. Table 1.1 in Chapter 1 gives descriptive values of the average hearing losses.

The term 'hearing level' has a specific meaning, which is the difference between the level at which threshold is measured and audiometric zero, effectively 0 dB on the HL dial on the audiometer. Therefore in terms of the audiogram, it is more correct to talk of HLs rather than hearing losses when describing the levels on an audiogram.

However, as can be seen from Figure 5.8(a), the audiogram has a zero represented by a straight line and not by a curve as would be expected from the SPLs given in Table 5.2 for audiometric zero and shown in Figure 5.8(b). The reason for this is that the equalizing circuit in the audiometer (Figure 5.4), automatically changes the output in keeping with Table 5.2. The tester is not normally interested in the SPLs but wishes to know how the hearing of the person being tested differs from the norm. Consequently a straight line for zero makes that task simple.

It should be noted that there are a number of standardized symbols used to represent the ear being tested and the type of test. Symbols for air- and bone-conduction thresholds and uncomfortable loudness levels, are shown in Figure 5.8(a). Figure 5.8(b) shows examples of typical audiograms.

**Masking**

When bone conduction audiometry is being undertaken, the vibrator is usually placed on the mastoid process, although for some tests it may be placed on the forehead. The vibrations from the vibrator cause the whole head to vibrate and consequently the signals that arrive at the cochlea of the test ear are at almost the same level as those at the other ear. Therefore, without asking, the tester does not know in which ear the subject is hearing the sound. Technically, the interaural attenuation, which is the difference in level that occurs when an acoustic signal is applied to one ear of an individual and measured at the other ear, is very small for bone conduction.

It is obviously important for the tester to be sure that he or she is testing the intended ear. To ensure this is the case, a masking noise is fed into the non-test ear. The purpose of this noise is to drown out, or mask, the test tone so that the subject is prevented from hearing the tone in the non-test ear and only responds to the sound in the test ear. For pure-tone testing the masking noise should be a narrow band of noise, usually one third of an octave, centred on the test frequency. A narrow band of noise will mask the test signal while keeping the loudness of the masking signal to a minimum.

# Pure tone audiogram

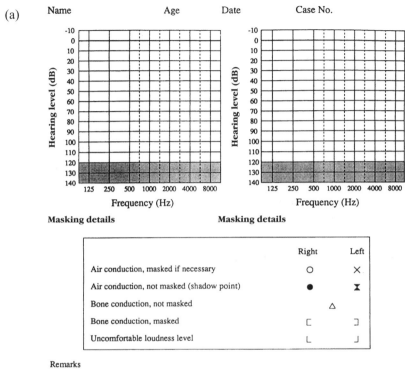

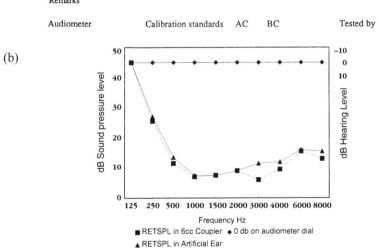

**Figure 5.8(a)**: Pure tone audiogram form.
**(b)**: Relationship between pure tone audiogram and SPL. While 0 dB on the audiometer HL dial remains constant, the SPL varies considerably with frequency for that setting. The SPL also varies with the type of ear simulator used to measure the output from the same earphone.

Apart from bone conduction, masking becomes necessary in audiometry when there is a significant difference in the level of hearing in each ear by air conduction. The interaural attenuation for air conduction is far higher than by bone conduction, but when the difference between the ears is some 40 dB or more, sound will be conducted across the head and be heard in the non-test ear. The effect of this is that, without masking, the true level in the test ear may not be measured, for example when one ear is profoundly or totally deaf there may be an impression of hearing when none is there.

Masking is not a simple procedure and if the correct level of masking is not applied it may produce incorrect thresholds. Fortunately in clinical audiometers the masking control is normally calibrated in effective masking. Effective masking provides the correct amount of masking to mask a signal at the level set on the masking control. The level of the signals required for effective masking are specified in ISO 389-4. For speech, broad band noise is required and is specified in IEC 60645-2.

## Subjective audiometric tests

Figure 5.9 shows the range of subjective hearing tests that are normally undertaken. As may be seen, these are divided into those using either pure tones or speech as the stimulus. They are then further divided on the basis

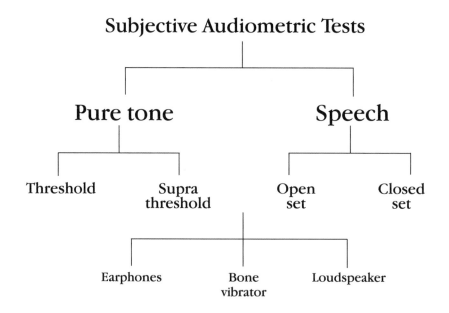

**Figure 5.9:** The range of subjective hearing tests possible and the means of presenting signals to the patient.

of whether the tests are used to determine the threshold of hearing, for screening at a fixed level or for measuring some aspect of hearing above threshold, e.g. loudness perception. Finally the figure shows the transducers used to present the stimulus to the subject, i.e. earphones, bone vibrator or via a loudspeaker.

## Pure-tone thresholds

The first audiometric subjective test that is carried out is a pure-tone audiogram. This requires the co-operation of the subject and can be carried out on children from the age of three or four as well as with most adults. The test produces in the first instance a chart – an audiogram – of the sensitivity of the ear to air conduction across the required frequency range. The number of frequencies used will depend on the type of test and the audiometer used. For clinical and rehabilitation purposes the number of frequencies used will vary between four and eight.

High-frequency audiometry for the detection of very early signs of hearing loss has recently become of interest. High frequencies are defined as ranging from 8 to 16 kHz. There are, however, still considerable technical difficulties in providing standardized equipment and measurements in this frequency range.

To differentiate between a conductive and a sensorineural hearing loss, bone conduction audiometry must be undertaken after the air conduction measurements are made. Bone conduction is normally limited to frequencies between 250 and 4000 Hz because of the practical problems of providing a suitable bone vibrator to go beyond those frequencies. Bone conduction also requires masking of the non-test ear as described above. The results from tests using air and bone conduction are shown in Figure 5.10.

## Screening tests

A hearing screening test is normally undertaken at a limited number of frequencies, e.g. 1000, 2000 and 4000 Hz and at a fixed level of say 30 dB HL. The subject is only required to determine if the test signal is there or not, still using the 50% criteria for detection. If the subject fails to detect the presence of the sound then he or she is referred for further investigation. Screening tests are undertaken in schools and noisy industries on a routine basis. Where screening is being undertaken in environments where the background noise is high, the earphones may have noise-excluding covers over them making them look like ear defenders.

## Self-recording audiometry

All the above tests use manual audiometry, where the tester pressing an interrupter switch makes the presentation of the test tone. An automated

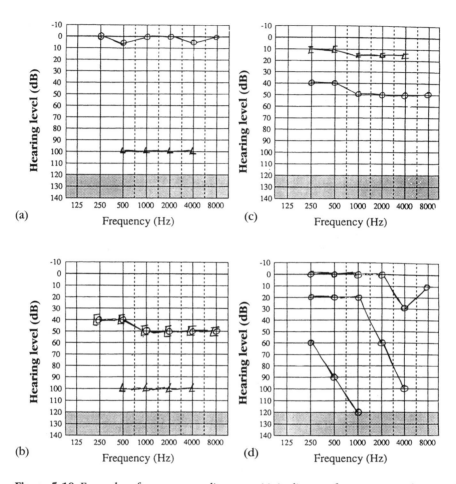

**Figure 5.10:** Examples of pure tone audiograms. (a) Audiogram for a person with normal hearing. Note the LDL at around 100 dB HL. (b) Audiogram of a person with a sensorineural hearing loss. The air- and bone-conduction levels are the same and the LDL is as for a normally hearing person. The dynamic range of the ear is therefore considerably reduced. (c) Audiogram of a person with a conductive hearing loss. Note that the bone-conduction levels are near normal whereas the air-conduction levels are reduced showing an 'air bone gap'. (d) Three typical audiograms. Top: a slight noise-induced hearing loss; middle: a ski slope loss; bottom: a corner audiogram for a profound hearing loss.

form of audiometry where the subject controls the level of the test tone is often used for screening purposes and in some clinical applications. This is called self-recording or Békésy audiometry and requires the use of a self-recording audiometer.

In this procedure, the test tone is pulsed automatically at a fixed rate and, for screening purposes, at a fixed frequency. The subjects have a button, which they are told to press when they hear the sound and to keep it pressed all the time they hear the sound. The audiometer reduces the level of the test signal in small steps until the subject no longer hears the sound, and the subject is instructed to release the button when they can no longer hear the sound. The effect of this is for the audiometer to increase the level of the sound until the subject hears it again. The subject then presses the button again and the level of the sound is reduced. The effect of this is to produce a repeated crossing of the threshold that is plotted against time, as in Figure 5.11. In screening self-recording audiometers the pulsed tone is presented for a fixed period of time before moving to the next frequency in the sequence. Once the testing is complete on one ear the audiometer will automatically switch the test signal to the other ear and repeat the procedure. This form of audiometry is particularly useful in industrial audiometry where large numbers of people are to be tested.

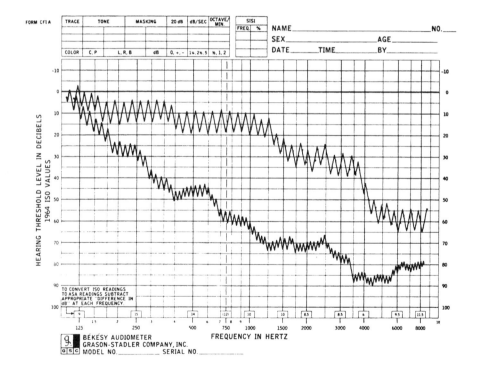

**Figure 5.11:** A record from a continuous frequency sweep self-recording audiometer. The upper curve shows a hearing loss with no recruitment and a near normal range of signal level for crossing the threshold. The lower curve shows marked recruitment and a very small range of excursions.

# Sound field audiometry

Most testing is undertaken using earphones, but this is not possible when evaluating people wearing hearing aids or for very young children. Figure 5.4(b) shows how signals can be fed into a loudspeaker and controlled from the audiometer. While it is possible to use pure tones for sound field testing, the effects of the room in which they are used creates problems. Consequently warble or frequency modulated tones are used, which reduce the effect of the environment.

To calibrate a sound field test facility it is necessary to measure the SPL with a sound level meter at the test point where the patient will be sitting. Requirements for the sound field are specified in ISO 8253-2. Provided that the test position is well-marked and maintained and that the sound field is properly calibrated, reliable measurements can be made. The results may be expressed as SPLs or as HLs if corrections are made for the standardized values for free field threshold contained in ISO 389-7.

### Supra threshold tests

One of the most commonly performed audiometric tests above threshold is that of measuring the loudness discomfort level (LDL) or uncomfortable loudness level (UCL). This test is designed to show on an audiogram the upper level of loudness that a subject can tolerate and indicates the dynamic range of the ear when compared with the level at threshold. Figure 5.10 shows typical audiograms for a normal ear and one with sensorineural hearing loss showing how the LDL hardly changes.

The test is performed after a pure-tone threshold is obtained. The subjects are told that they will hear the sound getting louder and louder and that they should say when the sound becomes uncomfortably loud, that is when they would not like to listen to it for any length of time. The test is undertaken at one frequency, then repeated to cover the range of frequencies that are of interest to the tester.

While the LDL test shows the dynamic range of the ear it does not show how the perception of loudness changes with increasing level between threshold and LDL. This is achieved by loudness balance tests such as the alternate binaural loudness balance (ABLB) test.

# Speech audiometry

While pure-tone audiometry is an indicator of the sensitivity of the ear across the measured frequency range, it is not a good indicator of a subject's ability to recognize speech. There is obviously a correlation between the degree of hearing loss and the ability to recognize speech; the greater the hearing loss the more likely it is that speech will be more difficult to recognize even if it can be heard clearly. However, for any degree of hearing loss there is a wide spread of ability to recognize speech from subject to subject.

Speech audiometry was used in the past to diagnose the cause of a sensorineural hearing loss, especially to indicate the presence of acoustic neuromas. Modern imaging techniques, especially magnetic resonance imaging (MRI) (see Chapter 7), have superseded this use of speech audiometry. The main use of speech audiometry today is for rehabilitation purposes (Green 1997). It is also used to identify cases when the conductive component of a 'mixed' conductive and sensorineural hearing loss appears worth rectifying by surgery. In a case when speech audiometry shows a good speech recognition score with sufficient amplification, the patient may benefit from successful middle-ear reconstruction surgery. However, if there is poor speech recognition ability, the patient is less likely to be helped by such surgery, since even if speech becomes louder after the operation it will not become clearer.

Speech audiometry has the limitation that the test material must be recognizable to the person being tested and is therefore language-dependent. It is also dependent on the intellectual ability of the person being tested to understand the test and also to be able, in the case of open set audiometry, to have sufficiently good speech production to repeat the words heard. The tester has also to be able to hear and recognize what has been said by the test subject in order to be able to record the result correctly.

Pure-tone audiometry is largely about the detection of pure tones and is cognitively the simplest of tasks. However, in speech perception there is a hierarchy of tasks as indicated in Figure 5.12. Speech audiometry can be used to measure the patient's ability to *detect* the presence of speech, to *distinguish* one word from another, to *recognize* words or to *understand* the meaning of a sentence or phrase. In audiology speech audiometry is normally performed at the recognition level.

In pure-tone audiometry there are standards for equipment and thresholds of hearing. In speech audiometry the equipment is standardized (IEC 60645-2) but because of the nature of speech there are no international standards for speech test material. This material has to be evaluated by the designers of the tests and detailed information should be provided with the recording of the speech material. However, there is a standard for speech audiometry procedures (ISO 8253-3) which also specifies what information should be available on any recording of speech test material and the relevant calibration signals. Recordings of speech test material must contain calibration signals and information on their relationship

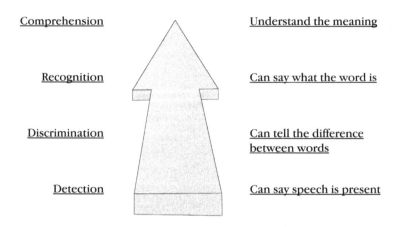

Comprehension — Understand the meaning

Recognition — Can say what the word is

Discrimination — Can tell the difference between words

Detection — Can say speech is present

**Figure 5.12:** The upward path to speech comprehension. At the detection level it is only possible to say that sound is present. At the discrimination level it is possible to say that the test material is speech and that there are differences between two stimuli. It is not possible to recognize the speech and say what the words are. At the recognition level it is possible to say what the word is. At the comprehension level it is possible to recognize words and understand the meaning of any speech presented.

with the speech test material. Without calibration signals it is not possible to set the correct level of loudness for speech audiometry.

A distinction has to be made between 'live voice' speech audiometry and that using recorded test material. Live voice speech audiometry is where the tester produces the test material by reading out loud from a prepared list. Because of the difficulties involved in producing speech in a constant manner, live voice speech testing is subject to greater variability and therefore should only be used where it is not possible to use recorded material.

**Speech test material**

The problem in speech audiometry is that due to the nature of speech, different speech test material will give rise to different results. Speech test material may be single words, sentences, meaningless speech sounds called logotoms or nonsense syllables. Results may also vary with different speakers presenting the material and with the quality of the recording and replaying equipment.

It is normally recommended that only recorded speech test material be used, because this gives a good degree of repeatability and reliability. However, live voice speech audiometry has to be used in some circumstances and the variability involved in this form of presentation has to be taken into account when evaluating results.

One of the first distinctions to be made with regard to speech test material is whether the material is produced in the form of an open or a closed set. Open-set material is that which gives no information to the person being tested; they have to rely on their knowledge of the language to determine if they can recognize the words being presented.

In a closed-set test, the subject has to choose which word they heard from a small number of words that are placed in front of them. This method allows particular aspects of speech recognition to be evaluated and for the process to be automated with computer-controlled presentations and scoring.

The recording of the speech test material must contain a calibration signal to allow the audiometer to be set up correctly. There should also be a means for ensuring that the reproduction of the speech is up to standard (ISO 8253-3).

## Equipment for speech audiometry

Today, speech audiometers as separate instruments are rarely made and most speech audiometry is undertaken using a pure-tone audiometer with a speech channel. Figure 5.4(b) shows a typical arrangement when using a pure-tone audiometer. The means of monitoring and controlling the input level to the audiometer is very important as this determines the calibration of the speech signals. The calibration signal on the recording should be set to a reference point on the audiometer level indicator at the start of each test session.

Where speech audiometry is being conducted with the patient in a separate audiometric booth or room it is essential for the tester to be able to hear the verbal responses of the patient by means of an effective communication system.

## Speech audiogram

A speech audiogram is obviously very different from a pure-tone audiogram, as may be seen in Figure 5.13. The x-axis is the level of the speech signal and the y-axis the percentage of words or sounds recognized correctly. The method of scoring for speech audiometry uses either the number of whole words correctly recognized or the number of phonemes recognized in each word. Table 5.3 shows a typical set of results from a list of words using phoneme scoring.

For each point on the audiogram one complete list of the test material must be used.

Figure 5.13(a) also shows the effect of using different types of material. In general, it is more difficult to recognize unfamiliar short words than longer words and sentences. The effect of this is that the curves produced

**Table 5.3:** A typical set of responses from a subject who is achieving a good speech recognition score. A score of 1 is given for each phoneme recognized correctly and 0 for each error. The total score is calculated as a percentage

| Test word | Response | Score |
|---|---|---|
| Fish | Dish | 0,1,1 |
| Duck | Duck | 3 |
| Gap | Gap | 3 |
| Cheese | Cheat | 1,1,0 |
| Rail | Hail | 0,1,1 |
| Hive | Hide | 1,1,0 |
| Bone | Born | 1,0,1 |
| Wedge | Wed | 1,1,0 |
| Moss | Moss | 3 |
| Tooth | Tooth | 3 |
| | **Total score out of 30** | **24** |
| | **% Correct** | **80%** |

from different test materials tend to be steeper the easier the material is to recognize.

## Terminology for speech audiometry

Unlike pure-tone audiometry where there are very few terms used to describe the results, in speech audiometry there are a number of terms, which are described below and illustrated in Figure 5.13. These terms are based on ISO 8253-3.

### Speech level

The SPL of the speech signal, measured in an appropriate ear simulator or in a sound field with specified frequency weighting and specified time weighting.

### Speech detection threshold level

The speech detection threshold level is that where speech is detected (i.e. just heard, but not understood). This level often corresponds well with the pure-tone threshold at 500 Hz because this frequency is the one that corresponds to the loudest part of the speech spectrum. This level is also very constant across many types of speech test material.

### Speech recognition score

The percentage of correctly recognized test items, e.g. phonemes, words or sentences, at a stated speech level.

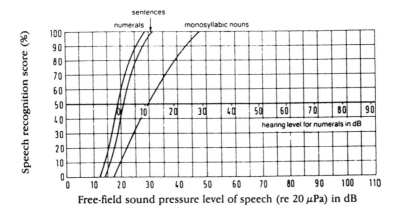

(a)

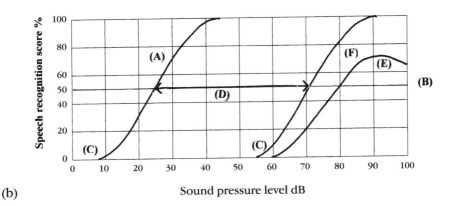

(b)

**Figure 5.13:** (a) A typical speech audiogram showing the difference between reference curves for different speech test materials. (b) A speech audiogram illustrating terms used in speech audiometry. (A) reference speech recognition curve; (B) speech recognition threshold level, 50% level; (C) speech detection threshold; (D) HL for speech; (E) maximum speech recognition score; (F) speech recognition curves illustrating a conductive hearing loss and a sensorineural loss where 100% score is not achievable.

## Speech recognition threshold level (SRT)

The speech recognition threshold level is that at which 50% of the test material is recognized correctly. This value varies with the type of test material, speaker, etc., as may be seen in Figure 5.13. In the past this was called speech reception threshold.

*Maximum speech recognition score*

The maximum score that a subject can obtain regardless of level.

*Optimum speech level*

The speech level at which the maximum recognition score is obtained.

*Half-optimum speech level*

The speech level at which half of the maximum speech recognition score is obtained. This level is used where subjects do not reach above the 50% level required for SRT.

*Speech recognition curve*

A curve that describes, for an individual subject, the speech recognition score as a function of speech level.

*Reference speech recognition curve*

For specified speech test material and a specified manner of presentation, a curve that describes the median speech recognition score as a function of speech level for a sufficiently large number of otologically normal persons of both sexes, aged between 18 and 25 years inclusive, for whom the test material is appropriate.

*Hearing level for speech*

The speech level minus the appropriate reference speech recognition threshold level.

## Uses of speech audiometry

As has been already mentioned, speech audiometry is not generally used today for clinical diagnostic purposes. However, it has great value in indicating the presence of speech recognition problems that cannot be identified from the pure-tone audiogram alone. It must be appreciated that speech audiometry is a time-consuming process and therefore is not undertaken routinely with all patients.

Figure 5.14 shows the pure-tone audiograms for a number of patients who have similar audiograms in each ear but very different speech recognition capabilities. These differences are most likely to be described by the patients, but without speech audiometry it would not be possible to quantify the problem.

A major use of speech audiometry has been for identifying the benefits derived from hearing aids. While the use of speech audiometry has

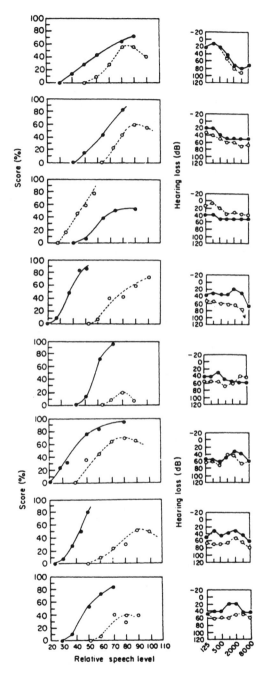

**Figure 5.14:** A comparison of pure tone and speech audiograms of patients with similar pure tone audiograms in each ear. Note the marked difference in speech audiograms between the ears. From Hood (1984).

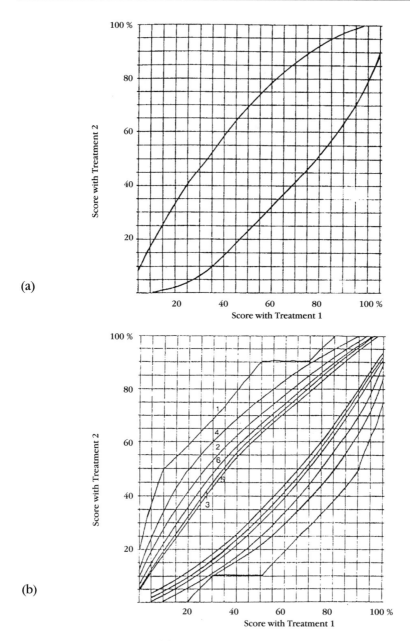

(a)

(b)

**Figure 5.15:** (a) Minimal differences between treatment scores for statistical significance (95% confidence limits). If the score for treatment 2 falls within the boundary of the curves at the points of intersection with the score for treatment 1, then the difference between scores cannot be attributed with any certainty to a difference between treatments. From Green (1997). (b) Minimal differences for a range of speech test material and the number of tests; the larger the number of tests the smaller the difference required for significance.

considerable merit in identifying the overall value of a hearing aid, or any other intervention, it is very poor in determining differences between different aids, etc. Figure 5.15 shows the differences that are required to ensure a statistical difference between two aids/treatments. It can be seen that very big differences are required in terms of the recognition scores to achieve statistical significance. Improvements can be made but only by conducting many more tests. Caution should therefore be shown in interpreting the differences between treatments based on speech audiometry alone.

To obtain recognition scores, monosyllabic words are commonly used, as well as sentences. However, running or conversational speech can be used for setting both comfortable and uncomfortable listening levels when assessing the benefits of hearing aids.

Speech audiometry is essential in assessing the ability of children to recognize speech and may have considerable implications for their education. For very young children 'toy tests' and other techniques may be used to determine a child's ability to hear and understand speech (see also Chapter 11 for a further description of hearing tests for children).

On assessing an adult patient's suitability for a cochlear implant, sentence recognition tests using hearing aids play a vital part in deciding whether an implant is likely to be of greater benefit than the use of a hearing aid.

# Chapter 6
# Objective audiometry

RICHARD T RAMSDEN AND PATRICK R AXON

In a sense, the term 'objective audiometry' is a bit of a semantic contradiction. Hearing, which audiometry purports to measure, can only be a subjective sensation or experience, as can vision, touch, taste and smell. It can only be enjoyed and recalled at an intimate, personal level, at a cortical plane of emotion and cognition that defies objective analysis. Nevertheless, scientists who are interested in such matters recognize that there are certain mechano- and electrophysical events, epiphenomena perhaps, which accompany the passage of a sound stimulus from the ear to the auditory cortex, that can be recorded and measured; from these, intelligent inference may lead to certain conclusions regarding the subjective experience of hearing.

When a sound wave enters the ear canal it sets into vibration a relatively crude system of levers – the ear drum and the ossicular chain – which deliver the stimulus to the oval window and on to the cochlea. The cochlea is a transducer, it converts sound waves into electric currents, which are then passed through the auditory nerve to the brainstem and from there to the higher centres. The process of transduction takes place in the hair cells of the organ of Corti. They are bathed in endolymph, a fluid that carries a strongly positive electric charge compared with the hair cells themselves. It is thought that the shearing forces exerted on the hair cells by the incoming sound wave, in the presence of the endolymphatic potential, initiate the process of electrical depolarization in the hair cells, which then proceeds to activate the neurons of the auditory nerve and so, via a series of relay stations or nuclei, on throughout the auditory pathway to the cortex. The activity initiated by these events can be recorded in a variety of ways, which allow us to speculate with varying degrees of success as to the integrity of the auditory system, and to the normality of hearing itself.

A series of tests that record events that occur in the auditory system in response to sound will be described.

# Middle-ear compliance measurements

### Tympanometry

The eardrum separates the middle ear from the external ear canal. Normally the middle-ear air pressure is the same as the atmospheric pressure in the ear canal, because of the action of the eustachian tube, which opens many times a day as we talk, swallow and yawn, and which equalizes the pressures. Aeronauts and scuba divers are familiar with this action. In the normal ear, there is no pressure differential across the drum, which therefore presents little resistance to the passage of sound. Only a small proportion of an incoming sound wave will be reflected from its surface. To put it another way, the drum has very little acoustic impedance, or conversely the system is very compliant. A number of middle-ear conditions occur which, at the same time as causing a certain degree of hearing loss, are responsible for measurable alterations in the middle-ear compliance.

If there is a relative vacuum in the middle ear, the eardrum is sucked inwards, or retracted, and as a result becomes slightly more taut. A sound wave entering the ear canal will strike a membrane which will tend to reflect a higher proportion of the energy than normal. The system has therefore lost compliance. The subject experiences a sensation of muffled hearing, which may be easily corrected by swallowing or by popping the ears (the Valsalva manoeuvre). Compliance may be further reduced if there is fluid in the middle ear, and also by any condition which reduces the mobility of the ossicular chain (e.g. otosclerosis, tympanosclerosis). It may be increased if there is loss of the continuity of the ossicular chain, or if there is a thin segment of the eardrum, perhaps a healed perforation.

Tympanometry is a technique that allows one to measure the compliance of the eardrum and ossicular chain. An airtight probe is fitted into the ear canal. It emits a low-frequency tone, and contains a sound pressure level meter that measures the proportion of the probe tone that is reflected back from the drum. In addition, it is connected to a pump, which allows the pressure on the eardrum to be increased or decreased. Compliance is measured by studying the proportion of the probe tone reflected under differing conditions of pressure. Figure 6.1 shows the reading from a normal middle ear. The peak on the graph (the point of maximum compliance) occurs when the eardrum is in its normal position (i. e. no pressure is being applied to it by the pump in the ear canal). Compare this with Figure 6.2, which is the tracing from a patient with negative middle-ear pressure. Here a negative pressure of 200 mm $H_2O$ has to be applied by the pump in order to suck the drum back to its position of maximum compliance.

In Figure 6.3, glue ear, the surface tension of the exudate is so great that the pump cannot pull the drum away back to its normal position: a flat graph with low compliance therefore results. Figure 6.4 shows the trace from a middle ear with normal pressure, but high compliance (ossicular discontinuity), and Figure 6.5 illustrates the result from a patient with normal middle-ear pressure and low compliance (ossicular fixation).

It is important to realize that tympanometry only tells us about the mechanics of the middle ear. It provides no information about inner-ear function. Any one of these traces could be obtained from an ear with a sensorineural hearing loss or even a 'dead ear'.

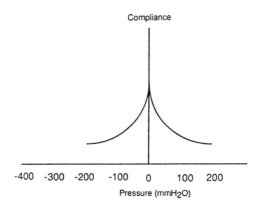

**Figure 6.1:** Tympanonetry: normal curve.

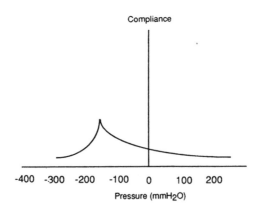

**Figure 6.2:** Tympanometry: negative middle-ear pressure.

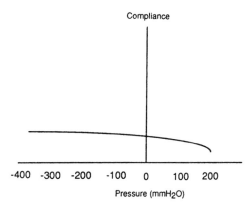

**Figure 6.3:** Tympanometry: flat curve indicating presence of glue ear.

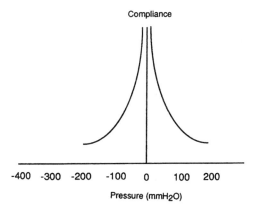

**Figure 6.4:** Tympanometry: ossicular discontinuity.

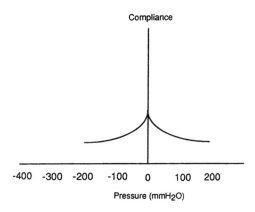

**Figure 6.5:** Tympanometry: ossicular fixation.

## Stapedial (acoustic) reflex measurements

When a sound of approximately 85 dB SP above threshold enters a normal ear, it causes the small stapedius muscle, which is attached to the neck of the stapes, to contract and dampen the vibration of the stapes in the oval window, thus protecting the cochlea from excessive stimulation. The afferent fibres for this reflex travel via the cochlear nerve to the cochlear nucleus in the brainstem, where they relay the stimulus to the efferent fibres in the facial nerve. The reflex is 'crossed', i. e. stimulation of one ear produces a bilateral response. The contraction of the stapedius muscle is accompanied by a transient decrease in middle-ear compliance. Study of the stapedius reflex (SR) can therefore yield information on the state of the middle ear, the cochlea, the auditory nerve, the brainstem and the facial nerve. The stapedius reflex threshold (SRT) is usually measured at frequencies between 500 and 4000 Hz. In cochlear deafness, the SRT is usually less than 85 dB above the hearing threshold because of recruitment.

In neural deafness, e. g. acoustic neuroma, the difference between the hearing threshold and the SRT is usually normal or increased. Some lesions of the brainstem, e. g. multiple sclerosis, are associated with abnormalities of the reflex even though the hearing is normal. In stapedial fixation due to otosclerosis, the reflex may not be recordable because the inability of the stapes to move means that the reflex is not associated with any change in compliance. The other clinically useful aspect of the reflex is the rate at which it decays or fatigues with sustained stimulation. Lesions of the auditory nerve are associated with an increase in the rate of stapedial reflex decay. The presence or absence of the SR may help to localize the site of the lesion in cases of facial paralysis, for example, following skull base fracture or in the investigation of idiopathic facial palsy. If the SR is normal this implies damage to the nerve distal to the nerve to the stapedius muscle, perhaps from a tumour in the parotid gland. If the SR is absent but tear production is normal this implies a lesion proximal to the nerve to stapedius but distal to the branch of the facial nerve to the tear gland. If both the SR and tear production are absent, the site of the injury is proximal to the nerve to the lacrymal gland.

Electrically elicited SR is a modification of the test which has been introduced since the development of cochlear implantation. The test is carried out during surgery after the insertion of the electrode array into the cochlea. The surgeon places the external stimulus coil over the receiver antenna and delivers a series of electrical stimuli to the intracochlear electrodes in turn. He may then observe under high magnification the contraction of the stapedius muscle (the anaesthetist must avoid the use of muscle-relaxing drugs). This observation tells him several things. The cochlear implant is functioning and is in the right place; the auditory nerve is present and can transmit current; the facial nerve is functioning and has not been damaged during the surgery. It is reassuring for the patient or his or her parents to receive this confirmation immediately after surgery.

The other possible application of the electrically evoked SR is in predicting a safe level of stimulus when it comes to eventual tuning and switch-on of the implant. Peroperative testing allows one to establish the SRT, and this level should not be exceeded when planning the current levels at switch-on, otherwise unpleasant or even painful sensation may be experienced. This is clearly of special importance in young children.

# Electric response audiometry (ERA)

Each level of neuronal activity in the auditory pathway, from the cochlear hair cell to the cortex is associated with an electrical potential or a number of electrical potentials that are evoked by the sound stimulus. Depending on their latencies, these responses are classified as early, middle or late. The potentials are small but techniques of electric response averaging or time domain averaging allow them to be summated so that they can be displayed on the oscilloscope screen and extracted from random background electrical activity. Some of these responses have become established as having value in the objective assessment of hearing threshold as well as in the differential diagnosis of deafness and other neuro-otological syndromes. Each has its own advantages and limitations, and often the tests may be employed in combination to provide complementary information.

## Electrocochleography (ECochG)

This technique records the electrical events in the cochlea and first-order auditory neurons. For large, easily identifiable responses, the active electrode is best sited on the medial wall of the middle ear – the promontory – which overlies the basal turn of the cochlea. A fine stainless steel needle electrode is passed under local or general anaesthesia through the drum. Some workers employ the less invasive extratympanic electrode, but the responses are smaller and a larger number of averages, and therefore more time is required to obtain them. A reference electrode is placed on the mastoid process and a ground electrode on the forehead. Wideband click stimuli (spectral average of approximately 3.5 kHz) are usually employed, although more frequency-specific tones may also be used.

Three potentials are recorded. The cochlear microphonic (CM) in a normal ear is an exact electrical 'mirror' of the acoustic signal stimulating the ear. Many of its features suggest that it is a non-neural potential, and it seems probable that it arises from the hair cells prior to the generation of the neural compound action potential (CAP, see below). What is not clear is whether it is essential to the process of transduction, or merely a coincidental phenomenon. The summating potential (SP) is another non-neural potential seen as a direct current (DC) shift in the baseline of the CAP, particularly at high stimulus intensity. The CM and the SP are unpredictable in magnitude and have no place in the estimation of hearing threshold, although abnormalities of both may be seen in certain disease states.

The CAP represents the synchronous depolarization of a large number of fibres in the auditory nerve (Figure 6.6). It has a latency of between 1.5 and 4.5 ms depending on the intensity of the signal. As can be seen, the magnitude of the response decreases as the signal intensity lessens. CAP measurements are accurate to within 15 dB in estimating the true hearing threshold. Its main disadvantage, and this is shared by most ERA techniques, is that it does not provide accurate information at frequencies below 1 kHz. Abnormalities of the shape of the CAP occur in certain disease states, and may provide help in diagnosis, especially of Ménière's disease. The responses are not affected by sedation or general anaesthesia.

### Auditory brainstem response (ABR)

The synonym for ABR is brainstem-evoked response (BSER) and this technique is one of the most useful in neuro-otology. Recording from scalp electrodes, a series of five or six potentials can be detected in the auditory nerve and brainstem in the first 10 ms after presentation of a sound stimulus (Figure 6.7). As the electrodes are more remote from the generators of the potentials than in ECochG, a larger number of averages is required, but this disadvantage is outweighed by the value of the information acquired.

The potentials (NI-NV) are thought to have the following sites of origin, although there is still much continuing debate about the details: NI, auditory nerve; NII, cochlear nucleus; NIII, superior olivary nucleus; NIV, nucleus of the lateral lemniscus; NV, inferior colliculus. These responses and their latencies are very reproducible from test to test and from person to person. They may be used for threshold estimation or in neuro-otological diagnosis. Delay in the later waves may be seen in tumours of the auditory nerve (vestibular schwannoma), or in brainstem disorders such as multiple sclerosis. As the test is non-invasive it can be carried out by staff who are not medically qualified. The thresholds of the responses are not affected by sedation or general anaesthesia. Accurate thresholds cannot be obtained at frequencies below 1 kHz.

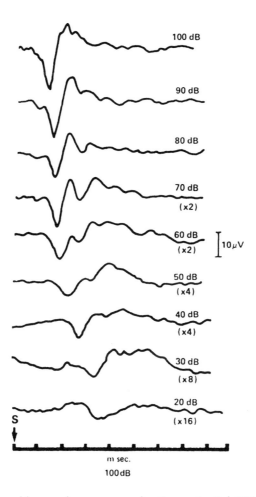

**Figure 6.6:** Electrocochleography: compound action potential (CAP). Note that the magnitude of the response decreases and its latency increases as the intensity of the stimulus decreases.

As with the stapedial reflex described above, the ABR can be elicited by an electrical stimulus (EABR), and this variant of the test has become important since the advent of cochlear implantation. The test can be performed as a preoperative means of confirming that the implant is functioning and correctly located, that the auditory nerve is functioning and that stimuli from the implant are reaching at least the level of the mid-brain. In addition, information about threshold levels of stimulation may be obtained. EABR is also a useful tool in the preoperative assessment of certain individuals for cochlear implantation when there is uncertainty as to the status of the cochlear nerve.

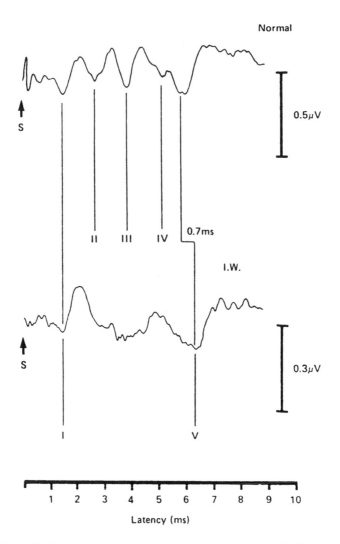

**Figure 6.7**: ABR: the upper trace shows a normal response with five negative waves (NI–V) at normal latencies. The lower trace illustrates how the technique can be of value in the diagnosis of disease. There is significant delay in the latency of NV, a finding suggestive of a tumour of the audiovestibular nerve (acoustic neuroma).

The presence of a functioning cochlear nerve is of course essential for successful implantation. In some congenitally deaf children, there may be some doubt as to whether the cochlear nerve has been properly formed (see Figure 7.16, Chapter 7); it may on occasion be totally absent. In some adults deafened after skull base injury, the possibility of avulsion of the auditory nerve from the cochlea must be considered. The stimulus is delivered through an electrode in the region of the round window, and in the case of children the test is performed under a general anaesthetic. If no response is obtained the individual may be turned down for implantation.

Simpler variants of this technique are the promontory and round window stimulation tests. No objective recordings are made. The subject simply reports whether or not he or she can hear sounds when current is delivered to the ear. The test requires a conscious and linguistically competent subject and is clearly not suitable for small children.

A form of the EABR can be obtained by stimulation at the level of the cochlear nucleus in the brainstem. This has emerged since the development of the auditory brainstem implant (ABI). This device is very similar to a cochlear implant but is used in certain people with total bilateral deafness with loss of the auditory nerves for whom a cochlear implant would be contraindicated. In practice, such persons are nearly all sufferers from the familial condition of neurofibromatosis type 2, which is characterized by the presence of bilateral tumours of the audiovestibular nerves (vestibular schwannomas). Some useful hearing may be restored by inserting an implant device on to the surface of the cochlear nucleus. The surgeon is helped in the accurate location of the device by peroperative recording of the later part of the EABR (Figure 6.8).

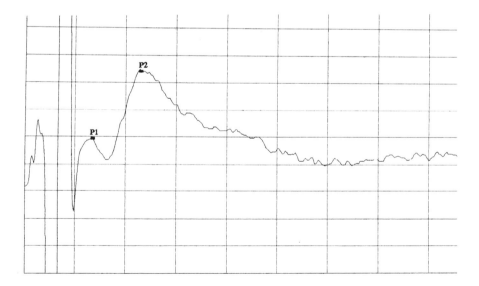

**Figure 6.8:** EABR recorded through an auditory brainstem implant, showing a large stimulus artefact followed by the waveform showing two positive peaks.

### Cortical-evoked response audiometry (CERA)

In this technique, late responses from the auditory cortex are recorded from scalp electrodes. It is used for testing older children and adults and has become of great importance in the assessment of medico-legal and compensation claims. The stimulus is a frequency-specific tone burst and has a duration of 50 ms. It is repeated at intervals of 1–2 s. About 50 repetitions are necessary for response acquisition at each frequency. The response, which is known as the slow vertex response (SVR), shows two positive and two negative peaks and occurs between 50 and 250 ms after delivery of the stimulus (Figure 6.9). It is possible to determine thresholds to an accuracy of around 10 dB, and it is this degree of accuracy combined with its frequency specificity that makes the test so valuable. The test has some shortcomings. It is time-consuming and requires a conscious subject, because the responses are abolished by sleep, sedation and general anaesthesia.

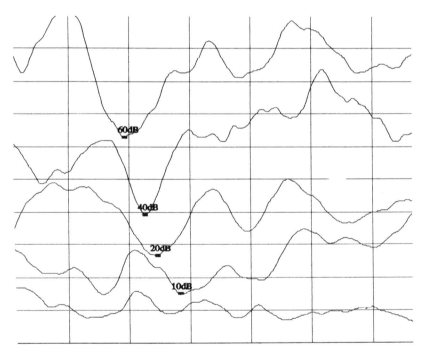

**Figure 6.9:** CERA, showing progressive increase in latency of N1 as threshold is reached. Latency, 50 ms per division.

### Endogenous potentials

There are two potentials that come closer than any others to representing the cognitive processes involved in hearing. These are the P300 and the contingent negative variation (CNV). These emerge as variations in the pattern of the SVR when the subject is given a task to concentrate on during the presentation of a sound stimulus. P300 is recorded when the subject has to concentrate on listening for a transient change in the frequency of the test tone, and the CNV occurs when a sound stimulus conditions a sense of expectancy for another stimulus, which may not necessarily be acoustic, e. g. a flash of light.

# Evoked otoacoustic emissions (cochlear echoes)

Earlier in this chapter we sketched an outline of cochlear physiology (see also Chapter 3). The cochlea has been recognized since the work of von Békésy as being a transducer and frequency analyser. The travelling wave produces maximal displacement of the basilar membrane at a distance from the oval window that depends on the frequency of the incoming wave. It was accepted until the late 1970s that the hair cells of the organ of Corti were entirely passive, that they awaited the arrival of the travelling wave, were depolarized and initiated neural transmission in the auditory nerve fibres. If this were the case it would be a very inefficient system because friction of the cochlea would damp the wave and prevent it from travelling the full length of the cochlea.

It is now recognized that the incident wave stimulates the inner hair cells only, which are the primary sensory cells of the cochlea. The majority of the hair cells, the outer hair cells, have a mainly efferent innervation and they contribute to the sensitivity and sharp frequency resolution of the cochlea. They are mechanically active and contract in response to the incoming wave. This motility is probably the result of the contractile properties of the actin and myosin filaments found in the outer hair cells. The effect is to assist the passage of the wave along the cochlea, by physically nudging it along the cochlea, as Kemp (1978) has so graphically described it. One of the concomitants of this active process in the cochlea is the emission of energy, the so called otoacoustic emission (OAE).

There are in fact several types of otoacoustic emission classified into two groups, spontaneous and evoked. Evoked OAEs are further subdivided into three main variants depending on the methods of stimulation of the ear:

- transient evoked emissions (TEOAE)
- stimulus frequency emissions (SFOAE)
- distortion product emissions (DPOAE).

Spontaneous OAEs are quiet signals, which can be recorded from the ear canal from about 40% of normal individuals with normal pure-tone audiograms in the absence of any external stimulus. They are usually inaudible to the subject. For some reason they are twice as common in females as males. They have no real role as a clinical tool in the investigation of deafness, although their relationship to tinnitus has been the subject of some speculation.

Of the evoked emissions, TEOAE and DPOAE have been most extensively studied and have the greatest clinical value. User-friendly, relatively inexpensive equipment has been developed to allow measurement of OAEs in a clinical setting. An insert is placed in the ear canal with a stimulus emitter and a microphone. The stimulus is applied and the ensuing TEOAE is detected by the microphone. In fact the TEOAE has to be separated from the stimulus because both are picked up by the microphone, and this is made possible because there is a slight delay (1/100 s) in the onset of the TEOAE due to the time taken for the travelling wave to pass along the cochlea. It is this delay that led to the TEOAE being known as the 'cochlear echo' or 'Kemp echo'. The response is displayed on a small computer screen (see Figure 6.10). The use of a broad-band click stimulus yields information between 500 and 5000 Hz and thus covers most of the speech frequency spectrum.

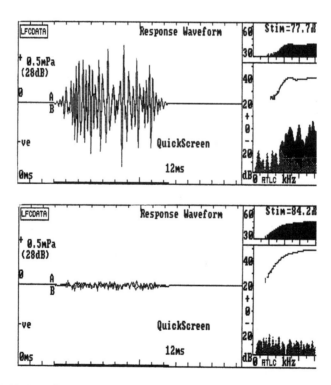

**Figure 6.10:** TEOAE showing (a) normal response and (b) an absent response.

TEOAE are present in almost 100% of normal ears and are not measurable in ears with a hearing loss of more than 25-30 dB. They are detectable in the neonate and their reliability, ease of detection, objectivity and the non-invasive nature of the test procedure are the basis of their increasing role in neonatal screening programmes. Because TEOAE does not depend on averaging techniques, the responses are obtained much more quickly (less than 5 min for both ears) than ABR and can be recorded at the cotside by nonmedical personnel. The detection of a normal TEOAE means that the baby has a hearing level that is within 30 dB of normal at the frequencies tested. Repeated failure to obtain a response suggests that the child has a hearing loss greater than 30 dB, and should be referred for further, more detailed assessment of the hearing, such as ABR.

The main problem with TEOAE is that the response may be absent in the presence of middle ear pathology such as glue ear. However, the effect of this is an error in the right direction, in that a false negative response will simply mean that more children will be investigated further. A false positive response could mean that some cases of deafness could be missed. A recent report commissioned by the Department of Health recommended the introduction of a national screening programme for congenital hearing impairment and the aim of early identification of all children with a permanent hearing impairment of at least 40 dB. It seems likely that the use of TEOAE will be central to that programme when it is eventually established.

The role of DPOAE in the differential diagnosis of sensorineural deafness is arousing increasing interest at the present time but remains largely in the realm of research.

## The role of objective audiometry

Why should investigators want to develop a series of 'objective' tests of hearing? There are two main reasons: threshold estimation and neuro-otological diagnosis.

### Threshold estimation

Threshold estimation is important in those groups of individuals who are unable or reluctant to cooperate in behavioural audiometry. The former include the very young, especially if they are felt to be 'at risk' of hearing loss, and the multiply handicapped. There is a need for simple screening tests that can be used easily and with a high degree of sensitivity by non-medical staff, e.g. otoacoustic emissions in neonates and tympanometry in the preschool age group. Objective threshold estimation using ABR or ECochG and occasionally EABR is essential in the assessment of the very young child for cochlear implantation. Cochlear and brainstem implantation programmes rely heavily on the availability of good-quality objective measures of function of the auditory pathways. CERA has become the investigation of choice in suspected functional or non-organic hearing loss, whether psychogenic or, in cases with medico-legal and compensation implications, due to exaggeration or frank malingering.

## Neuro-otological diagnosis

Analysis of deviations from the norm of certain waveforms, particularly of the ABR and ECochG, can lead to speculation as to the probable cause of the hearing loss. Thus the delay in N1-NV on ABR can suggest vestibular schwannoma, although it is true that with the increasing availablity of high-quality magnetic resonance imaging (MRI), the role of ABR in diagnosis of these tumours is becoming less important. Alterations in the shape of the CAP and SP, and the magnitude of the CM in ECochG can point to a diagnosis of Ménière's disease.

As a final observation on 'objective' audiometry we should not lose sight of the fact that all test results have to be interpreted by the tester. Despite the fact that the subjectivity of the patient may have been reduced or eliminated, the fallibility of the tester or the programmer of the test equipment remains. Furthermore, equipment must be correctly maintained and calibrated and the test environment must be as close to ideal as possible so that electrical interference and artefact are minimized. Thus even 'objective' results may be subject to error.

# Chapter 7
# The radiological assessment of hearing loss

Richard T Ramsden and Patrick R Axon

Deafness is not a single nosological entity. It may arise as a result of pathology at any point in the auditory pathway from the most peripheral to the most central, from the external auditory meatus to the auditory cortex. Depending on the site of the lesion there will be different patterns of impairment and handicap, and sophisticated audiological and psychoacoustic tests may reveal unique patterns which allow the clinician to locate the probable site of injury with a reasonable degree of accuracy. Additional insights into the pathological processes associated with hearing loss may be provided by ever-more-detailed imaging techniques now available, especially computerized tomography (CT) scanning and magnetic resonance imaging (MRI).

This chapter deals with the radiological techniques now in common use in the evaluation of hearing problems.

## Radiology of deafness

The radiological assessment of hearing loss has evolved at an extraordinary pace since the introduction of computer technology into clinical practice in the mid-1970s. Until then, plain films, tomography and radioisotope scans were the only resources at the disposal of the clinician, and when one looks back at such films with 20 years' hindsight it really is remarkable that they were able to provide any meaningful information. In fact, a distinguished neurosurgical colleague of the authors laconically but accurately referred to these images as 'hintograms'. The work of Godfrey Hounsfield in the early 1970s led to the introduction of CT scanning, a technique which soon found an application in the imaging of the temporal bone as well as the posterior cranial fossa (Hounsfield 1973). The 1980s saw the introduction of MRI, and as a result of these two innovations,

117

plain radiology of the ear and its pathways has rapidly passed into history. Such was the impact of the imaging revolution that clinico-audiological assessment of deafness in many situations became relegated by the new gold standard of imaging.

CT and MRI each produces a derived cross-sectional image of the target tissue, and computerized manipulation of the derived data allows reconfiguration of images in other planes. Each technique has its peculiar advantages. CT tends to produce clearer images of bony structures and abnormalities than MRI (e.g. details of temporal bone anatomy and destruction). MRI, on the other hand, permits highly detailed study of the non-bony components of the auditory system, the fluids of the inner ear, the auditory nerves in the cerebellopontine angle and the brainstem, and higher neural centres in the brainstem and auditory cortex. CT utilizes the differential absorption of an X-ray beam through tissues, whereas MRI exploits the complex interplay of tissue protons when exposed to an applied magnetic field. The short summary that follows is intended to be a simple introduction to the complexities of image production, a full description of which is beyond the scope of this chapter.

CT emits a narrow X-ray beam that is directed through the patient's body. X-rays are differentially absorbed by the various tissues in their pathway, so that only a proportion of them is detected on the other side of the body and thus recorded on a photographic film. The beam is rotated through 360 degrees around the patient in multiple steps. At each step the proportion absorbed varies, depending on the type of tissue through which the beam has passed. The absorption characteristics of a complete two-dimensional slice are thus obtained, and computer analysis allows a cross-sectional image to be constructed. Figure 7.1 shows the bony detail of the temporal bone, middle and inner ears revealed by high quality CT imaging.

In MRI, the body is surrounded by a large magnetic field which causes the protons in the body to vibrate. The protons in different nuclei vibrate at different frequencies (resonant frequencies), which can be increased or decreased by varying the strength of the magnetic field. MRI utilizes the resonant frequency of the hydrogen nucleus, which is chosen because of its abundance within the body. Localization of hydrogen nuclei within a particular tissue requires that their frequency is unique, so that they 'stand out in the crowd'. MRI therefore graduates the magnetic field throughout the body, with the result that hydrogen nuclei vibrate at different frequencies. By tuning to a particular frequency while knowing the magnetic strength that was required to create that frequency, the location of the hydrogen nuclei can be ascertained. This information together with the amplitude of the signal allows spatial characterization and enables an image to be formed. Figure 7.2 demonstrates the inner ear and its central connections on MRI.

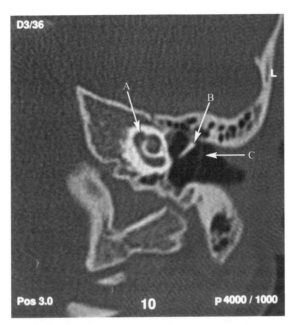

**Figure 7.1:** High-definition CT scan of normal left temporal bone, coronal view. The cochlear lumen can be clearly identified surrounded by the dense bone of the otic capsule (A). The long process of the incus (B) is seen within the aerated middle-ear cleft, which is separated from the external auditory meatus by the tympanic membrane (C).

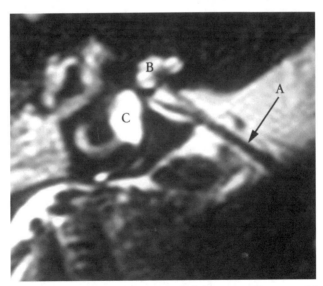

**Figure 7.2:** Magnetic resonance image (MRI) of the normal temporal bone demonstrating the vestibulo-cochlear nerve (A) traversing the cerebellopontine angle from the brain stem to the cochlea (B) and vestibule (C).

There are many congenital and acquired abnormalities of the ear and temporal bone, the details of which have become more clear since the introduction of CT and MRI.

# Congenital hearing loss

Congenital abnormalities of the auditory system may occur in the external ear, the middle ear and the inner ear. Congenital external ear abnormalities may affect the pinna alone, in which case the defect is largely cosmetic, or there may be atresia of the external canal, in which case there may be a conductive hearing loss. CT scanning will tell the surgeon if the canal occlusion is bony or soft tissue. Congenital middle-ear anomalies may involve the ossicular chain at various points. The wide variety of abnormalities need not be covered here, but CT imaging has reached a degree of sophistication such that ossicular chain defects including hypoplasia and fusion can often be diagnosed with a high degree of certainty. Severe external-ear deformities are not uncommonly associated with congenital abnormalities of the middle ear. However, it is less common for these anomalies to occur together with inner-ear developmental abnormalities, because the inner and middle ears are derived from different embryological sources.

Congenital anomalies of the inner ear are often bilateral and may be associated with a profound hearing loss present at birth, or one which progresses throughout childhood to become total or subtotal by adolescence or early adult life. The normal structure of the cochlea has been described in Chapter 3. It has the shape of a coiled tube, similar to a snail's shell. It comprises three parallel, fluid-containing tubes and in the middle tube, or scala media, is the organ of Corti where the mechanical energy of sound is converted into electrical impulses, which pass down the cochlear nerve to the brain. Differentiation of the cochlea and indeed of the semicircular canals of the balance organ may be arrested by agents largely unknown at an early stage of intrauterine development. Total aplasia associated with a total absence of hearing may occur (the so-called Michel deformity, Figure 7.3). Intermediate forms between total aplasia and a normally formed cochlea are more common. One of the most frequently recognized is the Mondini deformity, in which there is a normal basal turn to the cochlea but a fusion of the middle and apical turns, associated with a severe to profound hearing loss (Figure 7.4).

A dysplasia that is recognized more and more thanks to the sophistication of modern imaging, is the large vestibular aqueduct syndrome (Figure 7.5). In this condition there is a wider-than-normal passage between the intracranial space and the inner ear so that normal pressure changes in the skull may be transmitted to the inner ear with consequent damage to the organ of Corti. It is interesting that there may be exacerbations in the deafness following relatively minor degrees of head injury.

Many of these children with congenital inner ear abnormalities are candidates for cochlear implantation.

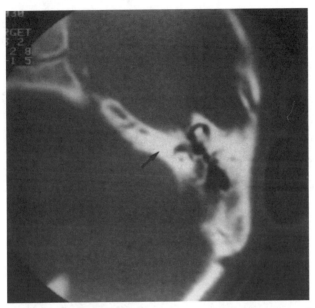

**Figure 7.3:** CT image of the left temporal bone, illustrating the Michel deformity. There is complete absence of any inner-ear structure. The arrow indicates where the cochlea should be.

# Cholesteatoma

Cholesteatoma is a condition characterized by the abnormal accumulation of skin cells within the middle ear or temporal bone. This may lead to a potentially dangerous erosion of bone and poses the threat of damage to important structures such as the ossicular chain, the facial nerve, the balance organ, the cochlea and, most important of all, the intracranial contents, with the risk of meningitis or brain abscess.

Cholesteatoma may be congenital, with skin cells trapped in the temporal bone from birth, or acquired, when there is an ingrowth through the eardrum of skin cells into the middle ear and mastoid. CT scanning will demonstrate the degree of bone erosion caused by the process and MRI may allow the soft tissue of the cholesteatoma to be differentiated from other less common pathologies (Figures 7.6 and 7.7)

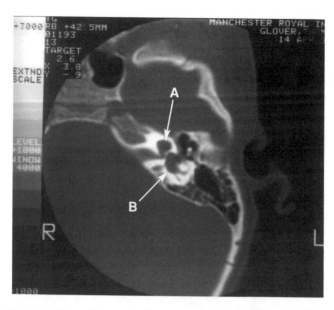

**Figure 7.4:** High-definition CT image of the left temporal bone. The patient had severe hearing loss from birth with further deterioration during early adult life. There is a Mondini deformity of the cochlea with fusion of its middle and apical turns (A). The vestibule is also dysplastic (B).

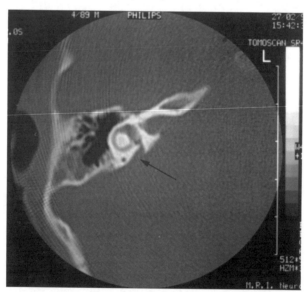

**Figure 7.5:** High-definition CT scan of the right temporal bone. The patient had mild hearing loss from birth, with stepwise deterioration in childhood often associated with minor head injuries. The image clearly shows a wide vestibular aqueduct (arrow).

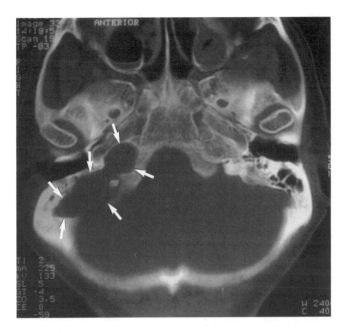

**Figure 7.6:** CT image of temporal bone showing widespread destruction due to acquired cholesteatoma (arrows). Note the loss of the normal anatomical features compared with the normal opposite side.

## Otosclerosis

This condition is one of the commonest causes of hearing loss in man. The cardinal abnormality is the production of metabolically abnormal bone in certain sites of predilection in the ear. This new bone is most commonly seen in the oval window where it encroaches on the stapes, impairs its vibration and causes a conductive hearing loss. Additionally, there may be altered bone in the region of the cochlea and a sensorineural (cochlear) deafness may result. The bony changes round the stapes are difficult to image at present but the demineralization round the cochlea is often quite dramatically shown on CT imaging (Figure 7.8).

## Tumours

Tumours of the ear are not common. The most frequently encountered is the vestibular schwannoma with an annual incidence of 1: 80 000. This benign tumour takes origin on the audiovestibular nerve for reasons that are not understood. When small, they cause symptoms of deafness,

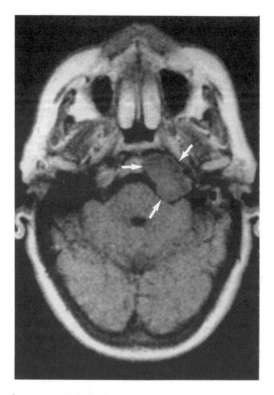

**Figure 7.7:** MRI of a congenital cholesteatoma (arrows) of the petrous apex and the cerebellopontine angle.

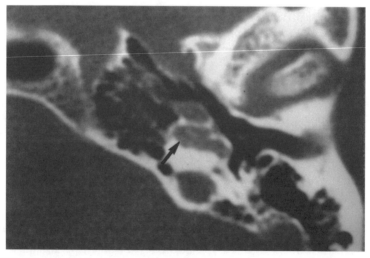

**Figure 7.8:** High-definition CT image illustrating marked demineralization of the right temporal bone, a feature of advanced otosclerosis (arrow).

tinnitus and imbalance, but as they grow inwards towards the brain they may cause facial numbness, ataxia and loss of coordination from local pressure, and headache, failing vision and eventual death from raised intracranial pressure. The early use of MRI, especially with enhancement from the paramagnetic agent Gadolinium GDPA, as an investigation in patients with unilateral audiovestibular symptoms which are not readily explainable, has resulted in the early diagnosis of these tumours and a more favourable outcome from surgery (Figures 7.9 and 7.10).

In a minority of individuals, vestibular schwannomas occur on both sides. This is the condition neurofibromatosis type 2, a dominantly inherited condition which is the result of mutation on chromosome 22. In addition, there may be other intracranial tumours (e.g. schwannomas on other cranial nerves, or meningiomas) and tumours of the spinal nerves. MRI has allowed the clinician an accurate assessment of the distribution of tumours and has helped considerably in the planning of surgery (Figure 7.11).

Other tumours of the ear are very rare, but mention should be made of the glomus jugulare tumour, which arises in the receptors at the top end of the internal jugular vein responsible for detecting changes in the blood chemistry (chemoreceptors). These tumours are extremely vascular and are highly destructive to the temporal bone and the bone of the skull base

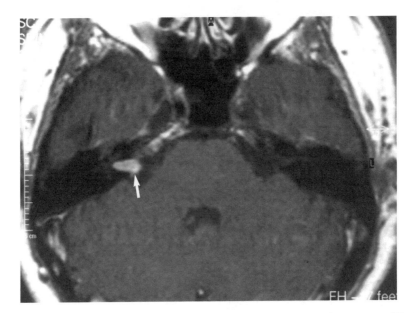

**Figure 7.9:** MRI with contrast enhancement. A small vestibular schwannoma fills the right internal auditory meatus without significant extension into the cerebellopontine angle (arrow).

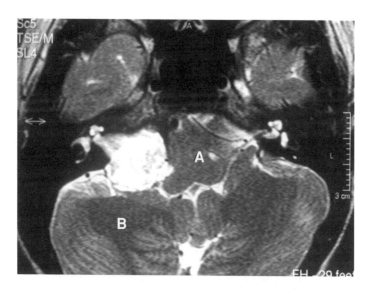

**Figure 7.10:** MRI of a large vestibular schwannoma filling the right cerebellopontine angle. There is widening of the internal auditory meatus and compression of the brain stem (A) and cerebellum (B).

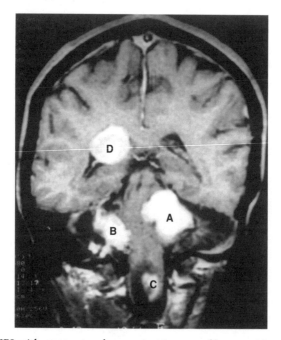

**Figure 7.11:** MRI with contrast enhancement in neurofibromatosis type 2. Tumours can be seen compressing the brain stem (A, B,) and spinal cord (C). A further tumour lies in the left lateral ventricle (D).

(Figure 7.12). Their blood supply is well demonstrated on angiography, and the radiologist can often help the surgeon by reducing the vascularity of the tumour by blocking off the main arteries supplying the tumour using the technique of embolization (Figure 7.13).

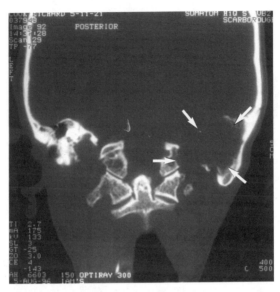

**Figure 7.12:** CT image of a large glomus tumour that has destroyed most of the right temporal bone (arrows).

# Head injury

Severe head injury may impair the hearing by damage to the middle-ear sound-conducting mechanism or to the inner ear by causing fracture through the temporal bone and cochlea. The commonest injury to the ossicular chain is dislocation of the incus, which is displaced, usually inferiorly but sometimes laterally through the eardrum with a consequent severe conductive hearing loss. The loss of the normal configuration of the ossicular chain can be demonstrated on CT imaging (Figure 7.14). Fracture through the inner ear is usually associated with a total or subtotal hearing loss. Sometimes these fractures involve the facial nerve, causing paralysis of the facial muscles. Such fractures can usually be seen on good quality CT scanning (Figure 7.15)

# Cochlear implantation

Cochlear implantation has, in the past decade, been the biggest and most exciting advance in the treatment of profound deafness resulting from

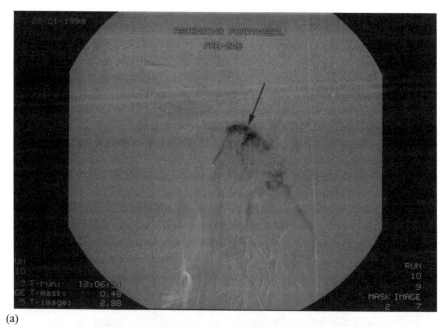

(a)

(b)

**Figure 7.13:** Digital subtraction angiography of left glomus tumour. Tumour blush (arrow) is seen on injection of contrast into the ascending pharyngeal artery (a). After successful embolization, contrast is unable to enter the tumour and no blush is seen (b).

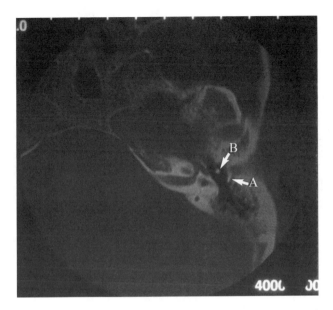

**Figure 7.14:** High-definition CT imaging demonstrating a traumatic dislocation of the ossicular chain. The incus (A) can be seen in the external auditory meatus lateral to the malleus (B).

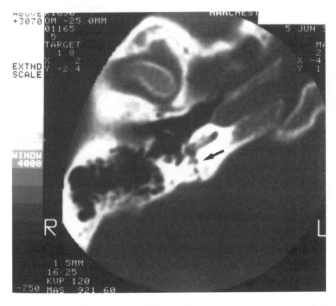

**Figure 7.15:** CT image of a temporal bone fracture passing through the vestibule (arrow).

damage to the cochlea. The theoretical basis and practical aspects of cochlear implantation are described in Chapter 19. One of the prerequisites for cochlear implantation is a cochlear lumen into which to insert the electrode array. Congenital deafness may be associated with varying degrees of inner ear dysplasia, some of which (e.g. the Mondini abnormality and the large vestibular aqueduct syndrome) do not preclude cochlear implantation. CT is the investigation most likely to reveal structural abnormalities of the inner ear. Figures 7.1, 7.3 and 7.4 show normal and dysplastic cochleas. Rarely, CT scanning may reveal a developmental abnormality of the internal auditory meatus suggesting that the cochlear nerve may be absent, thus precluding the possibility of cochlear implantation (Figure 7.16).

Another role for imaging is in the assessment of the cochlea afflicted by a disease process likely to obliterate the cochlear lumen and thus make insertion of an implant difficult. Certain disease processes (e.g. meningitis) can stimulate new bone formation (labyrinthitis ossificans), which may narrow or completely obliterate the lumen. The presence of this new

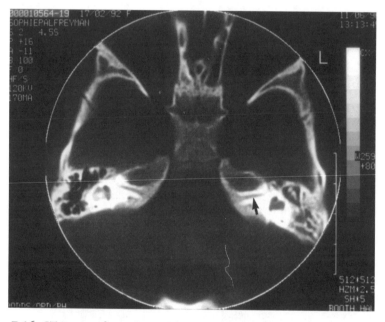

**Figure 7.16:** CT image of a patient with Feingold's syndrome. The internal auditory canals are very narrow (arrow) and can only contain the facial nerve. The cochlear nerve is therefore assumed to be absent; cochlear implantation is contraindicated.

bone may be suggested on CT imaging (Figure 7.17), but is more likely to be revealed on MRI, and in particular on surface rendered three-dimensional MRI using the so-called T2 sequence (Figure 7.18). Sometimes the prior knowledge of scala tympani obliteration will warn the surgeon that a scala vestibuli insertion may be necessary, or that he may have to drill an artificial gutter in the wall of the cochlea to accommodate the electrode array. Plain images are used as a routine postoperative measure to check the position of the electrode in the cochlea (Figure 7.19).

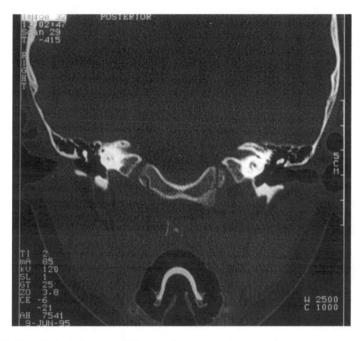

**Figure 7.17:** High-definition CT scan from a patient undergoing assessment for cochlear implantation, with a history of meningitis. The cochlear lumen has been almost completely occluded by new bone formation.

# The future

Functional MRI and positron emission tomography (PET) promise to reveal real-time activity in the auditory pathways and auditory cortex in response to acoustic signals. The research potential here is vast and should have a major impact on our understanding of the basic physiology of central auditory function and the auditory association areas.

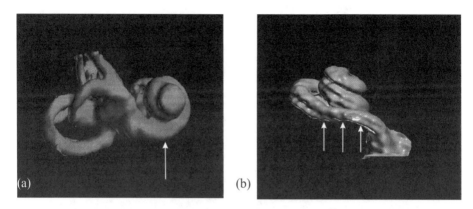

(a)                                        (b)

**Figure 7.18:** Surface rendered three-dimensional T2 weighted MRI of a normal cochlea (A). The white image is of the fluid in the cochlea and semicircular canals. The arrow points to a normal fluid signal from the basal turn of the cochlea. In (B) the arrows point out a portion of the basal turn of the cochlea where there is no fluid signal. This implies obliteration of that part of the cochlea by new bone and might warn of difficulties during the insertion of cochlear implant.

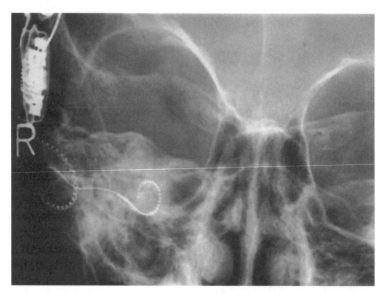

**Figure 7.19:** Plain radiograph of a cochlear implant fully inserted into the cochlear lumen.

# Chapter 8
# Causes of conductive hearing loss and their non-surgical management

## James Robinson

The human ear functions by collecting sound waves transmitted in the air and conducting them to the inner ear (Figure 8.1). These airborne waves are converted to waves in the inner-ear fluid at the oval window, which is the interface between the middle and inner ear. Anything that interferes with this conduction of airborne sound waves results in a conductive hearing loss. Problems occurring beyond the oval window interface are the subject of Chapter 10.

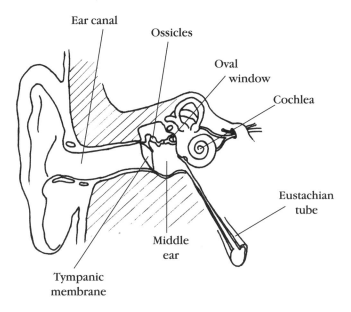

**Figure 8.1:** Anatomy of the ear.

133

# External ear canal

Any obstruction of the external auditory meatus causes a conductive hearing loss (Figure 8.2). The simplest way to demonstrate this is to try putting your finger in the opening of your ear canal. Any similar obstruction will have the same effect on hearing and the commonest condition of this sort is a collection of wax and skin debris in the ear. Wax is a natural product of modified sweat glands in the outer part of the ear canal and skin debris comes from the normal loss of surface skin cells from the lining of the ear canal. Under normal circumstances the wax and any other debris gradually works its way out of the ear because the skin cells in this part of the body have the unique ability to migrate outwards. Provided the ear is not interfered with, it usually has its own built-in self-cleansing mechanism. Unfortunately, people tend to interfere with their ears and disrupt this mechanism and some ears are naturally narrow and tortuous or the migration process is sluggish and does not cope with the problem adequately. Any other foreign body in the ear canal would also block incoming sound, and the range of objects which get inserted into ear canals by adults as well as children is quite astonishing.

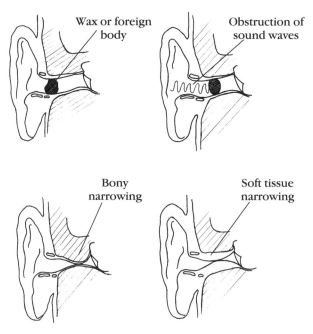

**Figure 8.2:** Causes of obstruction of the ear canal. Obstruction due to wax, foreign bodies or narrowing of the ear canal by bone, soft tissue or both will prevent sound waves reaching the tympanic membrane.

Swelling of the skin of the ear canal due to infection, bruising, allergy or various skin diseases is also not uncommon and when severe enough to close off the canal will cause a significant hearing impairment. The bone of the deeper part of the ear canal may occasionally start to grow again and narrow the lumen. This condition is known as meatal exostosis and has become more common in recent years due to the increasing popularity of watersports, in particular surfing and sailboarding. It seems that the combination of wind and water causes considerable cooling of the ear canal, which stimulates the bone to grow and eventually obstruct the passage of sound waves. There are also a number of cysts, masses and tumours, both benign and malignant, which can affect the ear canal. They are mostly quite rare and the malignant variety is especially uncommon.

Narrowing or stenosis of the ear canal can follow repeated infection or inflammation, accidental or surgical trauma, or may be congenital and present from birth. The narrowing may be of the soft tissue part of the canal or of its bony component or of both. On very rare occasions the congenital variety can be so severe that no ear canal is present at all. This variety is not infrequently found with abnormalities of the external ear or pinna.

## The middle-ear space

The tympanic membrane (Figure 8.3) collects the airborne sound waves and transmits them to the ossicles or middle-ear bones for conduction across the middle ear. Any malfunction of this mechanism results in a conductive hearing impairment. Defects in the membrane vary greatly, from pinholes to total loss. In most cases, perforations (Figure 8.4) result from infection, but they can also be caused by trauma. Fortunately, however, most traumatic perforations heal spontaneously, provided there

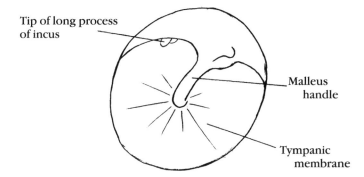

**Figure 8.3:** Normal right tympanic membrane.

is no associated infection, as this interferes with the healing process and is likely to result in a permanent defect.

Trauma can be caused by a slap or blast injury or by direct contact with the tympanic membrane from a foreign body being inserted down the ear canal. It is not infrequently self-induced while trying to clean the ear with objects such as cotton buds, hair grips or similar dangerous implements. The effects of such activity can be compounded if part of the offending object breaks away and is left behind. In general, the larger the perforation the greater the hearing loss, but results vary greatly and sometimes surprisingly good hearing is found in patients with substantial defects.

Scarring of the tympanic membrane follows infection or trauma when the ear has attempted to repair itself. This can take the form of a thickening or tympanosclerosis at one extreme, or thinning or atrophy at the

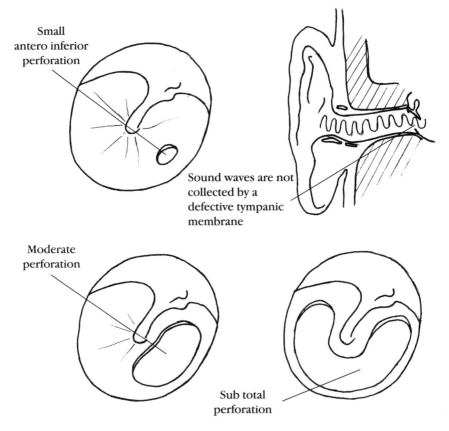

**Figure 8.4:** Perforation in a right tympanic membrane. Perforations of various sizes can occur and may affect different areas of the membrane. The damaged tympanic membrane does not collect sound waves efficiently.

other end of the scale. As with perforations, the effect of these changes on the hearing can be very variable and surprisingly large areas of sclerosis or thickening can be associated with excellent hearing, provided that the edges of the membrane have not become fixed, as this will allow sufficient vibration to take place.

The middle-ear space medial to the tympanic membrane (Figure 8.5) normally contains air at approximately the same pressure as the atmosphere and this allows the membrane to vibrate efficiently when exposed to sound, but even a slight change of middle-ear pressure can have a significant effect on hearing. The middle ear is therefore provided with a mechanism to maintain normal ear pressure. First, the lining of the middle ear and its connecting air cell system in the mastoid acts like the alveolar spaces in the lungs. Gases from the blood supply to this lining diffuse into the middle-ear space to provide an atmosphere similar in composition to the gases in venous blood. In addition, the middle ear is connected to the back of the nose via the eustachian tube, which enters the anterior part of the middle ear. Air can pass up this tube into the ear and fluids in the ear can drain out into the back of the nose through the same route. Many people are able to change the pressure in their middle ears by blowing their nose with their mouth closed: a useful trick when diving or flying to prevent the pain caused by changes in water or air pressure. These changes of pressure can affect hearing, as can anything that replaces the gas in the middle ear.

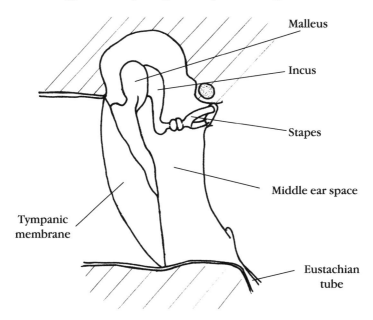

**Figure 8.5:** Normal middle ear.

Children frequently go through a phase when fluid collects in the middle ear: so-called 'glue ear' (Figure 8.6). This can cause a significant hearing loss at an important time in the child's development and, if it persists for a long time, can affect the acquisition of speech and language and so the ability to read and write. Fortunately the vast majority of children with this problem grow out of it spontaneously and require no treatment. Blood in the middle ear following trauma or surgery causes a similar loss but usually of short duration and, in a similar way, swelling of the lining of the ear due to infection or allergy can contribute to hearing impairment in these conditions. Very rarely a tumour may affect the post-nasal space area and cause problems with the eustachian tube and so present as a glue ear in an adult.

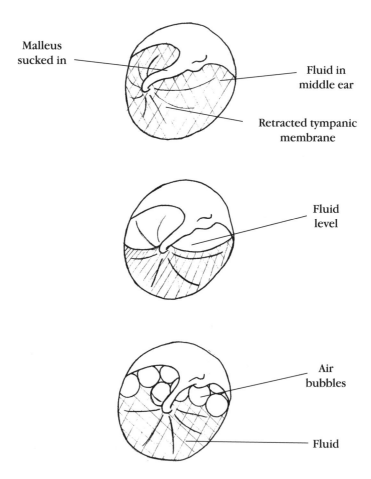

**Figure 8.6:** Glue ear or secretory otitis media.

# The ossicles

The three ossicles in the middle ear are a crucial component of the transfer mechanism which changes the airborne sound waves into waves in fluid. Any failure in the mechanism results in a conductive loss. The bones can be damaged by infection or trauma so that the continuity of the chain is lost (Figure 8.7). The incus in the middle of the chain is the most commonly damaged, probably because being furthest away from other structures, it has a vulnerable blood supply. Chronic ear disease due to infection or skin cyst formation (cholesteatoma) frequently causes erosion of the long process of the incus, which thus loses contact with the stapes.

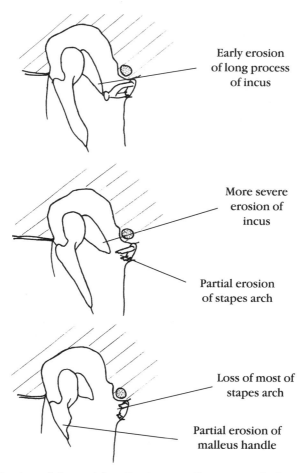

Early erosion of long process of incus

More severe erosion of incus

Partial erosion of stapes arch

Loss of most of stapes arch

Partial erosion of malleus handle

**Figure 8.7:** Erosion of the ossicles. Erosion usually starts with the tip of the long process of the incus and can progress, with time, to loss of a large proportion of the chain.

The stapes itself is the second most likely of the three bones to be damaged. The arch may be lost completely, but the footplate, which closes the oval window, nearly always survives. Erosion of the malleus is unusual, presumably because it derives a good blood supply from the tympanic membrane and its connections in the attic.

The ossicles are also vulnerable to traumatic damage from head injuries, insertion of foreign bodies and surgery. Blows to the head cause acceleration and deceleration of the middle ear-components and, as the incus and malleus have relatively much more massive bodies than their slim processes, considerable movement can take place, resulting in dislocation or subluxation of the joints between the ossicles and even fracture of the bones themselves, particularly of the stapes crura. Foreign bodies pushed down the canal can sometimes reach far enough to fracture or dislocate the ossicles and even drive the stapes into the inner ear, causing damage to the cochlea.

Surgery on the ear must be carried out with great care, because manipulation of the ossicles can result in excessive movement of the joints. Such subluxation can result in impaired function of these tiny joints, which can lead to disappointing hearing results postoperatively.

Congenital abnormalities of the middle ear also occur, often in association with the external ear canal deformities mentioned previously. These range from minor changes to a single ossicle, to major aplasia with fused, deformed ossicular remnants or even total absence of all the ossicles.

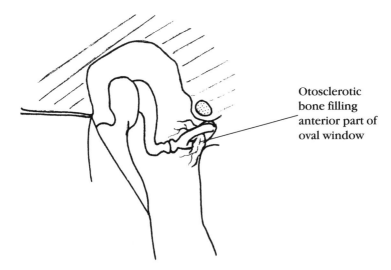

Otosclerotic bone filling anterior part of oval window

**Figure 8.8:** Stapes fixation by otosclerosis. The new bone formation usually encroaches on to the front part of the footplate initially, but on occasions can obliterate the oval window niche.

One of the commonest causes of middle-ear conductive loss occurring in adults is otosclerosis, which affects about 1% of the population. In this condition, spongy new bone grows into the oval window area and interferes with the free movement of the footplate of the stapes (Figure 8.8). It tends to present in early adult life and there is frequently a family history and a tendency for it to be somewhat more common in women than in men. The loss may affect one or both ears and tends to slowly progress until a significant handicap develops, particularly if it is on both sides. Provided the inner ear is not involved, the loss does not usually exceed 60 dB, but where the cochlea is also affected, severe or even profound deafness is possible.

## Non-surgical management of conductive hearing loss

Many causes of conductive hearing loss are amenable to surgical procedures. However, medical or non-surgical intervention does have a place (Figure 8.9). Obstruction of the external auditory meatus may be cleared

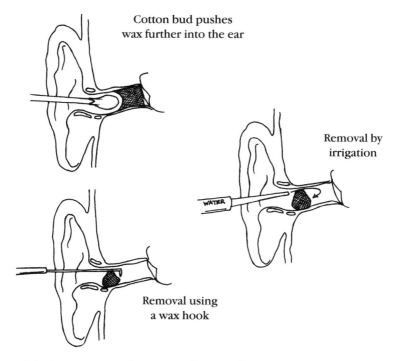

Cotton bud pushes
wax further into the ear

Removal by
irrigation

WATER

Removal using
a wax hook

**Figure 8.9:** Management of ear wax. The use of cotton buds is likely to push wax further into the ear. A wax hook, in the hands of an expert, can be passed beyond the obstruction to pull it out. Gentle irrigation with water at body temperture may be used to flush wax away.

by simple extraction of obstructing items such as foreign bodies or wax. Drops such as almond oil or bicarbonate of soda can encourage wax to be expelled naturally and if this does not occur, these drops will make any syringing that might be appropriate much easier. Infection in the canal responds to ear drops containing steroids with antiseptics or antibiotics, and in severe cases systemic antibiotics may be required. Similarly, infection in the middle ear often requires systemic antibiotics and when infections have gone on to perforate the tympanic membrane, topical treatment with ear drops may also be helpful. However, these drops need to be used with care because they may enter the middle ear through the defect and gain access to the round window membrane, which is the only protection to the delicate structures of the inner ear. Some antibiotics in ear drops may be toxic to the inner ear and may not be appropriate in such cases. Although such treatment may resolve middle-ear infections, damage may already have occurred which will result in some impairment, despite the body's attempts at repair.

Glue ear or secretory otitis media may be treated using decongestants and antibiotics but there is no convincing scientific evidence that this has much effect. Management of nasal allergy, however, has been shown to be more effective. There is evidence that secondary smoking is an aggravating factor and children should not be exposed to tobacco smoke.

Both children and adults with poor middle-ear function may be able to help themselves by autoinflation. This is achieved by holding the nose closed and blowing with the mouth shut to increase pressure in the back of the nose and force air up the eustachian tube. Nasal balloons or Otovents are available commercially to facilitate this manoeuvre and have been found to reduce the need for surgical management of glue ear. ENT surgeons sometimes make use of rubber bulbs attached to nasal nozzles to achieve the same object in adult patients, a technique known as Politzerization.

Most conductive hearing losses will respond well to amplification using hearing aids and, provided the ear canal is patent and there is no discharge, this can be a good form of management with no surgical risk. However, an aid causes obstruction of the meatus and therefore reduces the natural ventilation of the deep canal. This can sometimes destabilize ears that have dry perforations, mastoid cavities or a tendency to otitis externa. Some patients who are not suitable for conventional, in-the-ear hearing aids can be helped by various forms of bone conduction aids, which work by using a vibrating device against the mastoid bone behind the ear. These amplifying devices will be discussed in more detail in Chapters 18 and 20.

# Chapter 9
# Surgical management of conductive deafness

JAMES ROBINSON

## Glue ear

Surgical management of glue ear is the commonest surgical procedure carried out in this country at the present time. The simplest procedure is to carry out a myringotomy or incision in the tympanic membrane to drain the fluid from the middle ear. However, unfortunately this is only a short-term measure as the incision heals very rapidly and the fluid tends to recollect. To prevent the incision from closing so rapidly, a small plastic tube or grommet can be inserted into the incision (Figure 9.1). This allows

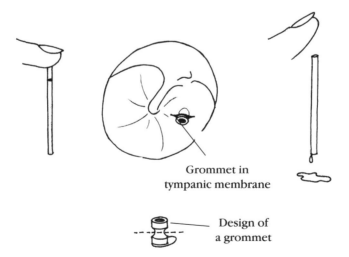

Grommet in
tympanic membrane

Design of
a grommet

**Figure 9.1:** Grommet treatment for glue ear. Inserting the grommet allows air into the middle ear, and in the same way that removing a finger from the end of a water-filled tube lets the water fall out, so the glue is able to escape down the eustachian tube.

air to enter the middle ear so that the fluid, which is the cause of the problem, can escape down the eustachian tube into the post-nasal space. This is a highly effective way of dealing with the problem, but only works as long as the ventilation tube is in situ and patent.

Statistical evidence suggests that the benefit to patients lasts approximately six months. After this time there is a tendency for the tube either to have become blocked or to have extruded. There is also quite a high spontaneous remission rate in this condition. In trials where a grommet is placed in one tympanic membrane and the other side is left untreated, within six months there is little difference in the hearing level between the two ears, partly because the treated ear has begun to deteriorate again and also because the untreated ear is beginning to improve.

The complications of the insertion of grommets include an incidence of discharge of fluid or pus through the ventilation tube of up to 20%. Many of these improve spontaneously, but about 4% of grommets need to be removed to prevent this discharge from persisting. There is a tendency for a tympanic membrane to become somewhat thickened in cases where grommets have been inserted. There is some disagreement as to whether this thickening causes any disadvantage to the patient. It seems likely that, provided it is limited to the tympanic membrane and does not extend to the ossicles within the middle ear, there is little disadvantage. If the grommet falls out, the resulting perforation usually heals spontaneously and quite rapidly, but depending on the type of grommet used, there is an incidence of persisting perforation, which may be as high as 4%. Some ventilation tubes have been designed to remain in position for much longer periods. The original version of this was the Goode T-tube and although this did remain in position for much longer, the incidence of residual perforation in these cases may be as high as 10–15%.

Adenoidectomy has also been considered a useful procedure in the management of glue ear. It is felt that the presence of the obstruction of large adenoids and the associated infection that these adenoids may carry, can have an effect on the ventilation through the eustachian tube where it enters the post-nasal space adjacent to the adenoid tissue. It has been shown that between the ages of four and eight years there is a long-term benefit in 60% of patients who have their adenoids removed in the presence of glue ear. It is important to understand that this is a naturally self-limiting condition, and therefore the choice of any surgical procedure must take this into consideration.

Problems arising from fluid in the middle ear are not limited to children, and may occasionally occur in adults. They are perhaps more common in the older age group. Adults do not have adenoids to be removed, but the use of ventilation tubes can be equally effective; unfortunately adults do not have the advantage that they are likely to grow out of the condition. Longer-term ventilation tubes may therefore be useful provided the increased risk of residual perforation is acceptable. Fluid may sometimes collect in the middle ear in adults following upper respiratory tract infections. A simple myringotomy does not always solve the problem. The use of a grommet seems to be somewhat excessive and recently a surgical laser has been used instead. This provides a small perforation in the tympanic membrane, which takes about one month to heal. This frequently allows enough time for the ear to settle down after the affects of the upper respiratory infection that caused the fluid to collect in the first place.

## Otosclerosis

Most patients with otosclerosis would normally be advised to try a hearing aid initially, as this approach has no surgical complications. However, if the patients feel that a hearing aid does not provide them with the hearing they require and that surgery would be a better option, then it is possible to bypass the fixed stapes using an artificial prosthesis. Access to the oval window area is obtained by lifting the posterior half of the tympanic membrane and entering the middle ear. The arch of the fixed stapes can be removed (Figure 9.2) using conventional manual techniques such as angled hooks and scissors or by using a surgical laser, which carries a very much smaller risk of undue mobilization of the stapes footplate. Having removed the stapes arch or crura, the footplate of the stapes can be fenestrated (Figure 9.2(c)) using a fine pick, by drilling, using the laser or a combination of these. Many surgeons today use a tissue graft of facia or vein to seal the small fenestration into the oval window. A piston of stainless steel or Teflon is then inserted into this fenestration and a loop from the end of the piston is attached to the long process of the incus thus re-establishing a mobile mechanism from the malleus incus assembly to the inner ear.

The results of these operations in experienced hands are excellent, with satisfactory results occurring between 85 and 95% of the time. The degree of success will of course vary, depending on whether the disease is unilateral or bilateral and the severity of the hearing loss that has occurred before surgery is undertaken. As in any operative procedure, there are a number of complications, the most important of which is severe sensory neural hearing impairment. In its severest form, this can result in total loss of hearing in the operated ear; but in the hands of experienced surgeons it

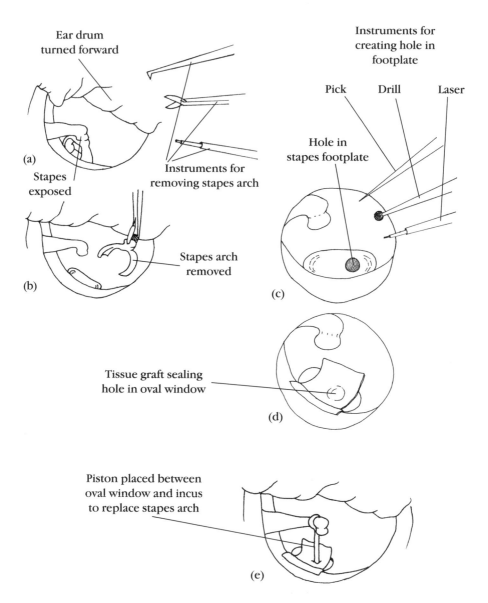

**Figure 9.2:** Surgery for otosclerosis. (a) The tympanic membrane is elevated to expose the stapes. The arch can then be removed. Various instruments can be used for this purpose, including micro-hooks, scissors or a handheld surgical laser. (b) The stapes crura have been divided and are removed with micro-forceps. (c) A small hole is created in the footplate using a micro-pick, diamond-encrusted drill or the surgical laser. (d) The small hole can be closed using a fine tissue graft, such as a piece of vein. (e) A Teflon piston is used to replace the stapes arch by placing it into the hole in the footplate and crimping it on to the incus.

occurs in only approximately 1–2% of cases. The reason for this loss is not understood and it is, therefore, not possible to select out patients who are at greater risk than others. Other complications that may arise are a period of loss of balance following surgery. This usually lasts only a few days, but on rare occasions it can be prolonged. Otosclerosis is, not infrequently, associated with tinnitus. In many cases, the tinnitus improves following surgery, but occasionally it is made worse or may even occur for the first time following an operative procedure.

One of the most frequent complications noted is some disturbance of taste. The reason for this is that the nerve to the tip of the tongue passes through the middle ear and may be stretched when the tympanic membrane is raised to obtain access to the oval window area. This is not a major complication, but nevertheless it is irritating and can last for many months before the symptoms disappear completely.

In a condition in which a non-surgical system of management is not an unreasonable alternative, careful selection of cases is essential and good preoperative advice mandatory. Some surgeons feel that if the disease affects only one ear then surgery should be withheld. However, there is no doubt this operation can provide excellent results and the advantages of having symmetrical hearing are considerable and should not be discounted. There is also considerable difference of opinion as to whether the operation should be carried out on the second ear of a patient who has the disease on both sides. The reason why some surgeons are reluctant to carry out a second operation is because there is a very small risk that a major sensory neural loss could occur on both sides, leaving the patient severely handicapped. If the surgeon intends to consider second-side surgery, it is absolutely essential that the patient understands this risk, that it has been properly discussed and that it is clear to the surgeon that the implications of the situation are fully understood.

## Reconstructive middle-ear surgery

Reconstruction of the hearing mechanism following chronic ear disease varies from the relatively straightforward reconstruction of a perforated tympanic membrane to the very much more difficult problems of dealing with major loss of ossicular components in the middle ear. Repair of the tympanic membrane or myringoplasty (Figure 9.3) is usually carried out using graft material from the patient. This is taken from a muscle, which is located just above and behind the ear. The lining of the muscle or fascia is used as this produces an excellent sheet of connective tissue that has a very low metabolic requirement. In other words, it requires a limited blood supply. If fascia is not appropriate, other connective tissue can be used, such as perichondrium, periosteum, vein or, where a particularly tough graft is required, a thin sheet of cartilage. In the past, tympanic membranes were transplanted from cadavers but unfortunately this has fallen out of favour as a result of the risk of infection from virus transmission of conditions such as HIV and hepatitis.

The remains of the tympanic membrane are elevated and a sheet of fascia is placed underneath the elevated material. The remnants of the eardrum are then replaced on top. In expert hands, this procedure has a take rate of around 95%. Hearing gain, however, may not be quite so satisfactory as a result of the irreversible changes from the disease that caused the perforation in the first place. It is important that selection of appropriate cases is made carefully and that the patient has realistic expectations.

There are a number of chronic ear diseases that can damage the bones of the middle ear – the ossicles – and some of these cases can be managed surgically by ossiculoplasty. The ossicles may be fixed by adhesions of

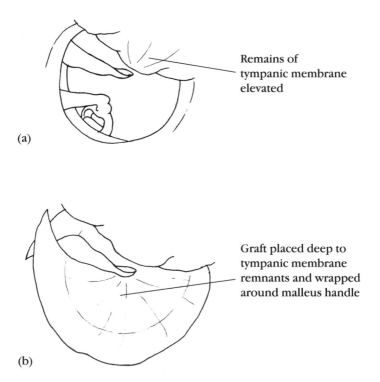

(a)

Remains of tympanic membrane elevated

(b)

Graft placed deep to tympanic membrane remnants and wrapped around malleus handle

**Figure 9.3:** Repair of tympanic membrane perforations. (a) The remains of the tympanic membrane have been elevated forwards. (b) A graft taken from the surface of a muscle behind the ear has been placed deep to the malleus handle and the drum remnants. These remnants will then be folded back on top of the graft.

fibrous tissue or thickening. The bone itself may fix to the adjacent bony structures. In more extreme circumstances, the bone is eroded and the ossicles may be damaged. The damage may be minor, with the loss of a millimetre or so, for example, of the tip of the incus; or more severe, with total disappearance of an ossicle. The techniques used to deal with these problems vary.

Fixation can be managed by very careful manipulation with micro-instruments, but this needs to be done with great care because excessive movement of the ossicles is transmitted to the cochlea and can cause permanent inner-ear damage. More recently, the surgical laser has improved the situation as the tissue is cut by light, which does not cause any movement and therefore considerably reduces the risk of cochlear damage. To prevent the bones from refixing, materials have been inter-posed between the bony components, using either plastic or natural material, such as fat. Where ossicles are damaged or missing they may be repaired or replaced using natural material such as parts of the patient's ossicular chain, pieces of cortical bone or cartilage (Figure 9.4). Alternatively, artificial materials such as plastics, metals or ceramics have been used to construct replacement ossicles. Technically, there appears to be no difference in the results between the homografts (natural materials) and the allografts (manufactured items). The difference in cost, however, is considerable.

In general, the results of ossicular reconstruction are disappointing. This is largely because the damage caused by the chronic ear disease produces a very poor surgical environment. Apart from the damage to the ossicles, the lining of the middle ear is in poor condition, the ventilation is impaired and there is generalized fibrosis within the middle-ear cleft. All of these produce almost insurmountable problems for the surgeon at the present time and, for this reason, a careful preoperative assessment and counselling of the patient are essential to prevent unreasonable expectations.

Much research work is being carried out in all of these areas and the prospects for the future are good. However, at present, it is necessary to be cautious and also to consider the alternatives. A patient with a dry, stable ear can make use of a conventional hearing aid when an ossiculo-plasty has not been effective.

Acute infections of the ear rarely cause damage that requires recon-struction, but the same principles as those applied to chronic ear disease would be effective, and less likely to be complicated by the scarring and fibrosis which is found after chronic disease. Trauma to the ear may result in a tympanic membrane perforation but the vast majority of these heal spontaneously. Where they do not, a myringoplasty as mentioned above is highly effective. Similarly, traumatic damage to the ossicles responds to

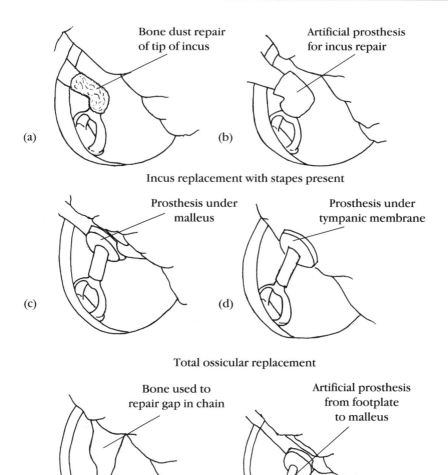

**Figure 9.4:** Techniques for repairing ossicular damage: (a) a small gap between the incus and the stapes has ben closed using a paste made of bone dust from the patient's ear canal, mixed with fibrin gel; (b) a similar defect has been closed using an artificial replacement made from hydroxyl apatite ceramic. Incus replacement with stapes present: (c) an artificial prosthesis has been placed from the stapes head to the under surace of the malleus handle; (d) in this case there is no malleus, so the prosthesis is placed under the tympanic membrane with a small piece of cartilage on top to protect the drum. Total ossicular replacement: (e) part of the patient's malleus has been fitted between the remaining stapes footplate and the under surface of the drum. No cartilage is required as the components of the repair originate from the patient and are therefore completely compatible; (f) an artificial prosthesis has been used between the footplate and malleus handle. A bone-to-bone repair does not require cartilage separation.

ossiculoplasty and this again is somewhat simpler in these situations as there is less chronic change in the middle ear: in other words the surgical environment is a little more friendly.

## Meatal stenosis

Narrowing of the external auditory meatus can be acquired or congenital. In acquired cases, it is due to infection, trauma or bony growth such as exostoses. The narrowing may be due to bone or to soft tissue or to both and can be handled by meatoplasty. This usually involves widening the bony component of the ear canal and reducing any redundant soft tissue, and trying to use the existing skin to recover the bony canal. On occasions it is necessary to use skin grafts to complete the covering of the exposed bone. More recently, the surgical laser has been found to be particularly effective in dealing with some cases of stenosis. The surgical problem is the tendency of the stenosis to reform; all tubular structures within the body if they are transected tend to stenose and attempts at surgical correction are frequently unsuccessful. In congenital stenosis, there may also be abnormalities of the middle-ear structures.

In the past, there has been considerable interest in attempting to reconstruct congenitally abnormal middle ears. However, more recently with the improvement in bone conduction hearing aids and, in particular, the development of the bone-anchored hearing aid, there is much less interest in surgical reconstruction because the hearing aid approach carries no surgical risk to the cochlea.

# Chapter 10
# Acquired sensorineural hearing loss

MARTIN J BURTON

Sensorineural deafness occurs when there is damage to the hearing mechanism within the cochlea or abnormal function of the cochlear nerve (Chapter 3). A small proportion of patients are born with such problems (Chapter 11) but in the vast majority sensorineural deafness is acquired in adult life.

## The extent of the problem

The prevalence of deafness has been considered earlier (Chapter 2). To reiterate, deafness is of a sensorineural rather than conductive type in the vast majority of patients with acquired deafness.

## 'Normal' deafness with ageing (presbyacusis)

Some cells in the body can be replaced when they die or if they degenerate due to any process, be it disease or simply the passage of time. The highly differentiated cells of the auditory system and the neural pathways of hearing do not belong to this group – from the moment of birth they age and die. The 'durability' of the auditory system depends on both genetic factors and the environmental factors to which the system is exposed.

With advancing age it is normal for hearing to deteriorate and this is termed 'presbyacusis'. It is not a disease, rather it is a term which acknowledges the association between ageing and hearing loss. In some elderly people with bilateral, symmetrical sensorineural hearing loss there will be a history of exposure to one of those factors discussed in the remainder of this chapter, which are known to produce such changes. In others, there will be a family history of progressive hearing loss. The majority will have neither and in the absence of any specific physical findings will be said to have presbyacusis.

Presbyacusis presents in a wide variety of ways. The disability caused by the reduction in hearing thresholds varies considerably. Two patients with the same thresholds measured with pure-tone audiometry may have quite different problems in terms of their abilities to communicate, to hear in the presence of background noise, use the telephone, etc. This may in part relate to differences in their ability to discriminate speech – something that can be measured with speech audiometry. But also, some patients develop better listening strategies than others. Those who have lost their hearing more slowly and gradually may compensate better than those who do so suddenly.

Anxiety is sometimes expressed about the lower age limit for making the 'diagnosis' of presbyacusis. If one considers it as a term that can be applied to 'idiopathic' (otherwise unexplained) bilateral, symmetrical sensorineural hearing loss in 'elderly' patients it becomes clear that this is just a question of semantics. It would probably be easier to drop the term altogether. The reason the question is posed is because there is a (mistaken) belief that below a certain age comprehensive investigation for other causes is warranted, and above that age it is not. While a pragmatic approach must be taken when making decisions about the usefulness, merits and costs of diagnostic tests, chronological age is only one of several factors to be considered.

Several studies have looked, post-mortem, at the inner ears of elderly patients with 'presbyacusis'. The pathological findings have been correlated with the clinical features of the patients' deafness. As a result, several different 'types' of presbyacusis have been described. This classification is of very limited clinical usefulness and some of the pathological changes described are also seen in patients with hearing loss due to other causes. What follows is a description of these types; some of the explanations offered are still conjectural.

In *strial presbyacusis* degeneration of the stria vascularis results in degradation in the quality of endolymph. All parts of the cochlea are thus affected and a 'flat' audiometric pattern is associated with excellent speech discrimination. The loss is of insidious onset, between 40 and 70 years of age, and progresses slowly.

*Sensory presbyacusis* is associated with loss of hair cells in the basal (high-frequency) region of the cochlea. The audiogram slopes steeply downwards in the high frequencies, usually those above the speech frequencies. Speech discrimination is preserved for this reason.

Progressive loss of neurones within the cochlea occurs at a rate of about 2000 per decade, from an initial 35 000 at birth. Neuronal degeneration usually follows damage to the sensory hair cells of the organ of Corti. In *neural presbyacusis*, neuronal loss occurs in a fashion disproportionate to the loss of sensory hair cells. The typical audiogram shows a downward-sloping, high-frequency loss but is flatter than that seen in sensory presbyacusis. Speech discrimination is impaired to a greater degree than would be expected from the pure-tone thresholds.

The term *cochlear conductive presbyacusis* has been applied to those patients with no histological evidence of cochlear disease but a gradually descending audiogram. This leaves a group which has been termed *indeterminate presbyacusis*. The late Professor Harold Schuknecht in his seminal text on ear pathology suggests that 25% of cases of presbyacusis fall into this category (Schuknecht 1993).

From a practical point of view, these descriptions serve to highlight the variety of patterns of auditory dysfunction that can be measured using standard audiometric tests in patients – usually the elderly but not necessarily so – in whom no other cause can be found for their sensorineural deafness.

Sometimes patients may ask if their hearing is 'normal' for their age. It is tempting to compare their thresholds with average values for people of different ages produced from population-based studies. In essence, this is what most practitioners do on the basis of their personal experience when looking at an audiogram. It must be borne in mind that there may be people included in these population studies who do have an identifiable cause of hearing loss. Consequently, a proper history should be elicited from each individual patient so that due consideration can be given to the need for further investigations.

## Deafness due to other causes

Important clues as to the cause of sensorineural deafness are obtained from the history of the deafness itself and from information about other symptoms of ear disease. Before discussing in detail the causes of sensorineural deafness it is prudent to consider a number of the important features of the history.

The onset of sensorineural deafness may be gradual or sudden. Both ears may be affected equally or one more than the other. Both these factors may provide clues as to the nature of the underlying disorder.

Most sensorineural deafness occurs gradually and equally in both ears. This reflects the fact that the underlying cause (such as the ageing process, industrial noise or an ototoxic drug) is: (a) not directed specifically at one ear alone and potentially affects both ears; and (b) exerts its influence over an extended period of time. Conversely, it is more likely that patients who have a unilateral problem have some localized disease process. For example, most patients who develop a benign tumour affecting the cochlear nerve do so on one side only. Some processes, such as trauma, may be directed at one ear only (surgery, for example) or at both (a major head injury).

Trauma is also a good example of a process likely to result in sensorineural deafness of sudden or rapid onset. Fluctuating sensorineural deafness is unusual but characteristic of Ménière's disease.

In addition to deafness, the other cardinal symptoms of ear disease are tinnitus, discharge (otorrhea), pain (otalgia), vertigo and facial weakness. The presence or absence of these provide further clues as to the specific diagnosis. While a full discussion of these symptoms is beyond the scope of this chapter, brief mention must be made of the term 'vertigo'. This should be used to describe a sense of movement of the surroundings (usually but not always a spinning sensation) when the patient and surroundings are in fact stationary. It is not the same as a feeling of faintness, light-headedness or 'swimminess', nor a sensation of wanting to veer or fall to one side. True rotational vertigo is often a sign of inner ear dysfunction; the other sensations rarely are.

The various causes of sensorineural deafness will be considered on the basis of the characteristic history as this is how the diagnosis is usually reached (Table 10.1). The headings serve as a broad outline only. In most cases it is impossible to be categorical and it would be wrong to say, for example, that vertigo does not occur in otosclerosis.

**Table 10.1:** Causes of acquired sensorineural deafness

| | |
|---|---|
| Progressive deafness with vertigo | Ménière's disease |
| | Syphilis |
| Progressive deafness without vertigo | Ototoxic drugs |
| | Vestibular schwannoma |
| |   Neurofibromatosis |
| | Disorders of bone |
| |   Otosclerosis |
| |   Osteogenesis imperfecta |
| |   Paget's disease |
| | Chronic otitis media |
| | Noise |
| | 'Presbyacusis' |
| Sudden deafness with trauma | Ear surgery |
| | Head injury |
| | Barotrauma |
| | Blast injury |
| | Perilymph fistula |
| Sudden deafness without trauma | Infections |
| | Idiopathic |
| | Immunological |

# Progressive deafness with vertigo

## Ménière's syndrome, Ménière's disease and endolymphatic hydrops

In 1861, Prosper Ménière published details of the disorder which bears his name. He recognized that a condition characterized by episodic vertigo, previously thought to arise from 'cerebral congestion', had its origin in the inner ear.

Although patients with the classical features of Ménière's disorder are readily identifiable, considerable problems have arisen surrounding the diagnosis of some patients and the terminology used to describe the disorder. Diagnosis is not straightforward as no 'gold standard' diagnostic test exists. As a result whenever anything is published purporting to deal with patients with Ménière's, one should be cautious about interpreting the results unless the criteria for making the diagnosis are explicit and are those which the reader accepts as reasonable. In 1995, the Committee on Hearing and Equilibrium of the American Academy of Otolaryngology – Head and Neck Surgery (AAOHNS) produced guidelines for the diagnosis of Ménière's and evaluation of therapy; although not universally accepted they provide a useful starting point for improving diagnostic rigour. They propose that the only 'certain' cases of Ménière's are those in which a clinical diagnosis of 'definite' disease (as defined – see below) is accompanied by histopathological (post-mortem) confirmation.

*Ménière's syndrome* consists of the following clinical features:

- recurrent episodes of spontaneous vertigo
- fluctuating hearing loss
- tinnitus
- a feeling of fullness in the ear.

*Ménière's disease* is the term used to describe idiopathic cases of *Ménière's syndrome*. Other causes of the syndrome are:

- post-traumatic
- post-infectious
- syphilitic
- classic Cogan's syndrome
- atypical Cogan's syndrome.

Some patients with Ménière's syndrome have specific histopathological findings in their inner ear: these are termed 'endolymphatic hydrops'. This refers to an apparent excess of endolymph in the scala media, with 'ballooning' of Reissner's membrane into the scala vestibuli. There has been a tendency to use the term endolymphatic hydrops interchangeably with Ménière's disease or syndrome as if there is an inevitable association between the two. This is a mistake for several reasons. Endolymphatic hydrops is found in a wide range of disorders, to the extent that it is seen in about 1 in 20 of all human temporal bones with otological pathology. The proportion of patients with Ménière's syndrome who have the histological changes of endolymphatic hydrops is unknown. Conversely, however, only about a third of patients with endolymphatic hydrops on histological examination are known to have had episodic vertigo in life.

The inference that some factor or factors produce endolymphatic hydrops, which in turn produce Ménière's syndrome, and that the syndrome can only occur by this mechanism, may be fallacious. Notwithstanding, the theory that hydrops is responsible for Ménière's syndrome is the dominant one in current thinking. The cochlear duct and saccule are initially affected. An increase in endolymphatic pressure is postulated as the cause for 'ballooning' of Reissner's membrane into the scala vestibuli. The saccular wall balloons outwards to contact the opposite wall of the vestibule, including, eventually, the footplate. Distension of the vestibular aqueduct or endolymphatic sac has not been reported. Dilations or out-pouchings of the membranous labyrinth are seen and ruptures in the membranes produce fistulae between the endolymphatic and perilymphatic spaces. With advanced disease, sensory cells (hair cells) are lost.

The increased pressure in the endolymph is said to be responsible for the feeling of fullness in the ear, distortion of hearing and loudness recruitment, and the dysequilibrium. The ruptures are said to be responsible for the acute episodes of vertigo. Time will tell if these theories are true. Endolymphatic hydrops may be an epi-phenomenon simply indicating inner ear dysfunction. It is likely that Ménière's syndrome is multifactorial in origin and hereditary elements may combine with a wide variety of external stimuli.

The natural history and clinical features of Ménière's disease are well documented but the reader should bear in mind the caveat above about diagnostic 'accuracy'. The incidence varies from country to country being reported as 150 per 100 000/year in the UK and 15 to 40 per 100 000/year in the USA. The symptoms usually start in middle age, the mean age being between 40 and 45 years. Men and women are probably affected equally, although women present slightly more often. There is a family history in about one patient in 20. Although there have been few formal studies of psycho-social factors it is commoner in the higher social classes and rare in developing countries. Patients are more commonly 'intelligent, introspective and somewhat obsessive'. Stress undoubtedly precipitates disease activity.

The 'classic' Ménière's attack consists of a feeling of fullness in the ear accompanied by increasing tinnitus, reduced hearing and the sudden onset of rotatory vertigo. This lasts from 20 minutes to several hours and may be accompanied by autonomic symptoms such as nausea, vomiting, sweating, etc. The patient does not lose consciousness. The attack can come on at any time even when asleep. After the acute vertigo has stopped the patients continue to feel unwell and their balance is poor, often for the rest of the day.

Between attacks it is not uncommon for patients to experience fullness in the ear, tinnitus or positional vertigo, or simply instability with quick movements. Alternatively they may be completely asymptomatic. There is great variability in the pattern of the disease. Some have only one or two attacks per year and their hearing is relatively stable. Others have periods of frequent attacks for weeks or months, then periods of remission. Some are totally incapacitated by their disease, becoming housebound and unable to work.

The hearing loss of Ménière's begins with sound appearing distorted and having a 'tinny' quality. The audiogram shows a low tone loss. Loudness recruitment is present so the patient may develop hyperacusis and be intolerant of loud noises. When the hearing drops during an attack, it will usually recover within a few hours in the early stages of the disease.

The AAOHNS criteria allow a diagnosis of 'definite' Ménière's disease to be made when two or more episodes of vertigo lasting more than 20 minutes are associated with audiometrically documented hearing loss and tinnitus or fullness in the affected ear. 'Probable' Ménière's disease requires all these features but only one attack of vertigo.

Diagnostic difficulties may occur when the full set of symptoms does not develop at the same time. The syndrome may begin with hearing loss, vertigo or tinnitus alone although the latter two presentations are unusual.

It will be clear from the above that the history is the most important factor in making the diagnosis of Ménière's disease. However, several diagnostic tests have been proposed and promoted by their enthusiasts. Two findings on ECochG (see Chapter 6) are said to be characteristic of Ménière's. These are an enhanced summating potential (SP) and an increased SP/AP (action potential) ratio. The poor test/re-test reliability, sensitivity and specificity of this test, even in cases where the diagnosis is in no doubt, make its usefulness questionable. It is of dubious value in establishing or refuting the diagnosis in patients with equivocal histories. The glycerol dehydration test evaluates changes in hearing thresholds in response to a dehydrating agent (glycerol). Some authors feel it may be useful in the diagnosis of Ménière's.

The aim of the medical treatment of Ménière's disease is to (a) reduce the number and severity of attacks and (b) limit the symptoms during an individual attack. To achieve the first aim the patient is encouraged to follow a low-salt diet, as this is believed to reduce inner-ear pressure. Betahistine hydrochloride (Serc) is prescribed. A mild diuretic can also be added. The acute attacks may be aborted by the use of a vestibular sedative such as prochlorperazine; sublabial versions or suppositories are available to avoid the problems of swallowing while feeling nauseous. In some patients, oral steroids may have a role.

If this medical regimen fails to control the patient's symptoms, more invasive treatment may be considered. It must be accepted that Ménière's disease is a disorder with a high natural resolution rate and that several placebo-controlled studies have shown some placebos to be remarkably effective in controlling symptoms. It has even been suggested that simply contemplating surgery may lead to a clinical improvement.

There are two alternative goals of surgery for Ménière's disease. Either it may aim to preserve hearing while modulating or abolishing vestibular function, or it may be destructive, destroying both hearing and balance in the affected ear. One of the least invasive surgical procedures is endolymphatic sac decompression. This is undertaken in the belief that raised endolymphatic pressure is responsible for the symptoms and that endolymphatic pressure is reduced as a result of the procedure. A cortical mastoidectomy is performed and the sac identified within the posterior fossa dura on the posterior surface of the temporal bone. It is incised and a drain may be inserted. The procedure does not affect hearing. If an initial improvement is not maintained the procedure can be revised.

Vestibular nerve section is a more invasive procedure. The nerve can be sectioned (preserving the cochlear nerve and hence the hearing) to prevent the vertiginous symptoms of Ménière's. This can be performed via a retro-labyrinthine route (opening into the posterior part of the cranial cavity) or via the middle cranial fossa in a manner similar to that described below for vestibular schwannoma removal. There is a risk of hearing loss and facial palsy with this procedure and if all the fibres of the nerve are not divided the results may not be wholly satisfactory.

If hearing is poor and unserviceable, a formal labyrinthectomy may be performed in which the inner ear is destroyed. This can be undertaken via the middle ear, with opening of the oval and round windows and disruption of the membranous labyrinth. Alternatively, via a mastoidectomy approach, the bony labyrinth can be removed entirely. All hearing is lost as a result of either of these procedures. Recently there has been an increase in popularity of medical labyrinthectomy with hearing preservation. The tendency for some ototoxic antibiotics to be more vestibulo-toxic than cochleo-toxic (see below) has led to the use of intratympanic gentamicin to perform a medical labyrinthectomy. This procedure has several advantages, including few side effects and the avoidance of any risks associated with major ear surgery. A grommet is inserted through the tympanic membrane to allow repeated injections of gentamicin into the middle ear. Various timing and dosage regimens have been proposed, including daily or weekly injections. It is important to monitor hearing on a regular basis and not to continue the series of injections if hearing thresholds fall. This technique of chemical labyrinthectomy has been shown to be both effective and safe if the appropriate precautions are followed.

### Syphilis

Syphilis is an infectious disease caused by the spirochaete *Treponema pallidum*. For many years this sexually transmitted disease was in decline; its incidence has increased again in recent years. It is an extremely rare cause of hearing loss, but cases do occur. If one considers the diagnosis in patients with unexplained deafness or vertigo, and performs the appropriate blood tests, one will occasionally be surprised at a positive result.

Early syphilis can present with a treponemal labyrinthitis. In these circumstances, deafness may be sudden and bilateral and accompanied by imbalance. Hearing loss may persist as the acute infection resolves spontaneously. Treatment is with penicillin. Late syphilis occurs up to 40 years after the primary infection.

Congenital syphilis often presents with a fluctuating, bilateral deafness with tinnitus and vertigo symptoms very similar to Ménière's disease. If this condition is not treated appropriately, the hearing loss progresses to become total or near total. The use of oral steroids, in addition to any appropriate anti-treponemal medication, will result in a reduction in the hearing loss in a proportion of patients.

## Progressive deafness without vertigo

### Ototoxic drugs

Drugs that are toxic to the ear ('oto-') and impair auditory and vestibular function, affecting hearing and balance either temporarily or permanently, are 'ototoxic'. The commonest groups of compounds are shown in Table 10.2.

The aminoglycoside group contains some very potent and useful antibiotics, albeit ones which are well known for their potentially toxic side effects. Some, such as streptomycin, dihydrostreptomycin and neomycin, are predominantly toxic to the cochlea rather than to the

**Table 10.2:** Drugs affecting auditory and/or vestibular function

| | |
|---|---|
| Commonly | Aminoglycoside antibiotics |
| | Quinine and related compounds |
| | Salicylates |
| | Loop diuretics |
| Occasionally | Erythromycin |
| | Cisplatin |
| | Nitrogen mustard |
| | Practalol |
| | Ampicillin |
| | Tetanus antitoxin |
| | Naproxen |
| | Potassium bromate |

vestibular system. In addition to the inherent toxicity of each individual aminoglycoside, other risk factors for toxicity may include:

- concomitant exposure to other ototoxic drugs
- noise exposure
- duration of therapy
- total dose, plasma level and level in the perilymph
- age
- sex
- liver or renal dysfunction
- bacteraemia
- dehydration
- hyperthermia.

The drugs damage the inner row of outer hair cells of the cochlea. Electrochemical changes in the cochlea have also been found. Minor disturbances may be responsible for the reversible changes sometimes seen clinically.

To minimize the risk of developing ototoxicity, great efforts are made to keep the plasma levels of the most frequently used aminoglycoside antibiotics within a 'safe' range. The fact that the drugs continue to be used at all reflects their usefulness in certain clinical situations when, for example, their potential life-saving properties have to be weighed carefully against the risk of side effects. Gentamicin is excreted via the kidneys and may produce renal damage as well as ototoxicity. In all patients, but especially in those with compromised renal function, serum levels must be carefully monitored and the doses administered are adjusted in the light of 'peak' and 'trough' serum levels. Prospective studies have demonstrated some degree of hearing loss in 7–15% of patients receiving 'safe' doses of gentamicin and tobramycin. The hearing loss may progress after the treatment has been discontinued. The loss is usually in the high frequencies and may be unilateral or bilateral. In about half the patients, hearing recovers. Despite these observations, gentamicin is usually regarded as being more toxic to the vestibular system than the cochlea.

Much attention has been focused on the possibility of hearing loss resulting from the use of ear drops which contain aminoglycoside antibiotics. There should be no problem in patients with an intact eardrum as the drops will not reach the inner ear. The situation is different if there is a hole in the drum and drops enter the middle ear. In these circumstances, the drops may reach the round window niche where the only barrier between them and the inner ear is the round window membrane itself. In theory at least, the aminoglycoside could diffuse through the membrane, enter the inner ear and have a toxic effect.

The evidence that this occurs in practice is extremely limited, especially when one considers the vast number of patients worldwide who take potentially ototoxic ear drops of this type in this manner. In the presence of active middle-ear infection or inflammation, when the mucosa is swollen and oedematous, the medication may have difficulty diffusing through the round window membrane. In any event, such patients run a risk of developing inner-ear dysfunction as a result of this infective process and so treating this with aminoglycoside may be the lesser of two evils. However, the question remains, is it safe to give aminoglycoside-containing ear drops in the presence of a perforation with little or no middle-ear inflammation? As always, the treatment should be titrated against outcome and if the infection settles quickly, treatment can be discontinued. Being pragmatic, it may not be possible to see the patient sufficiently frequently to assess improvement. It would seem prudent in these circumstances to limit treatment to, say, 5 days or less. Before using aminoglycoside drops the necessity for the combination of steroid and antibiotic should be reviewed: is the antibiotic component necessary? Is there a bacterial infection present? In some situations, drops containing steroid alone may be equally appropriate. When infection is present, the infecting organism is often *Pseudomonas* and in the future a topical form of ciprofloxacin may become available for use in the ear.

The therapeutic use of the vestibulotoxic effect of gentamicin in patients with Ménière's disease has been mentioned above.

Quinine and related compounds are used to treat malaria and night cramps. Toxic doses may produce a syndrome known as cinchonism. This includes deafness, tinnitus, vertigo, headache, nausea and visual disturbance. The auditory disturbances are usually temporary but may be permanent.

The salicylate group includes acetylsalicylic acid – aspirin. In high doses, it can produce deafness, tinnitus and occasionally vertigo. These changes are reversible.

Frusemide and ethacrynic acid are 'loop diuretics' used to increase fluid excretion from the body. They may produce permanent or temporary hearing loss, the latter being more common. Patients most at risk are those with impaired renal function and premature infants.

Reversible hearing loss, tinnitus and vertigo has been described with large doses of the macrolide antibiotic erythromycin. Several anti-neoplastic agents are ototoxic. Cisplatin has been used to treat a variety of malignancies. It produces an irreversible, high-frequency hearing loss related to the dose of drug administered. Tinnitus may be a warning sign of impending hearing loss.

**Vestibular schwannoma – 'acoustic neuroma'**

Tumours of the ear and temporal bone are not common. They are extremely important, however, for several reasons, not least because prompt diagnosis and treatment are likely to lead to the most favourable outcome for the patient. For many years the commonest tumour of the temporal bone, and hence the commonest tumour diagnosed by otologists, was known as an 'acoustic neuroma'. This name is in fact a misnomer; the tumour in question arises not from the acoustic (cochlear) nerve but from the Schwann cells covering the superior or inferior vestibular nerves. The preferred name is vestibular schwannoma.

Vestibular schwannomas account for between 6 and 10% of all intracranial tumours and 80–90% of all tumours in the cerebellopontine angle – the angle between the cerebellum and the pons. They occur in approximately two people per 100 000 population per year. The tumours arise in the internal auditory canal at the point where the vestibular nerve covering changes from glial cells to Schwann cells. They are slow-growing, benign tumours and do not infiltrate local tissues or metastasize (spread to other organs of the body). However, as they grow they compress adjacent tissues and produce their clinical effects in this way. As is the case with other intracranial benign tumours, these pressure effects may be extremely serious because of the inability of the bony cranial cavity to expand. While they lie within the internal auditory canal the tumours only affect the vestibular and cochlear nerves (the facial nerve is extremely resistant to pressure). When the tumour starts to grow out of the internal canal it pushes medially, superiorly and inferiorly. With time it presses on the brainstem, produces a rise in intracranial pressure and death may ensue.

The reason why patients develop vestibular schwannomas is unknown in most cases. Men and women are affected equally and the mean age at diagnosis is about 50. The advent of an accurate and efficient means of diagnosing these tumours (the MRI scan, discussed below) may be responsible for an apparent increase in the 'incidence' of tumours noted in recent years. It is probable that a large number of tumours are asymptomatic and are still 'missed', remaining undiagnosed during the patient's lifetime. In the past, histopathological studies of temporal bones have shown tumours to be present in a much larger proportion of such bones than expected from the numbers of tumours diagnosed in the general population. There may be several reasons, but it has been suggested, not unreasonably, that many stop growing or shrink without producing symptoms.

The most common clinical presentation of a patient with a vestibular schwannoma is progressive unilateral sensorineural deafness, due to slowly increasing compression on the cochlear nerve. However, the hearing loss may be sudden in 15–25% of cases. Other features include unilateral or asymmetric tinnitus (occasionally the only symptom) or balance disturbance. The latter is often not a prominent feature. The slow growth of the tumour results in a gradual, progressive loss of vestibular function. In most patients, neural plasticity allows the process of central compensation to occur; the abnormal input of vestibular signals is compensated for and the patient is unaware of the deteriorating peripheral vestibular function. The only sign may be a sense of imbalance when the balance system is stressed, for example when moving and turning quickly. If the tumour becomes large, more sinister symptoms can develop: cerebellar symptoms of motor incoordination, pain or paraesthesia in the face due to involvement of the trigeminal (Vth cranial) nerve, headaches, diplopia and vomiting due to raised intracranial pressure.

The audiogram classically shows asymmetrical sensorineural hearing loss worse in the higher frequencies. Usually this is a difference of at least 15 dB between thresholds at 1, 2 and 4 kHz; sometimes the difference is much smaller. Speech discrimination is reduced to a greater degree than would be expected from the audiogram. Occasionally the audiogram appears normal.

The 'gold standard' diagnostic test is an MRI scan, with appropriate contrast injection, unless the full length of the audiovestibular nerves can be clearly visualized without contrast in a scanner with appropriately high resolution. The test is non-invasive and free of the risks of exposure to X-rays. CT scanning may detect large tumours and those arising in the internal canal which have widened the latter. However, with CT, small intracanalicular tumours will be missed.

In the past, a range of audiovestibular tests have been used as a screening tool to select those patients in whom MRI scanning might be most appropriate. These include brainstem-evoked response audiometry and caloric testing. There is always a significant false-positive and false-negative rate with these tests and, if at all possible, MRI scanning is preferable. The high cost of such an investigation is often cited as a reason for being selective in its use. However, it has been clearly shown that MRI can be used as a screening tool at an overall cost that is less than that incurred by using the various screening protocols first and only scanning selectively. A protocol is required in which the MRI department allocates one entire session or day for scanning these patients at regular intervals, with the machine configured specifically for scans of the posterior fossa. The resulting cost per patient is very low. Implementing such a protocol may mean that some patients have to wait some weeks for a scan, but given the 'screening' nature of the test and the slow-growing nature of the tumours this is acceptable. Clearly, if the suspicion of a tumour being present is extremely high, an urgent scan can be arranged.

The management of a patient with a vestibular schwannoma depends on several factors, most importantly the size of the tumour and the patient's general medical condition. In patients whose medical condition and/or age make the risks of surgery greater than usual, it may be appropriate to monitor the growth of the tumour with regular scans and defer treatment, potentially indefinitely. The factors which influence the growth rate of tumours are not well understood. The 'average' tumour (if such a thing exists) grows at a rate of 0.1–0.2 cm diameter per year, but 10–15% of tumours grow at more than 1 cm per year. In contrast, growth may be self-limiting in some patients and a tumour may even shrink. The arguments for operating on these tumours once they have been diagnosed are: first, that the rate of growth can be unpredictable; second, that the risk of surgical complications increases as the tumour grows; and third, that as the patient becomes older they may be less able to withstand major surgery.

Radiotherapy treatment with the 'gamma knife' is another non-surgical option. The merits or otherwise of this treatment modality are still being debated.

Surgical treatment aims to remove the tumour and prevent the risks associated with continued tumour growth. These tumours are generally on the vestibular nerve and deafness is caused by compression of the adjacent cochlear nerve, so if the patient still has serviceable hearing, a secondary aim of surgery may be preservation of this, by leaving the cochlear nerve intact. Similarly, whenever possible the function of the facial nerve, which also lies in the internal auditory meatus, should be preserved. The proximity of the nerve to the tumour (it may be intimately applied to it, even stretched over it) puts it at risk during surgical removal of the tumour.

Several different surgical techniques are available and the use of one rather than another depends on several factors, including the size of the tumour, the desirability of trying to preserve hearing and the experience of the surgical team. A team approach involving otologists specializing in this type of surgery, neurosurgeons, neuroanaesthetists and intraoperative neurophysiological monitoring personnel is desirable.

In the translabyrinthine approach the internal auditory canal is reached via the mastoid by removing the bony labyrinth. Hearing is inevitably destroyed but this is an approach that is suitable for many tumours, especially when there is already profound deafness. The retrosigmoid approach provides excellent exposure to the tumours in the cerebello-pontine angle and it is possible to preserve hearing using this approach. However, it is a more invasive procedure, involving opening the skull with a craniotomy and retraction of the cerebellum. There may be long-term sequelae of this. The internal canal can be approached from above via the middle cranial fossa approach. The temporal lobe of the brain is gently retracted through a craniotomy above the ear, and the roof of the internal auditory canal is opened. Hearing preservation results are said to be superior with this approach but difficulty reaching the cerebellopontine angle makes it unsuitable for larger tumours.

## Neurofibromatosis

Two related genetic disorders, neurofibromatosis types 1 (NF1) and 2 (NF2) are associated with vestibular schwannomas. NF1 is inherited as an autosomal dominant disorder but sporadic cases are common. The clinical manifestations are variable but characteristically consist of 'café au lait' spots and multiple neurofibromas on peripheral nerves. Unilateral involvement of the cochleovestibular nerve occurs in probably less than 2% of patients. In contrast, in NF2, bilateral vestibular schwannomas are common. This disorder is autosomal dominant and is associated with other neoplasms of the central nervous system (especially meningiomas). The tumours develop in childhood or early adult life and are more aggressive than other vestibular schwannomas, growing rapidly and eroding and enveloping local tissues. Management of an individual patient with NF2 may be extremely taxing and require a series of difficult decisions on the part of the surgical team and of the patient and his or her family. Apart from the risks to life and health associated with the growth of existing (and potential future) tumours in the skull and spinal cord, there are the risks of bilateral damage to facial nerve function and of damage to hearing, associated both with the tumours themselves and with their surgical removal. Genetic counselling is an important part of management of the affected patient.

## Disorders of bone

### Otosclerosis

This is a hereditary disorder in which the bone of the otic capsule (the hard, compact bone surrounding the structures of the inner ear) is replaced by bone of greater cellularity and vascularity. Usually the disease occurs just anterior to the oval window at the fissula ante fenestrum. The abnormal bone in the active phase of otosclerosis has been likened to lava from a volcano. Its presence at the edge of the oval window results in fixation of the stapes footplate within the window and consequently a conductive hearing loss results. There is contradictory evidence about the damage that otosclerosis may cause to the inner ear with the production of a sensorineural hearing loss. Some authors have suggested that the abnormal bone produces toxins, which damage the inner ear structures; others have disputed this, stating that the sensorineural loss observed is no greater than one would expect in unaffected patients of the same age, etc. There is particular disagreement about the entity known as 'cochlear otosclerosis' – otosclerosis affecting the inner ear without signs and symptoms of fixation of the stapes. While this is recognized by some clinicians, there is little pathological evidence to support its existence.

Surgery may correct the conductive deafness (see Chapter 9). It will not improve any coexisting sensorineural deafness. Moreover, profound sensorineural deafness is a potential complication, either at the time of surgery or many years later.

The surgical procedure for otosclerosis is stapedectomy (see p. 146). Deafness is possible because opening into the inner ear may lead to damage to the delicate structures therein. Although surgical technique is important, deafness can occur even when the most skilled surgeon performs this part of the procedure without any apparent excess trauma. Before the inner ear is entered, the region of the footplate should be well visualized. The area should be dry and blood or tissue fluid should be sucked away. Nowadays, a small hole (stapedotomy) is often made in the stapes footplate using a microdrill or laser. In the past, half or the whole of the footplate was removed. The defect is often covered with a vein graft before the prosthesis is inserted. These techniques, of using a small hole and covering that hole with a graft, help prevent perilymph leaking from the inner ear at the time of surgery or later and the incidence of a 'dead' ear following surgery has been reduced. In a small number of cases, opening into the inner ear produces a profuse and brisk flow of fluid. This is known as a 'gusher'. The fluid is initially perilymph but then quickly becomes cerebrospinal fluid (CSF) as the entire volume of perilymph is rapidly lost. The gusher results from a defect in the fundus of the internal auditory canal (or possibly, but less certainly, an enlarged cochlear aqueduct), which establishes an abnormally large pathway between the intracranial CSF in the subarachnoid space and the perilymph in the cochlea. The potential for gushers is greater in children, and stapes surgery is contraindicated in this age group.

In the days following stapedectomy, hearing loss may develop due to perilymph leakage or infection or, rarely, to a reparative granuloma. Postoperative vertigo after stapedectomy is usually very short-lived, so increasing vertigo, increased tinnitus and hearing loss, and discomfort in the ear are warning signs of potential problems. Granulomas were said to occur in approximately 1% of cases, usually between the 6th and 15th postoperative day. The characteristic findings are of oedema and thickening of the tympanic membrane and skin flap associated with hearing loss and imbalance. Removal of the granuloma, graft and prosthesis has been recommended. However, with modern prostheses and vein-grafting techniques the incidence of granulomas appears to have fallen.

Sensorineural deafness may occur many years after stapedectomy. Sometimes there is a definite history of barotrauma (see below), on other occasions the loss is apparently spontaneous. Various factors have been implicated, including a perilymph fistula through an area of deficient graft or secondary endolymphatic hydrops (see p. 157). The prosthesis may become pulled inwards, into the cochlea, by fibrous adhesions and damage the underlying membranous labyrinth. When a potential fistula is present the ear may be explored. There are dangers associated with removing a prosthesis if there is no graft between its bottom end and the inner-ear contents. In these circumstances, it is impossible to know whether or not there are fibrous attachments between the prosthesis and parts of the membranous labyrinth. Removal may result in rupture of the latter and immediate total deafness. Removing and replacing a prosthesis known to be resting on a vein graft is associated with a much smaller risk of inner ear damage.

It will be clear from the above comments that all patients undergoing stapes surgery should be aware of the possibility of total sensorineural hearing loss following the procedure. Stapedectomy is a purely elective procedure. In the light of this, it is important that the patient is fully aware of the risks of surgery before giving his or her informed consent to proceed. What is the risk of sensorineural deafness following stapedectomy? A figure of 1–2% is widely quoted, but for most patients this may not be an accurate assessment of the risk they themselves run as it refers to the past results of those international authorities who have published their own series. Some surgeons will have better results, others worse. The surgeon's experience and skill are important. To a degree, the surgeon's selection of patients and his or her intraoperative decision making about continuing the procedure when faced with a difficult or unusual situation will determine overall 'success' rates. Individual surgeons should audit their own results and be able to give the patient a good estimate of the chances of success in their own hands. This strategy has clear implications for training. However, all surgeons who undertake stapedectomy surgery have to start at some point. A broad and thorough training in microsurgical techniques, together with close personal supervision by an experienced mentor during the initial procedures, should allow selected trainees to develop experience in the technique without compromising the quality of patient care.

## Osteogenesis imperfecta

Osteogenesis imperfecta is a disorder characterized by fragile bones, blue sclera (the 'whites' of the eyes) and deafness. This condition is due to defects in the synthesis of type I collagen – an important component of bone. It is quite distinct from otosclerosis, although the two conditions could coexist. The diseased bone may obliterate the oval and round windows. Sensorineural hearing loss may develop.

## Paget's disease

Paget's disease is a disorder of bone; it often presents late in life. The cause may be hereditary or a slow virus of the paramyxovirus group may be responsible. Classically, the patient has an enlarged skull and a progressive kyphosis (curvature of the spine) resulting in a loss of stature, but more often a subclinical form of the disease is present. It is estimated to occur in 3–4% of individuals over 40 years old. The skull is involved in about 70% of cases of Paget's disease and hearing is affected in 50% of these. The hearing loss is of a mixed type and several pathological processes have been advanced as potential causes. Given that the disease is not uncommon, the otological diagnosis of deafness due to Paget's disease is made rather infrequently. The underlying disorder can be diagnosed on the basis of a skull radiograph and blood tests for alkaline phosphatase (an enzyme involved in bone metabolism) and determination of the level of hydroxyproline in the urine. Other features of Paget's disease include pain and neurological symptoms. These can be treated with aspirin or non-steroidal anti-inflammatory medication. The use of calcitonin and etidronate may stabilize hearing loss in the long term.

**Chronic otitis media**

Sensorineural deafness may arise in patients with chronic otitis media by
two distinct mechanisms. First, it has been shown that there is a higher
incidence of high-frequency loss in such patients when compared to
normal. However, no differences were found when the inner ears were
examined histologically. It has been suggested that alterations in the
mechanics of the cochlea (such as stiffening of the basilar membrane)
might be responsible.

Chronic otitis media with cholesteatoma may produce sensorineural
deafness if the cholesteatoma erodes the bone of the otic capsule. The
most usual site for this is the lateral semicircular canal (then superior
ampulla, posterior canal and promontory). The expanding cholesteatoma
may produce a fistula into the canal by pressure erosion or as a result of an
erosive osteitis. Vertigo is the usual initial symptom, but deafness may
ensue. The diagnosis of a fistula is made clinically by applying pressure to
the air in the external auditory canal, commonly by pushing the tragus
over the meatal opening and applying firm pressure. The increased
pressure in the canal is transmitted via the fistula to the inner ear and the
patient is briefly dizzy. With modern CT scanning techniques the fistula
can usually be visualized.

The presence of a fistula is usually an indication for prompt surgical
intervention. Any infection in the middle ear or mastoid (such as that
associated with the cholesteatoma causing the fistula) can more readily
spread to the inner ear via the fistula. A course of intravenous antibiotics
should be instituted to eradicate infection prior to surgery. A decision
must be made during the surgical procedure about what to do with the
fistula. At the very least, the region of the fistula must be exteriorized, that
is left uncovered as part of the wall of a mastoid cavity. The cholesteatoma
matrix over the fistula may be left alone, untouched, and the remainder of
the walls of the cavity grafted around it. Alternatively, some surgeons will
try and remove the matrix, peeling the layer of epithelium off the underlying exposed endosteum of the canal. The advantage of doing this is that
a thicker graft can then be placed over the fistula, protecting it for the
future. The risk of peeling off the matrix is that the inner ear will be
entered and a total sensorineural loss ('dead ear') will ensue.

# Sudden deafness with trauma

### Ear surgery

The deafness that may follow stapedectomy surgery for otosclerosis has
been discussed above. Sensorineural deafness may arise following any

otological procedure and the patient should be warned of this preoperatively. In some instances, the risk is extremely small.

Very little has been published about the risk of deafness following the most minimally invasive of procedures – insertion of a grommet (ventilation tube). Sensorineural deafness and otitis media with effusion often coexist in young children and occasionally it is not possible to quantify the degree of sensorineural loss until the effusion has been treated. The proportion of patients in whom sensorineural deafness following grommet insertion occurs as a direct result of this procedure is undoubtedly extremely small. This risk must be balanced against the risk of patients with otitis media with effusion and/or recurrent acute otitis media acquiring such deafness as a result of their underlying disease. The use of aminoglycoside antibiotic-containing drops in patients with grommets has been mentioned above. However, it should be noted that they are widely used in this situation and are sometimes the only treatment that is effective in controlling middle-ear infection in patients with grommets in situ. The risk is undoubtedly extremely low and probably arises from prolonged use of such medication.

The risk of sensorineural deafness from other surgical procedures on the ear depends on the nature of the procedure, the underlying disease and the skill of the surgeon. As discussed above in respect of stapedectomy, a surgeon should be able to tell a patient the expected outcomes of the procedure, both the benefits and the risks, based on his or her experience of similar cases. It is likely that the appropriately trained otologist will expect sensorineural deafness following a straightforward myringoplasty in fewer than 1% of cases. The risks are greater in mastoid surgery. The commonest injury resulting in deafness is inadvertent opening into the lateral semicircular canal. This is more likely to occur if the bony covering has been eroded by cholesteatoma and a fistula is present (see above). Overmanipulation of the ossicular chain may result in dislocation of the ossicles or subluxation or fracture of the stapes footplate. If a rotating burr being used to drill the mastoid comes into contact with an intact ossicular chain, the vibrations transmitted to the inner ear may produce a high-frequency sensorineural hearing loss.

While the risk of sensorineural deafness must always be considered prior to ear surgery it takes on particular importance when the ear to be operated on is either the better-hearing or the only hearing ear. The potential benefits of surgery must be balanced carefully against the risks to the patient's overall hearing ability.

## Head injury

It has been estimated that trauma to the temporal bone occurs in between 30 and 75% of head injuries. This trauma can affect the inner ear in several ways. However, it must be borne in mind that the temporal bone is very hard and dense and a large amount of force is required to fracture it. For this reason the majority of such fractures are associated with multiple injuries at other sites and, as such, the temporal bone fracture can easily be overlooked. Blunt trauma is the usual cause. A blow to the head, which is severe enough to cause a fracture, will almost certainly result in a period of loss of consciousness. Traditionally temporal bone fractures have been divided into two types, longitudinal (70–90%) or transverse (20–30%), depending on the direction in which the fracture runs through the temporal bone. However, very few fit neatly into one or other category and 50–70% could probably be categorized as 'mixed'.

Longitudinal fractures run along the axis of the temporal bone. They result from blows to the side of the head (parietal and temporal regions). Clinical features include a conductive hearing loss (due to dislocation of parts of the ossicular chain with or without a perforation in the tympanic membrane) and bleeding from the ear. In about 15% of cases, there is weakness of the face due to involvement of the facial nerve. The onset of this is usually delayed and hence in trauma patients it is vital to record facial function as soon as possible after the injury so that a delayed weakness can be recognized as such. The weakness usually recovers. Leakage of CSF is common because the fracture crosses the roof of the middle ear, but often subsides spontaneously as the fracture heals. Sensorineural hearing loss affecting the high frequencies and most severe at 4 kHz is common. Some improvement may occur in the first three weeks after injury.

A transverse fracture runs across the axis of the temporal bone. It usually results from a blow to the occiput at the back of the head. Bleeding from the ear is not common, but bleeding into the middle ear produces a haemotympanum and consequently the tympanic membrane appears blue. The facial nerve is torn in 50% of cases and produces paralysis of immediate onset. Profound sensorineural hearing loss and vertigo are common as the fracture passes through the inner ear. This may be due to a perilymph leak (see below).

Temporal bone fractures are diagnosed on the basis of high-resolution CT scan images.

A head injury may result in damage to the inner ear without producing a temporal bone fracture. Both sensorineural deafness and imbalance can occur. The cause may be damage to the central nervous system or the inner ear itself. Even a relatively moderate blow may produce sensorineural deafness. It has also been suggested that Ménière's disease may arise in some cases as a long-term consequence of head injury.

Other injuries around the head and ear may damage the inner ear, producing sensorineural deafness. Foreign bodies poked into the ear may not only lead to disruption of the tympanic membrane and ossicular chain but may produce subluxation or fracture of the stapes footplate with consequent perilymph leakage from the oval window.

## Blast injury

A nearby explosion may produce a blast injury as a result of both the high intensity of noise and the shock wave. The damage occurs as the pressure rises in the ear and the rapidity of this rise seems important. Pressure changes of less than one atmosphere may produce damage. The commonest form of damage to the ear is conductive deafness from perforation of the tympanic membrane; this may improve if the membrane heals, but there may be an additional conductive deafness from damage to the ossicles, which can be repaired. Sensorineural deafness following blast injuries can range from total deafness in one or both ears to a relatively minor high-frequency loss; some degree of spontaneous recovery may occur.

## Barotrauma

Barotrauma may occur when the ear is exposed to sudden pressure changes, such as those experienced when flying or diving. At sea level the ambient pressure is one atmosphere. In flight, as one ascends the pressure falls, halving with each 18 000 feet of ascent. In 'pressurized' aircraft the cabin is usually pressurized to 8000 feet. When diving the pressure increases by one atmosphere for every 33 feet of descent. As pressure decreases during ascent when flying or diving, the volume of gas in the middle ear and mastoid increases. The pressure will be dissipated by the release of gas down the eustachian tube into the nasopharynx unless there is total tubal obstruction, which is very unusual. During descent, however, the reverse occurs and the volume of air in the middle ear decreases. If the eustachian tube does not open, intense negative pressure in the middle ear results in the tympanic membrane, round window membrane and stapes footplate being pulled into the middle ear and swelling of the middle-ear mucosa with bleeding or tissue fluid leakage occurring in the middle ear. The tympanic membrane may rupture. A forceful Valsalva's manoeuvre in these circumstances will lead to an increase in CSF and perilymph pressure and the pressure differential between the inner and middle ears will become even greater. Whether or not a Valsalva's manoeuvre has been performed, the round window membrane may rupture in these circumstances producing a perilymph leak. Inner-ear decompression sickness is another possible cause of audio-vestibular dysfunction following diving. This may be related to gas-bubble formation or hypercoagulation within the inner ear.

## Perilymph fistula

A perilymph fistula is an abnormal communication between the perilymphatic space and the middle ear. The usual sites are (a) a defect in the round window membrane or (b) a breach in the ligament between the stapes footplate and the oval window itself. The leakage of perilymph, which may also be associated with the entry of air into the inner ear, is usually associated with sensorineural deafness and vestibular symptoms of sudden onset.

Fistulas are discussed in this section because there is little disagreement about their existence as a result of certain types of trauma. Postoperative fistulae have been discussed. Direct trauma to the ossicular chain (from a cotton bud poked into the ear canal for example) or indirect trauma to the head may produce a fracture or dislocation of the stapes and consequent leak. There are patients with congenital abnormalities of the middle ear in whom recurrent meningitis arises as a consequence of a congenital fistula. In all these cases, exploration of the middle ear and the plugging of any defect with soft tissue are appropriate.

Controversy surrounds the concept that more minor trauma, such as barotrauma or the trauma associated with physical exertions such as straining, lifting, coughing, laughing, vomiting, etc., may produce a fistula. Still more controversial is the notion that a 'spontaneous perilymph fistula', unprecipitated by any stress, can be a cause of sudden sensorineural deafness.

There are several difficulties in evaluating the literature (which is not inconsiderable) surrounding this topic. The chief difficulty is that there is no 'gold-standard' diagnostic test to establish or disprove the diagnosis. This may seem surprising because it is a relatively simple matter surgically to elevate the tympanic membrane and inspect the round and oval window regions. Unfortunately the middle-ear cleft is almost never completely dry and the presence of tissue fluid compromises the assessment of whether or not perilymph leakage is present. This has been studied scientifically and a group of surgeons were invited to assess the same ear and decide whether or not a leak was present. Satisfactory agreement was not obtained. Second, many authors have described seeing 'tears' or 'perforations' in the round window membrane. These claims must be disputed; it is anatomically impossible to see the round window membrane without drilling away the edge of the round window niche. What is seen is a fold of mucous membrane covering the opening of the niche and not the relatively thick membrane itself.

The individual otologist will make up his or her own mind about this controversial diagnosis. If there is a clear history of a sudden onset of sensorineural deafness and vertigo occurring synchronously with an episode of exertion it seems reasonable to entertain the diagnosis. The author is much more sceptical about the concept of spontaneous fistulae.

When the diagnosis is in doubt, a period of conservative treatment is advised. This should comprise bed rest with the head raised. A significant proportion of cases will settle spontaneously. Progression of symptoms or failure to improve should prompt consideration of surgical exploration.

## Sudden deafness without trauma

Sudden sensorineural deafness is a medical emergency. Unfortunately this is not always appreciated and all too often patients present for specialist treatment too late for intervention to be effective. One reason perhaps is that sudden hearing loss is often assumed to be due to a conductive cause, such as middle-ear fluid. This can lead the patient's general practitioner to prescribe decongestants, sometimes for several weeks, delaying the correct diagnosis, which could often have been suspected had the simple basic tuning fork tests of hearing been performed. Patients who are suspected of suffering sudden sensorineural deafness, or in whom conductive deafness has been excluded by tuning fork tests, should be referred urgently to an otolaryngology clinic.

It may be considered semantic to ask what is *sudden* sensorineural deafness? Most otologists would feel that they know it when they see it. It has been defined as 30 dB or more loss in three contiguous audiometric frequencies occurring within 3 days or less. A slower loss is termed 'rapidly progressive'.

In some cases, the cause of the hearing loss is immediately apparent, such as those described above in association with trauma. The deafness may also be a presenting feature of an acoustic neuroma or may mark an initial attack of Ménière's disease. There are many case reports and short series describing sudden hearing loss in a variety of systemic disorders affecting the vascular, haematological, immune, metabolic and skeletal systems. The imputed cause of deafness is cochlear damage. Similarly, there is a long list of disorders of the peripheral and central nervous system in which sensorineural deafness has arisen. However, there remains a large group in whom no cause can be found and this is considered below under the heading 'idiopathic'. It will be appreciated that this is a diagnosis of exclusion and one which can only be reached after a comprehensive series of investigations has excluded other causes.

**Infections**

Bacterial infection of the inner ear (labyrinthitis) is an uncommon complication of acute otitis media when infection spreads into the labyrinth. In
contrast, serous labyrinthitis occurs when bacterial toxins spread to the
labyrinth. The characteristic clinical features are sensorineural hearing
loss and vertigo, which recovers partially or completely as the infection
subsides.

Bacterial meningitis may be a complication of otitis media or sinus
disease, but in many cases the disease follows an upper respiratory tract
infection and the mechanism by which the offending organism (usually
*Haemophilus influenzae*) reaches the meninges is unknown.

Meningitis can lead to sensorineural deafness when the labyrinth is
infected. It is one of the commonest causes of severe or profound
acquired deafness in infants and children. The pathway by which the infection spreads is usually via the cochlear aqueduct, but it may be through the
internal auditory canal. The deafness is usually bilateral and may be associated with other problems, such as mental handicap, blindness, epilepsy,
spasticity and ataxia. The risk of developing these complications is greater
the younger the child and the more prolonged the delay in treatment. The
prognosis is also dependent on the causative organism, the
*Meningococcus* and *Pneumococcus* having a particularly bad prognosis.
The incidence of hearing impairment following meningitis has been
estimated at between 4 and 40%. Ossification of the basal turn of the
cochlea often follows meningitis. This process continues even after the
hearing has been destroyed.

All patients who have suffered from meningitis, especially children,
should have their hearing tested as soon as possible after recovery. In
adults, pure-tone audiometry is appropriate. In small children, it may be
necessary to use an objective technique such as brainstem electric
response audiometry. The appropriate hearing aids should be fitted as
soon as possible to optimize the patient's auditory rehabilitation.
Consideration should be given to providing a cochlear implant. There are
several important and specific issues surrounding the use of implants in
post-meningitis patients. First, any patient being considered for an
implant should initially have a reasonable trial with optimally fitted
hearing aids. Second, however, it has been shown that the earlier a
profoundly deaf child who cannot derive significant benefit from hearing
aids is implanted, the better the long-term results. Third, a very small
number of children with hearing loss after meningitis recover some or all
of their hearing within 6–12 months following infection. Finally, the
implant can be inserted into the cochlea most easily when there is no
obliteration of the basal turn by new bone formation. In delaying the

implant procedure, one may be making the insertion more difficult or even preventing a full insertion.

Many cases of acute deafness or vertigo or both cannot be attributed to a specific cause and a viral infection is often implicated. This is partly because on many occasions upper respiratory symptoms or an influenzal type of illness are associated with the episode. When viral labyrinthitis does occur it can involve the inner ear or the audio-vestibular nerves. The symptoms and the resulting long-term deficits may affect the cochlea or labyrinth or both, producing deafness or vertigo alone or together.

The effects of some viruses have been more clearly defined. Herpes zoster oticus (Ramsay Hunt syndrome) is caused by the virus that also causes chickenpox. The main features are facial weakness on the same side as a severe pain in the ear. Vesicles can be seen in the ear canal. In the current context, this infection is important because sensorineural deafness, tinnitus and vestibular symptoms may also occur. The hearing loss is usually high-frequency and unless severe, some recovery is usual. Treatment is with appropriate antiviral agents such as acyclovir, with or without steroids.

Measles and mumps, childhood illnesses caused by paramyxoviruses, are both associated with sensorineural deafness. In measles, the loss is usually moderate to profound and bilateral. In mumps, bilateral loss is extremely uncommon, the patient usually developing a unilateral loss varying form a mild high-frequency loss to profound deafness. There does not appear to be a relationship between the severity of the mumps and the development of hearing loss. Encephalitis may complicate both measles and mumps. In the former, the chance of developing hearing loss is increased. The prognosis for the latter is better and carries no greater risk of deafness.

There can be little doubt as to the cause of hearing loss or vertigo when these symptoms develop during the course of an infection and the latter is confirmed by rising titres of antibodies in the bloodstream. However, it is not uncommon for a patient (often a child or teenager) to present with unilateral profound deafness and a past history of mumps. In these circumstances, it is difficult to be categorical about the cause of the deafness. The incidence of mumps and measles is changing with the intro-duction of measles, mumps and rubella (MMR) immunization. Although there are case reports of sensorineural hearing loss after immunization, these must be treated with the usual caution and the risk must be weighed against the potentially fatal consequences of infection in the unimmu-nized patient.

Many other viruses have been implicated as causes of sensorineural deafness, including herpes simplex, Epstein–Barr virus, influenza and parainfluenza viruses.

There is a high prevalence of otological symptoms, including sensorineural hearing loss, vertigo, tinnitus and aural fullness, in patients with HIV infection and AIDS. These patients often receive multiple medical therapies, some of which may be ototoxic, and are also prone to opportunistic infections.

### 'Idiopathic sudden sensorineural hearing loss'

It has been estimated that the incidence of this problem is 15 000 cases per year worldwide. The condition is equally common in men and women. About half of the patients also experience some vestibular symptoms. In about a third of patients, spontaneous recovery occurs. If this happens it normally does so in the first two weeks. A third have a partial recovery and a third have no recovery in hearing. Unfavourable prognostic features include a severe loss, a downwards sloping audiogram showing a high-frequency loss and the presence of vertigo.

Several possible causes of idiopathic sudden sensorineural hearing loss have been advanced. The high incidence of symptoms suggestive of a previous viral illness (rates up to 65% have been quoted) puts a viral aetiology near the top of the list. Seroconversion to a wide variety of viruses has been described. Reduced cochlear blood flow is another popular hypothesis, while primary or secondary immunological causes are particularly favoured in some parts of the world (see below).

It will be clear from the above that the patient with sudden sensorineural deafness requires careful management. It is important to realize that the patient is often extremely distressed about his or her misfortune and the possible cause of it, particularly if the loss is severe. They are often worried that they may have some sinister intracranial problem and are anxious about the future, especially about losing their hearing altogether. A thorough history and physical examination must look for symptoms and signs of any systemic or local disorder. In idiopathic cases, none is found. A baseline audiogram will record the extent of the hearing loss. The focus of further investigations is the exclusion of a treatable underlying cause.

A number of blood tests are usually recommended, but the yield of these is not great. A 'standard' battery of tests might include a full blood count and erythrocyte sedimentation rate (ESR), syphilis serology, random glucose, thyroid function tests, serum lipids and possibly viral titres (with a repeat specimen 2 to 3 weeks later). An MRI scan should be obtained to exclude a vestibular schwannoma or demyelination.

Treatment is often initiated before all the results of these investigations are available. There are few randomized controlled trials with conclusive results on which to base a rational treatment protocol. Many different regimens have been proposed based on 'evidence' of variable quality. At this time, there is no treatment which one can categorically state to be effective. As the patient must implicitly accept any risks of the treatment proposed, the empirical nature of the treatment should be made clear during the process of obtaining consent to it. Most patients will accept the proposed treatment in the spirit in which the recommendation is being made. Some will decline it for a variety of reasons. It is important that their decision is respected and, particularly if they turn out to have a poor outcome, that they are supported in understanding that their decision was a reasonable one. No matter which treatment strategy is followed, it is mandatory to follow the patient up and arrange the appropriate auditory rehabilitation for those whose hearing does not improve.

Various medical treatments have been proposed; many of these are thought to improve intracochlear blood flow. Those with the greatest 'acceptance' and which the author favours include:

- a short course of oral steroids (e.g enteric-coated prednisolone 60 mg/day for 3 days, then 45 mg/day for 3 days, then 30 mg/day for 3 days, then 15 mg/day for 3 days, then stop. If necessary, combined with a proton pump inhibitor or $H_2$ antagonist).
- regular inhalation of carbogen (95% oxygen: 5% carbon dioxide).
- betahistine hydrochloride (Serc) 16 mg three times a day.
- if the differential white cell count suggests a possible viral aetiology the addition of an anti-viral agent such as acyclovir should be considered.
- bed-rest is often recommended.

Treatment should be initiated as soon as possible after the hearing is lost, and certainly within 2 to 3 weeks. Treatment after this time is less likely to be rewarding.

### Immunological

The notion that immunological mechanisms might be responsible for inner-ear disorders including sensorineural deafness is not new. However, it is only relatively recently that these mechanisms have been investigated and there is still not widespread acceptance of the diagnosis of 'autoimmune inner-ear disease' in all those situations in which its protagonists would like us to accept it. The term 'autoimmune inner-ear disease' covers a variety of different clinical syndromes in which cell-mediated or humoral-mediated mechanisms produce inner-ear dysfunction. Two distinct types are recognized: organ-specific and non-organ-specific.

The concept of organ-specific inner-ear disease relies on establishing that auto-antibodies or cell-mediated immune responses directed against inner-ear antigens are present and result in inner-ear disease. A clinical syndrome comprising rapidly progressive bilateral sensorineural deafness occasionally associated with dizziness has been described and attributed to such an autoimmune process. Many laboratory tests have been proposed to look for evidence of response(s) to inner-ear antigens. None has achieved wide acceptance, although proponents of this diagnosis believe that they have identified a protein (HSP-70) that is either the target of the autoimmune response or a substance produced as a result of inner-ear damage. A Western blot immunoassay has been used to identify this protein and it is proposed that the presence of this protein is diagnostic (in patients with progressive deafness) of an immune-mediated cause and predicts sensitivity to treatment with steroids.

Non-organ-specific autoimmune inner-ear disease is diagnosed in patients with a similar clinical presentation to that outlined above, but in whom a systemic immune disease coexists. The disorders in question include polyarteritis nodosa, Wegener's granulomatosis, Beháçet's syndrome, relapsing polychondritis, systemic lupus erythematosus and rheumatoid arthritis. Cogan's syndrome is a disorder of young adults characterized by interstitial keratitis and audio-vestibular dysfunction. Acute episodes of hearing loss associated with tinnitus and vertigo progress over a period of a few months to total deafness. 'Atypical Cogan's syndrome' is a term used to describe similar audio-vestibular symptoms but ocular problems other than keratitis, such as episcleritis, uveitis or conjunctivitis.

The importance of recognizing cases of autoimmune inner-ear disease lies in the possibility of treating those patients with disabling symptoms with immunosuppressive medication. There is no satisfactory evidence from controlled trials on which to base recommendations for treatment. One regimen which has been proposed utilizes 1 mg/kg/day of prednisolone for an initial 4 weeks, thereafter tapering treatment according to the response. The potential side effects of this regimen are not insignificant. Even more powerful immunosuppresive medications such as cyclophosphamide have been suggested, as has serum plasmapheresis in some resistant cases. Hopefully, the development of clear diagnostic criteria (in particular the advent of a simple serological test which is both sensitive and specific) may lead to the appropriate randomized controlled trials to determine the most effective treatment.

# Chapter 11
# The causes of childhood deafness and its identification and confirmation

## PETER WATKIN

Even though a 'cure' in the medical or surgical sense is not possible, establishing the cause of childhood deafness is important both for the child and his or her family. Is the deafness associated with an illness, which may have implications for the child's health or development? Is it genetic with a chance of recurrence in other family members? Parents need to know answers to these questions early after diagnosis, and eventually every child asks the inevitable question 'why me?'. Establishing causation is also important for the community. Primary prevention, which aims to reduce the occurrence of avoidable deafness, depends on local epidemiology. In the UK, preventative measures have markedly reduced the incidence of certain associated illnesses. Congenital rubella and rhesus haemolytic disease are now rare. Improved antenatal care has also reduced maternal illness, and aetiologies such as attempted abortion with quinine only remain to be recalled in the literature. Measures of secondary prevention also depend on an understanding of those conditions and illnesses associated with deafness. Secondary prevention reduces the progression of a condition by detecting it early. This is facilitated by the recognition of risk factors. To be forewarned is to be forearmed.

These preventative measures have resulted in rapid changes in the epidemiology of childhood deafness. Despite the changes, it remains useful to classify causes of deafness as in Figure 11.1. The relative proportions of each category within a population vary according to enrolment bias. Causes may also not always be correctly attributed, with aetiologies becoming fashionable – at least for a time. At one time it appeared that the blitz was responsible for much childhood deafness; later the aetiological finger pointed to congenital rubella; and today perinatal illness or meningitis are often implicated – even though there may be no real substantiating evidence. Multifactorial aetiologies may also be unrecognized.

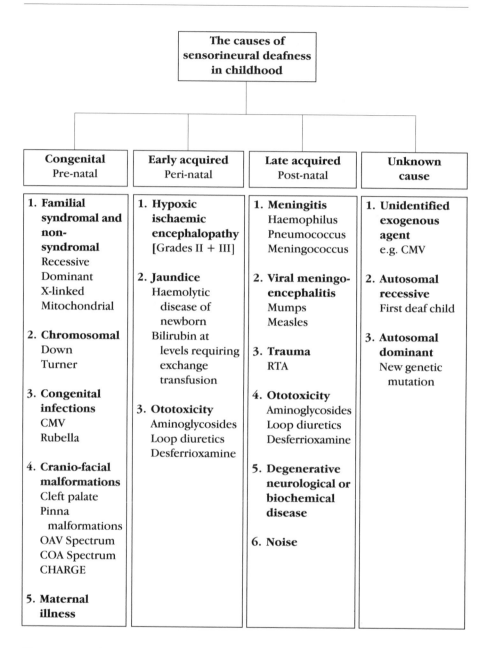

**Figure 11.1:** The causes of childhood deafness.

Another difficulty is that even after complete investigation, in up to one-third of cases the cause may remain unknown. While an unidentified exogenous factor may be causative in some, hereditary factors are probably responsible in the majority. Such diagnostic imprecision will be reduced by the rapid progress in identifying and localizing the mutations in the many different genes that can cause deafness. Molecular diagnosis for deafness genes is currently just emerging for clinical use. Its routine availability is the key required to unlock most of the remaining aetiological uncertainties.

# Inherited deafness

It is quite impossible to remain indifferent to the explosion in our understanding of the role played by our genes. Inheritance seemingly affects every aspect of human existence. Unravelling genetic mechanisms is thus fundamental to understanding the cause of deafness. Around half of those children with a permanent deafness have inherited it from one or both of their parents. The genes responsible are usually transmitted in accordance with Mendelian rules of inheritance. The deafness may be syndromal or non-syndromal. Children with syndromal deafness have a characteristic combination of features, with deafness being but one of them. Non-syndromal deafness is clinically undifferentiated, without associated abnormal physical features.

There has been considerable progress in identifying the genes responsible for both types of deafness. Initially the deafness gene has to be localized or mapped to a site on the chromosome. The gene sequence then has to be identified and cloned. As well as facilitating prenatal diagnosis and accurate counselling through molecular testing, this understanding may have knock-on consequences, allowing the mysteries of the molecular processes underlying hearing to be unravelled. Once the gene sequence has been identified it is possible to predict the type of protein produced by the gene, and to replace defective proteins produced. This raises the tantalizing and provocative, futuristic possibility of therapeutic rather than prosthetic interventions.

## Familial non-syndromal hearing loss

Hearing loss is an isolated symptom in over two-thirds of children with a familial deafness. It is usually inherited as an autosomal dominant, autosomal recessive or X-linked condition. Recessive inheritance accounts for some two-thirds of those children with a severe familial deafness, with dominant inheritance being relatively more common in those children with more moderate impairments. It has long been recognized that there is heterogeneity, with different gene mutations causing familial clinically undifferentiated deafness. Thus rather unexpectedly, children where both parents are recessively deaf often have normal hearing. If the parents had the same mutant genes, deafness in their children would be obligatory. Analyses of the pedigrees of such families almost half a century ago suggested that there were at least 36 different genes for recessive deafness. To date 24 different genes responsible for recessive non-syndromal deafness (DFNB genes) have been localized, with six gene sequences having been identified.

Similar heterogeneity occurs in dominant deafness. Genes for autosomal dominant hearing loss (DFNA genes) have already been localized to 20 different sites, with nine genes having been identified, and although X-linked deafness is clinically rare, responsible genes have already been mapped to eight sites on the X chromosome, with two gene sequences having been identified. Although X-linked deafness occurs in males, in some pedigrees the carrier females also have a hearing disability. Other families with this mode of inheritance have a clinically distinct, progressive, mixed hearing loss. The conductive component to their hearing loss often appears to be due to stapes fixation, but an inner-ear malformation allows cerebrospinal fluid to flow freely into the perilymphatic space, and disastrously a perilymph 'gusher' occurs if stapedectomy is undertaken.

Deafness transmitted through the maternal line is also a feature of mitochondrial gene mutations. The mitochondria each have a variably small number of chromosomes that are transmitted solely through the mother. Pedigree analysis usually readily distinguishes X-linked from mitochondrial inheritance where maternal transmission occurs to children of either sex. To date, two mitochondrial deafness genes have been identified. However, among all these genetic discoveries, one seems set to have far-reaching clinical impact. The first DFNB gene was localized to a mutation on chromosome 13. The gene (known as GJB2) encodes the connexin 26 molecule. This mutant gene may be involved in up to half of those with a familial non-syndromic childhood deafness. There are no distinguishing features associated with the deafness and it may vary in severity. Importantly it can be detected by a simple laboratory test – opening up the possibility of cost-effective gene screening in those where no other exogenous or syndromic causation is apparent.

**Familial syndromal hearing loss**

There remains disagreement about the contribution that syndrome identification plays in establishing the cause of deafness. Some consider syndromes to be present in only a very small number of hearing-impaired children. Others claim that at least one third of those with a familial deafness have a syndrome. It seems that their identification depends very much on the diagnostic acumen of the examiner. Twenty years ago, around 100 clearly delineated Mendelian syndromes with deafness as a major component were detailed. This number has now quadrupled. Table 11.1 lists some of the conditions, with those more commonly encountered being further detailed.

**Table 11.1:** Examples of the more common genetic deafness syndromes illustrating classification by associated system abnormality

| System disorder | Syndromes in which deafness is associated with system disorder |
|---|---|
| Eye abnormalities | • Retinitis/Retinal degeneration and deafness syndromes – Usher, Alstrom, Cockayne, Refsum syndromes<br>• Myopia and deafness syndromes – Marshall, Stickler syndromes<br>• Oculoacousticocerebral dysplasia – Norrie Syndrome |
| Renal abnormalities | • Progressive deafness and chronic nephritis – Alport syndrome<br>• Renal tubular acidosis and deafness syndromes |
| Skin abnormalities | • Deafness and depigmentation syndromes – Waardenburg, Tietz syndromes<br>• Deafness and abnormal hair syndromes – Pili-torti, alopecia syndromes<br>• Deafness and hyperpigmentation – lentigines, ECG, ocular, pulmonary stenosis, abnormal genitalia, retardation of growth, deafness syndrome |
| Endocrine and metabolic abnormalities | • Deafness and inborn error of thyroxine synthesis – Pendred syndrome<br>• Diabetes insipidus, diabetes mellitus, optic atrophy deafness syndrome<br>• Deafness associated with the mucopolysaccharidoses |
| Nervous system abnormalities | • Motor and sensory neuropathies and deafness – Charcot–Marie–Tooth syndrome<br>• Mitochondrial myopathies and deafness – Kearns–Sayre syndrome<br>• Neurofibromatosis type II |
| Skeletal abnormalities | • Deafness associated with sclerosing bone dysplasias – osteopetrosis and Albers Schonberg syndromes<br>• Deafness associated with dwarfing dysplasias – Achondroplasia<br>• Deafness associated with craniosynostosis – Apert, Crouzon, Pfeiffer syndromes |
| Cardiac abnormality | • Deafness associated with prolonged QT interval – Jervell and Lange–Nielsen syndrome |

## Usher syndrome

This syndrome reportedly occurs in 3–6% of severely deaf children and is even more prevalent among certain deaf populations. It is recessively inherited and characterized by congenital sensorineural deafness and visual problems resulting from retinitis pigmentosa. The retinitis causes progressive night blindness and loss of the peripheral visual fields. At least three types of the syndrome exist. The Usher type I gene has been localized to the long arm of chromosome 14 and is characterized by profound congenital deafness with absent vestibular function. Night blindness and visual field loss generally commences just as the child is about to embark on secondary education. Unfortunately, vision slowly deteriorates, often progressing to blindness in later adult life. Usher type II is less common. The gene has been located on the long arm of chromosome 1. The hearing loss is more moderate in degree and the onset of visual problems is slightly delayed. Type III is unusual and has been characterized by a progressive hearing loss with variable onset of retinitis pigmentosa. The assessment of Usher type is crucial to the outcome and to providing communication skills that will remain appropriate.

## Waardenburg syndrome

The association of pigmentary disorders and deafness has been well recognized in a variety of animals for many years. The commonest human auditory pigmentary syndrome is an autosomal dominant disorder initially described by Waardenburg. It has been reported to be slightly less prevalent than Usher syndrome, but as the clinical features are often very subtle, it is very much under-recognized within the community.

Clinical, and subsequently genetic, studies have confirmed that at least four clinically distinct subtypes exist. Waardenburg types I (WS1) and II (WS2) are those usually encountered. They are clinically divided according to the presence of wide spacing of the medial canthi of the eyes (dystopia canthorum). This feature is invariably present in WS1 and absent in WS2. Pigmentary abnormalities are common to both types. They are often seen in the irides, with each iris being a different colour (heterochromia irides) or hypoplastic and a symmetrical startling blue. Another common feature is a distinctive white forelock. However, this may be very variable, consisting of but a few whisps of white hair present on the side or back of the head. The hearing loss is also variable. It is reportedly found in only 20% of those with WS1 but is present in 50% of those with WS2.

The gene responsible for type I has been mapped to 2q35 (band 35 on the long arm of chromosome 2) and identified as PAX3. In some families with WS2, the abnormality maps to the short arm of chromosome 3. The mutations seen in these families are in a gene identified as MITF. Interestingly, early editions of this book described a rare condition of deafness and oculocutaneous albinism, epononymously referred to as Tietz syndrome. Early after the original description there was nosological disagreement, with some considering the condition to be part of the Waardenburg spectrum. The current author recently investigated another family with these features. They were very distinctive and not at all typical of Waardenburg syndrome. However, there were grounds for the early nosological disagreements. Despite the distinctive phenotype, the family was found to have a mutation of MITF – as seen in Waardenburg type II!

**Treacher Collins syndrome**

This syndrome is a familial disorder of craniofacial development. It is transmitted by autosomal dominant inheritance. The abnormality of facial development is usually associated with a congenital conductive hearing loss. The auditory ossicles may be absent or severely malformed and unusually this may be associated with a malformation of the cochlea and vestibules. Those only mildly affected have nothing more than a slightly elfin facial appearance. Thus once again, the syndrome often goes unrecognized unless another family member is more severely affected. The facial dysmorphology is usually symmetric. The external ear may be small and malformed with complete stenosis of the external auditory meatus. The jaw is small (micrognathia) and this may be associated with a cleft palate. Depression of the cheekbones (malar hypoplasia) results in downsloping of the eyes. The gene mutation has been mapped to 5q32–33.1, and the actual gene (named Treacle) identified. Almost two-thirds of cases probably arise as a new mutation.

**Chromosomal disorders**

When one considers the subtle gene mutations that may result in deafness, it is not in the least surprising that a structural chromosome abnormality should result in deafness. Those born with a trisomy of chromosomes 13 or 18 almost always suffer from a severe sensorineural deafness, but the clinical relevance of the deafness is limited in these tragic babies, who rarely survive. In other children with a chromosomal aneuploidy, hearing loss may be a contributory disability. Down's syndrome (trisomy 21) is usually associated with conductive hearing loss caused by chronic serous otitis media. Poor aeration of the middle-ear cefts has been attributed to abnormal eustachian tube function. Occasionally, ossicular or cochlear abnormalities are present, and not uncommonly a progressive high-frequency loss resembling early onset presbyacusis commences in teenage years. Similar chronic middle-ear disease is seen in girls with Turner's sydrome (45XO). Once again this has been attributed to anatomical abnormalities of the eustachian tubes, but many also suffer a mid-frequency sensorineural hearing loss. Although this is more usual in Turner teenagers, it may first appear at a much younger age.

# Craniofacial abnormalities

Not all babies born with congenital malformations have a recognizable cause for their condition. Their chromosomes may show no structural abnormality – at least by currently available examination techniques – and the dysmorphology may not be determined by Mendelian inheritance. Such conditions may be associated with deafness, especially if there is a craniofacial malformation. Those children with a cleft palate are also at risk. Eustachian tube function is dependent on the palatal muscles. This mechanism is disturbed when the palate is cleft, and chronic middle-ear problems often ensue. The cleft may also be part of a syndromic phenotype, which includes perceptive deafness. Such an association is commonly seen in Stickler syndrome. Audiological and otolgical care are therefore routine in the multidisciplinary care of children with a cleft palate. Developmental abnormalities of the external ears may also be associated with deafness. Many of the structures in the external and middle ear originate from the same branchial arch embryonic cells. It is not surprising therefore, that pinna abnormalities may be the outward sign of an ossicular malformation, with unilateral external ear dysmorphology occasionally being associated with a bilateral permanent conductive deafness. Most external ear abnormalities are sporadic isolated defects, but they may be associated with renal tract malformations, or with a craniofacial syndrome. Two of the commoner syndromes are described.

### Goldenhar syndrome

This is the commonest of the so-called branchial arch syndromes and curiously usually occurs in males. The cause of the faulty embryonic development remains speculative, but is nearly always sporadic. The syndrome demonstrates a fine example of nosological confusion. The dysmorphology is usually unilateral, hence the alternative name of hemifacial microsomia. However, there is a very wide phenotype spectrum with many being mildly affected. The cardinal features are suggested by the more recent nosological term of oculo-auriculo-vertebral spectrum (OAV). Ocular abnormalities, including epibulbar demoids and unilateral upper eyelid colobomata, are common. Vertebral abnormalities with spinal fusions and hemivertebrae also occur. Auricular abnormalities consist of atretic external ear canals, grossly abnormal ossicles and underdeveloped inner ears. Despite the hemifacial appearance, these ear malformations may be bilateral and associated with a profound bilateral sensorineural impairment.

### Wildervanck syndrome

This syndrome shares many of the problems encountered with OAV. It is sporadic. It has a sex prediliction but in this case for females. Once again there is a wide spectrum of malformation and if possible even greater nosological confusion. It has been termed the cervico-oculo-acoustic spectrum of disorders (COA). Classically these children have deafness associated with fusion of the cervical vertebrae (the Klippel–Feil anomoly), and unilateral retrusion of the eye and abducens nerve palsy (Duane syndrome). The affected eye retracts when it looks inwards. Once again, there is enormous variability, with less severe forms being not uncommonly encountered.

### CHARGE association

Although the two previous eponoymous syndromes were both described half a century ago, CHARGE association was not recognized as a clinical entity until the 1980s. Yet this sporadic condition is very regularly encountered. CHARGE is a mnemonic describing some of the constellation of features. Cardinal features are Colobomata affecting the iris or retina, Heart defects, Retarded growth and development, Genital hypoplasia and Ear anomolies. The mneomonic could usefully be expanded to include other common features such as cleft palate, choanal atresia and facial palsy. Ear anomolies are almost always present. They consist of a wide spectrum of pinna dysmorphologies, often associated with a unilateral facial palsy. The external ear on the side of the facial palsy usually demonstrates the greatest anomoly, and thus the condition can superficially resemble hemifacial microsomia. Mixed deafness with impairments ranging from mild to profound are seen in nearly all affected children. The question remains as to why such a characteristic constellation was not nosologically identified many years ago.

# Congenital infections

Historically, deafness resulting from prenatal viral infection has been a common cause of childhood deafness. As recently as the 1970s, congenital infections were responsible in up to one-third of cases. Many different infections have been implicated, but there is often doubt about the relationship between the congenital infection and the deafness. No such doubts are harboured about prenatal infection with either German measles (rubella) or cytomegalovirus (CMV).

## Congenital rubella

Prenatal rubella is teratogenic and may devastate the unborn child. Before the introduction of rubella immunization programmes, around 10% of women of child-bearing age had not caught this innocuous illness and these immunologically unprotected women were at risk during pregnancy. The mildness of the maternal illness often left the expectant mother blissfully unaware of damage being wrought on her unborn child.

Prior to immunization, about 1 in 4000 pregnant women caught rubella, but epidemics occurred every eight or nine years. During these years the incidence increased 20-fold. In 1964, a rubella epidemic swept the USA leaving as its legacy some 20 000 handicapped children. The gestational age of the fetus at the time of maternal infection is a critical predictor of outcome. If the illness is caught during the first two months of pregnancy, the chance of the child being multiply-handicapped is almost 100%. The babies may be deaf and blind with severe learning difficulties, heart disease and cerebral palsy. With increasing gestational age, the probability of the fetus having multiple abnormalities is greatly reduced. With an infection in the second trimester there is a 75% chance of deafness but usually this is an isolated abnormality.

The devastation caused by this illness made it an important target for preventative measures and with the mass immunization of all children congenital rubella is now an unusual occurrence. Unimmunized women moving to the UK remain more at risk, with a small number of cases of congenital rubella resulting from maternal reinfection. There remain many other unexplained features of this prenatal infection. How was it possible that some prenatally infected were not clinically affected? Recent research has confirmed a genetic predisposition to deafness acquired by exogenous factors. A genetic predisposition to rubella deafness was clinically postulated by the Karolinska Institute in Stockholm many years ago. This linkage between our genes and acquired illness remains of tantalizing interest.

## Cytomegalovirus

CMV is another teratogenic intrauterine infection which causes congenital deafness. Primary CMV infection results in a mild glandular fever-type of illness. However, it is a typical herpes virus and, following the primary illness, a long-lasting infection is established in mesenchymal tissue. Reactivation may result in a mild systemic illness and is usually symptomless, although during pregnancy it may cross the placenta and infect the fetus. Usually the neonate is infected but not affected by the CMV. However, a minority of women catch CMV for the first time in pregnancy and, with no natural immunity, the fetus may be both infected and affected. Although the child may be symptomless, congenital CMV may result in a destructive infection of the central nervous system with deafness occurring as one of the sequelae or in isolation. Around one third of symptomatic cases, and 10% of asymptomatic but infected children, are deaf. The differentiation of those clinically infected and affected – or clinically infected but not affected – is taxing, but crucially important for the child. Those affected by CMV may suffer a progressive deafness and eventually be left profoundly deaf. This may be associated with microcephaly and severe learning difficulties. Despite the teratogenic devastation, immunization is not currently possible because CMV given prophylactically may reactivate.

## Perinatal illness

A neonate born with a beautifully formed and functioning organ of hearing, may have it irreversibly damaged during the struggle for life. Half a century ago this happened to one fifth of premature babies, but the intensive care of neonates has been revolutionized. Babies of a very low birth weight now survive with an excellent quality of life, and even in those units delivering a tertiary level of care, the overall incidence of sensorineural deafness is less than 1%. Several inter-related factors are involved.

### Birth asphyxia

Birth asphyxia may result in neurological and cochlear ischaemic damage. Although neuronal necrosis may result in central deafness, the cochlea is fed by a single-end artery, and this makes it very vulnerable to hypoxaemia. It is on a knife edge throughout pregnancy. Prenatal hypoxaemia may occur because of inadequate maternal oxygenation or placental perfusion. Compromisation of the umbilical circulation may occur during birth. Following delivery, the neonate may be unable to accomplish pulmonary inflation and there may be difficulties with the transition of the cardiopulmonary circulation. Maintaining adequate cochlear oxygenation is particularly difficult for the respiratory distressed premature baby suffering periods of apnoea.

Birth asphyxia itself often reflects a more prolonged intrapartum asphyxia, and although this may result in cochlear damage, prognostic indicators have been difficult to achieve. An Apgar score of 3 or less at 5 minutes, and the presence of an acidosis, are weak outcome indicators. A better prediction can now be made from the neonatal neurological examination and the presence of hypoxic ischaemic encephalopathy (HIE). Three levels have been defined, with stage I being the mildest. A minority of those with stage II, but the majority of those with stage III HIE have an adverse outcome. Around 10% of those surviving with stage III suffer a cochlear deafness.

## Jaundice

Historically, jaundice has also been a major cause of sensorineural deafness. The improvement in its management and prevention has had knock-on consequences for paediatric audiology. Jaundice occurs when there is excess bilribubin (hyperbilirubinaemia) circulating in the blood. The bilirubin is derived from the breakdown of red blood cells. It is bound to a protein (albumin) in the blood and carried to acceptor proteins in the liver where it is detoxified and excreted. However, for a variety of reasons, this complex detox programme may become stressed in the newborn. This occurs in haemolytic disease of the newborn, when there is a blood group incompatibility between mother and child. The commonest incompatibility is that of a rhesus negative mother and a rhesus positive baby. Maternal antibodies are formed but these break down the baby's blood cells, leaving him or her anaemic and jaundiced. With saturation of the blood's capacity for transporting it to the liver, free toxic bilrubin builds up. This attaches to fat membranes present in cells and is deposited in the cochlear nuclei and basal ganglia. A crucial factor therefore is the amount of toxic bilirubin that can be transported in the baby's blood. This binding capacity depends on the health of the baby. A small, pre-term, acidotic baby is less tolerant of rises in bilirubin than a robust full-term neonate. It is therefore not possible to give a single level of bilirubin that is damaging. Hyperbilirubinaemia at a level that may become deposited in the brain is now treated by exchanging the infant's blood for blood which will not be attacked by the maternal antibodies. Otherwise excessive brainstem deposition of toxic bilirubin results in kernicterus, with seizures and death ensuing. Survivors are left with a legacy of athetosis and sensorineural deafness. However, the prophylactic immunization of rhesus negative mothers with anti-rhesus antibody (anti-D) has been successful in protecting neonates from the hazard of haemolytic disease. Although kernicterus was responsible for around 10% of cases of childood deafness in the 1950s, it is now very rarely encoutered in the UK.

# Deafness acquired in childhood

### Bacterial meningitis

Bacterial meningitis is the single most common cause of late acquired deafness. It is generally caused by *Haemophilus influenzae* or by meningococcal or pneumococcal infection. Suppurative labyrinthitis results from the organisms spreading directly to the inner ear from the cerebrospinal fluid. Suppurative destruction of the organ of Corti predictably occurs with the acute illness, with deafness and imbalance presenting before the child leaves hospital. However, the stability of the deafness is conjectural. It has been suggested that the onset may be delayed by several months. Conversely some recovery of auditory function may take place, and threshold fluctuations may occur due to a secondary endolymphatic hydrops. However, this instability may be more apparent than real. Up to 10% of survivors can be left with neurological handicaps and deafness. With early diagnosis and treatment most children recover without sequelae. However, the reasons why only some children suffer sequelae, remains perplexing and recent attention has been focused on primary prevention. *Haemophilus influenzae* type B vaccine (HIB) and Meningitis C vaccine are now offered as part of routine infant immunization with Meningitis C vaccine also being offered in a special national catch-up programme.

### Mumps and measles

Mumps and measles are also often considered to have caused a sensorineural hearing loss. However, the link between viral meningo-encephalitis and sensorineural hearing loss has been much more difficult to establish. Mumps has been reported to be a common cause of unilateral deafness, with measles more usually considered to have caused a bilateral, symmetrical sensorineural loss, moderate in degree. In some, there is a definite temporal association between the illness and onset of deafness, and with the introduction of combined measles, mumps and rubella immunization, the prevalence of unilateral deafness in the school population has fallen.

### Other causes

Other causes of acquired deafness are less common. Trauma to the cochlea resulting from concussive head injury, often following a traffic accident has become a worrying problem. The administration of certain drugs may also damage the cochlea, but while the list of potentially ototoxic drugs is extremely long, a catalogue of incidents resulting from current therapeutic practice is short. In the case of certain drugs, such as quinine, aspirin and the loop diuretics, the deafness is reversible. The chelating agent desferrioxamine has been implicated in the onset of deafness in children with thalassaemia. However, throughout the world, by far the most commonly used ototoxic drugs are the aminoglycosides (e.g. streptomycin, gentamicin, etc.). These are antibiotics, which are administered by injection. Because of their known ototoxicity, dosage is carefully calculated and it is mandatory to monitor plasma levels. It has long been clinically apparent that there is considerable individual suscep-tibilty to the ototoxic effects of the aminoglycosides. Recently it has been shown that aminoglycoside deafness may in many cases be familial and associated with a particular mitichondrial gene mutation. This is the first definite link between genetic and exogenous causes of deafness and has far-reaching implications verifying a long-suspected association. Clearly there is still much to be understood before the enmeshed and inter-related causes of childhood deafness are entirely explained.

## Hearing screens and surveillance

Public health measures aimed at identifying hearing-impaired children have been implemented in the UK since 1867, when the Manchester and Salford Ladies Sanitary Reform Association employed 'respectable working women to go from door to door offering physical help and health advice'. However, it is only very recently that the need to implement programmes aimed at early identification has been scientifically under-pinned. The communication abilities of deaf children have been demon-strably improved by early habilitation. Optimal detection should be within the first half of infancy, but achieving this is difficult. Because other sensory cues are utilized, deafness presents with great subtlety and may be extremely difficult to detect until disability is obvious. The author investi-gated these difficulties and found that fewer than half the parents of severely or profoundly deaf children had recognized the presence of the deafness in infancy, with less than 10% recognizing a mild or moderate impairment at this age. While parental concerns about a child's hearing should always be taken seriously, secondary prevention in the form of hearing screens or surveillance is still required.

Hearing surveillance is undertaken at various ages within the programmes of child health promotion. Every health surveillance exam-ination should include a hearing evaluation. These require a diagnostic awareness of the effects of deafness on a child's development. They also involve working in partnership with parents. Detection may be facilitated by the use of a check list, which informs parents of the hearing responses that should be expected at certain ages. Such lists are now routinely included in parent-held records (Figure 11.2).

Hearing screens are a distinct and separate component of child health programmes. They consist of simple tests, which identify previously unrecognized impairments. They should be sensitive (able to identify those with a hearing impairment), specific (able to identify those with normal hearing),and practicable and acceptable so that there is high coverage. Three hearing screens are current in the UK. Each will be dealt with briefly.

### Pure-tone sweep testing

The audiometric screening of schoolchildren was advised in the 1931 Annual Report of the Board of Education. It is a modification of pure-tone audiometry, with different frequencies being 'swept' through at fixed intensities. Because adverse testing conditions exist in many schools, a sweep at 25 or even 30 dB hearing level (HL) is often accepted as a pass. Test specificity is thereby improved, but sensitivity is reduced. Those children with a very mild loss may be missed. The overwhelming majority failing the screen have otitis media with effusion (OME). However, a small minority have perceptive losses, and retention of the school sweep is required for identification of those with a unilateral or mild bilateral sensorineural deafness.

---

**How well can your child hear?**

These checks help you find out if your child is hearing as well as would be expected at a particular age. They help you answer the hearing questions on the review pages.

**At 6 weeks** your baby should be startled by loud sounds like a door slamming. Babies react by blinking or widening their eyes if they are awake.

**At 3 months** your baby should be starting to turn the head towards sound made to one side. Your baby should pause and listen to sounds such as the washing machine, and unless screaming should usually be soothed by your voice.

**At 7 – 9 months** infants should be turning their head round to look for quiet sounds or voices. By 9 months he or she should be babbling tunefully.

**At 18 months** your child should respond to quietly spoken instructions, such as 'wave bye-bye' or 'give me the .........', without you needing to point or gesture.

**At 2½ years and older** your child should answer simple questions when asked in a quiet voice and without needing to look at your lips. He or she should enjoy listening to stories, and should hear common sounds like birds singing and the phone ringing. Speech over the phone should be heard in both ears.

**Hearing**

Your child's hearing will be tested at intervals and the results will be recorded on the next page

If you have any worries you should not wait for the next routine test, but should discuss them with your health visitor as soon as possible

**Figure 11.2:** A check list included in the Parent-held Child Health Record which informs parents of the hearing responses which should be expected by specific ages.

## The infant distraction test

The distraction test was initially described by Sir Alexander and Lady Ewing in 1944. It is based on the infant's maturing auditory behaviour and is usually utilized from 7 months developmental age. By this age, quiet sounds are localized at ear level on the horizontal plane. The test was first employed as a public health screen in the 1950s. Widespread implementation as the health visitors' distraction test (HVDT) followed. However, although seemingly simple, the HVDT hearing screen has proven to be frustratingly difficult. The test is illustrated in Figure 11.3.

The infant is sat facing forwards on the parent's knee. Two trained screeners are required, with a 'distractor' situated in the front and a 'tester' positioned behind the parent's chair. The distractor controls the infant's attention, manipulating a brief window of opportunity within which the tester presents a sound stimulus. Localization of the sound is then observed. Valid responses must be repeatable, and false turns eliminated with 'no-sound trials'. As a screen of hearing, repeatable, reliable responses should be present at 30 dBA.

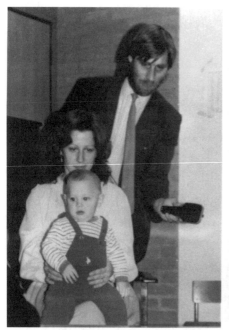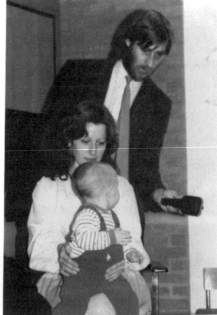

**Figure 11.3:** The infant distraction test undertaken with a hand-held warble-tone generator.

Traditional test stimuli have been high-frequency rattles, frequency-specific noise-makers and controlled vocalizations. However, frequency specificity is difficult to control and a more accurate stimulus can be delivered by a hand-held warble-tone generator. In practice, both sound sources offer different advantages. The distraction test is an indispensable technique for confirming infant hearing thresholds within the diagnostic clinic. Localization responses to frequency-appropriate stimuli are measured by a sound-level meter, enabling the hearing to be assessed over the speech-frequency range. However, despite this proven diagnostic value, the test has not been sensitively implemented as a screen. It requires a meticulous technique and is often implemented in less than ideal test conditions. Regular fieldwork training is required, but procedural errors remain problematic with stimuli being too loud and also broad-band in frequency composition. However, there is a more fundamental problem. Localization responses in deaf infants are difficult to assess. Hearing does not exist in isolation but is integrated with the other senses – and the deaf infant employs them all to detect almost imperceptible cues. Localization may occur when the tester is within the baby's peripheral vision, or when shadows, reflections, eye glances or even perfume cue the infant. Thus, the HVDT screen has not generally been effective and is no longer acceptable to many parents.

**Neonatal screening**

Even when the HVDT screen is operating effectively, habilitation is delayed until the second year of life. This is too late. In 1994, the National Deaf Children's Society recommended that 40% of bilateral congenital hearing impairments of moderate or worse degree be detected within the first six months of life. Neonatal screening is the only way to achieve this. At long last technological developments have made this possible. Currently three different technologies are available.

*The auditory response cradle*

The auditory response cradle, developed at Brunel University, is a microprocessor-controlled neonatal screening device. It automatically monitors the baby's head turn, head startle and change in body activity in response to a high-pass noise of 85 dB sound pressure level (SPL). Because behavioural responses to loud stimuli are monitored, it may less sensitively identify milder degrees of deafness.

*Auditory brainstem response (ABR)*

ABR testing has become the established method of measuring neonatal thresholds. Although traditional test methods are time-consuming, and can only be readily used to selectively screen a small percentage of the birth cohort, the development of automated ABR (AABR) has enabled this test to be used for universal neonatal screening. The AABR has an internally programmed template-matching algorithm, which measures for the presence of the ABR following the presentation of click stimuli at a pre-set intensity.

*Otoacoustic emission*

Otoacoustic emission recording offers another method for neonatal screening. The emissions were originally described in the late 1970s at the Institute of Laryngology and Otology, London (Kemp 1978). He subsequently developed simple non-invasive screening equipment for recording emissions evoked by a transient stimulus such as a click (transient evoked otoacoustic emissions or TEOAEs). A neonatal TEOAE test being undertaken as part of a universal screen is illustrated in Figure 11.4. The emissions are very quiet sounds produced by the outer hair cells of the normally functioning cochlea. As long as there is no blockage in the middle or external ear, they can be recorded by a microphone in the ear canal. The transducer required to deliver the click is sited alongside this

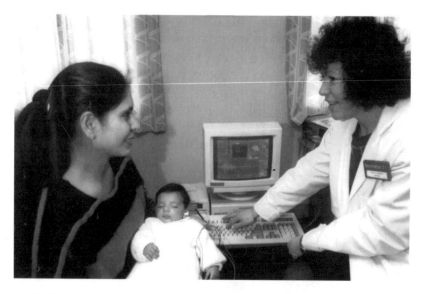

**Figure 11.4:** A transient evoked otoacoustic emission test being undertaken as part of a universal neonatal hearing screen (from Baldwin and Watkin 1997).

recording microphone. TEOAE recording tests the auditory system to the level of the cochlea. Emissions are absent even if there is a mild hearing loss, but their absence does not reveal the degree of impairment. Those without TEOAEs require a further threshold examination.

### Selective neonatal screens

The development of ABR allowed selective neonatal hearing screens to be undertaken. however the worth of selective screening has been questioned. This debate is by no means new. In the 1960s, much child health surveillance, along with the HVDT, was selective and restricted to those babies included on an 'at-risk' register. However, it was later concluded that such registers 'do no good and possibly do harm'. Despite this, neonatal testing by traditional ABR techniques has been feasible for only a selected cohort and the risk factors defined by the American Joint Committee on Infant Hearing have been widely adopted for use in the UK. It was optimistically thought that by selecting between 7 and 10% of the birth cohort, up to 70% of severe congenital hearing impairments could be identified. In the UK there has been further rationalization of the Joint Committee criteria. Admission of a baby for special care increases the risk for deafness by a factor of ten. These babies, plus those with a family history of permanent childhood deafness, or a craniofacial abnormality, have been targeted for testing.

### Universal neonatal screens

With the availability of new technology universal neonatal hearing screening (UNHS) has now been recommended on both sides of the Atlantic. It has already become well established in over 1000 programmes in the USA. Although it is being introduced cautiously in the UK, it is realistic to expect a UK-wide UNHS programme will be in situ by 2003 (National Deaf Children's Society 2000) Both TEOAE and AABR recording make this possible. The emission test is very sensitive to mild impairments, and the failure rate is therefore increased by vernix present in the ear shortly after birth. Specificity of the screen is improved to around 99% by implementing a second out-patient test, or by employing an AABR test before discharge from the maternity ward on those in whom a TEOAE was not recorded. Both tests are required to identify those babies where there is a pre-neural emission response, but an absent neural ABR. Such auditory neuropathies have generally been reported amongst those babies requiring special care. The introduction of UNHS has opened up a new and challenging era in paediatric audiology, enabling the detection in early infancy of the majority of children with a disabling hearing impairment. This is the essential prerequisite for effective management of the deaf child.

# Confirmation of childhood deafness

Confirming that a child has a permanent deafness has far-reaching implications. There are implications for the family, relatives and friends, those providing healthcare, speech therapists, teachers, nursery and playgroup staff, educational psychologists, education officers, social services, the voluntary agencies and, most of all, the child. Confirmation must therefore be unequivocal and correct. Small wonder that we put our faith in a 'paediatric test battery', even though there may be redundancy within the different tests. The battery includes, Otoadmittance, ABR and a variety of psychoacoustic tests. These have been detailed in Chapters 5 and 6. Additional tests confined to paediatric practice are further described.

## Behavioural observation audiometry

Behavioural observation audiometry (BOA) is an assessment of the behavioural responses to sound elicited when infants are tested under structured conditions. The responses observed may be categorized as being reflexive, attentive or autonomic. Reflexive behaviours include changes in head, body and limb movements, eye blinks, arousal and increased sucking. Autonomic responses include changes in heart rate and respiration, with attentive responses including quieting, breath holding, eye turning and cessation of activities such as sucking. BOA depends on many variables. Stimulus parameters such as bandwidth, rise time and rhythm affect the infant's behaviour, with speech being most effective and bands of noise being more effective than pure tones. However, stimulus intensity is also very important, with loud sounds being required to elicit reflexive responses and quieter sounds eliciting attentive behaviours. Unfortunately, problems arise with both. Suprathreshold stimulation is required to elicit reflexive responses and these may be provoked in the presence of a recruiting cochlear deafness. This problem is encountered with the auropalpebral reflex (APR), which is one of the most widely used behavioural observations. It is an involuntary eye-blink plus a startle or head jerk, in response to a signal of around 80–85 dB SPL. It is absent in severe or profound deafness, but present in milder recruiting impairments. It is elicited at louder levels when there is a conductive loss and is absent in some neurologically damaged babies. It is therefore very difficult to extrapolate from the observation of reflexive responses to sound.

However, hearing thresholds *may* be more realistically reflected by attentive behaviours. An important variable affecting the observation of attentive responses is the state of the infant. All behavioural responses depend on the infant's arousal state, and habituation is rapid. Attentive responses can best be seen when the infant is quiet and drifting in and out of sleep. When in this state, behavioural responses to quieter levels may be observed. Intra- and inter-subject variability also result from difficulties with observer interpretation. Reliability can be increased by the use of video recording or by applying auditory masking to the observers. Clearly many of the problems inherent in BOA cannot be readily overcome. Yet, unless electrophysiological tests are available, BOA may be the only test available for young infants and also for older, multiply handicapped children. Unfortunately the difficulties inherent in the method may prevent the accurate assessment of hearing by even the most astute and experienced.

**Visual reinforcement audiometry**

Much of our paediatric testing has been dictated by behavioural tests initially described by the Ewings in Manchester during the 1940s. More recently, testing by visual reinforcement audiometry (VRA) has been developed and refined. Its place in the routine paediatric test battery is now completely accepted in the UK. It allows the assessment of thresholds from around 6 months developmental age, until the age at which play audiometry is possible.

The child sits on the parent's lap, or at a small chair in front of a table in a soundproofed room. The tester is seated with the child and maintains his or her attention to the midline. A visual reinforcer, such as a colourful display (Figure 11.5), is illuminated at eye level when the auditory stimulus is presented. Sometimes it is more effective if the tester is in a separate room observing through a one-way mirror. However, activation of the toy and presentation of the stimulus can readily be undertaken by the tester seated in the same room as the child. A narrow band noise or warble tone is employed as the stimulus. Measurement of stimulus intensity with a sound level meter held at the ear is possible, but usually adds to procedural confusion, and the test is better undertaken within a calibrated sound field. The techniques are intuitive to anyone accustomed to paediatric testing.

The child is initially conditioned to associate the visual reinforcer with the sound stimulus. This must be presented at suprathreshold levels. This association is usually established after four or so presentations. The intensity is then reduced until threshold has been achieved. The visual reinforcer is only activated if the child responds to the stimulus. No-sound trials are used in the same way as for the infant distraction test. An advantage of VRA is that it can be undertaken using ear inserts. The 18-month-old child in Figure 11.5 is being tested with VRA and ear inserts. A foam eartip is inserted into the ear and connected by a tube to a sound

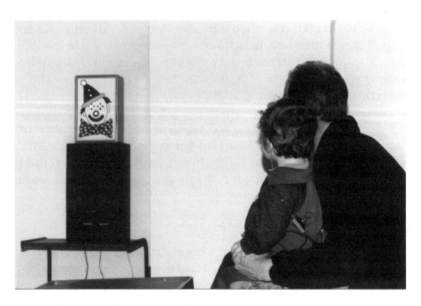

**Figure 11.5:** Visual reinforcement audiometry using ear inserts.

transducer, which is pinned to the clothing and plugged into the audiometer. The transducers may be connected directly to the earmoulds of a hearing-aid user. The use of insert earphones allows audiometric separation of the ears even in infancy – an advantage not shared by any other behavioural tests undertaken at this age. Unfortunately habituation to the reinforcer can occur before threshold is reached. The use of two or more reinforcers (e.g. stacked boxes with different arrays of toys that can be illuminated in turn), can delay this. Reinforcement with touch, vibration or even food can be used for children with learning difficulties, multiple handicaps or visual impairments. These procedures all have an established place within the paediatric test battery and are now being routinely used alongside the more traditional behavioural tests.

**Play audiometry**

Play audiometry is possible with most children aged 30 months and over, and even with some below this age. The child responds to sounds by performing a simple play task, but an ability to wait for the stimulus presentation before precipitately launching into the activity is essential. Initially the child needs to be conditioned to respond to the sound stimuli. Such conditioning is more usually accepted if sounds are delivered in a calibrated field. A hand-held sound generator or a speaker connected to an audiometer can be used. A variety of toys that facilitate the clear observation of a conditioned response should be available, e.g. men in boat, balls on stick, etc.

The tester gains rapport with the child through the toys and conditions appropriate responses to the stimuli: 'When the little man makes a noise he jumps into the boat' (Figure 11.6). Verbal explanations should be kept to a minimum. Long entreaties simply confuse and it is entirely possible to condition without any verbal explanation whatsoever. A visual demonstration of the association between stimulus presentation and play activity is the most effective method of explaining the task in hand.

Sound-field testing only reveals information about the better-hearing ear, but once conditioned, most children can be encouraged to use headphones. A single headphone can be employed, but the wearing of the headset allows masking to be employed and ensures audiometric separation of the ears. Modifications of the standard Hughson–Westlake audiometric technique may be required, with the achievement of thresholds to a low, mid and high frequency. It is essential that the initial conditioning should be well above threshold. Conditioning fails when the sound has not been heard and cannot be associated with the play activity. An impossible task has been asked of the child. Unreasonable demands, more than anything else, precipitate a downward spiral of non-cooperation during play audiometry. Even though a jaded tester may feel ready to capsize the little men in their boat, a test which entertains facilitates the completion of a reliable, masked pure-tone audiogram even in the young pre-school

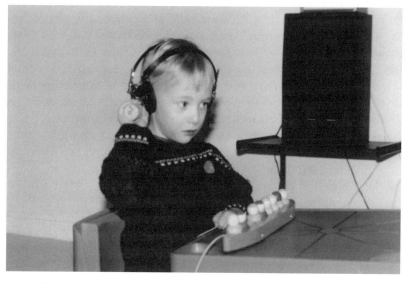

**Figure 11.6:** Play audiometry – 'When the little man makes a noise he jumps into the boat'.

child. This is an important milestone in the audiological management of any child.

## Paediatric tests of speech perception

Tests of speech perception are an integral part of the test battery. A child's hearing loss will almost always have been noted because of difficulties with the hearing of speech, and therefore these tests have a greater face validity than psychoacoustic or electrophysiological assessments. This may be more apparent than real. A large variety of tests exist, and the validity of any deductions depends on the test used. A test that makes available a large number of redundant cues reflects more realistically the child's hearing disability at a higher linguistic level. Audiovisual sentence tests offer this, but are very rarely used, even in older children. Paediatric speech tests generally use monosyllabic words. Such tests have low redundancy and reflect hearing impairment rather than any real-life disability. However, despite this limitation they have become a necessary part of the paediatric hearing examination.

The monosyllabic word lists compiled by Arthur Boothroyd (AB word lists) are those most commonly employed for older children. They can be delivered by speaker or headphone and performance/intensity function curves plotted. Toy tests are usually employed for younger children. Those constructed by Kendal and more recently McCormick are most popular. The tests consist of toys paired by vowel, e.g. house/cow; cup/duck; tree/key. Children with normal hearing can discriminate such monosyllables at voice levels of 40 dBA. Although the McCormick toy test consists of seven pairs of toys, the number may be reduced to test children as young as 18 months of age.

The toys are placed one by one in front of the child. They must be within the child's vocabulary, but the reticent should not be pressed into naming them. Live voice presentation is generally used with young children. The child is asked to point to the toy in response to the request 'show me the ...'. The tester's mouth should be completely obscured (Figure 11.7). Some prefer to administer the test from the child's side, although this by itself does not audiometrically separate the ears. The tests can be flexibly delivered, and as long as the basic rules of their administration are understood, they provide a very useful impairment measure. The toy tests have now been automated with speaker presentation of digitally stored speech waveforms. This ensures greater reliability of presentation for the inexperienced. There is inevitably some loss of the flexibility, which is so important in engaging the taciturn and the developmentally delayed, but generally child participation is good.

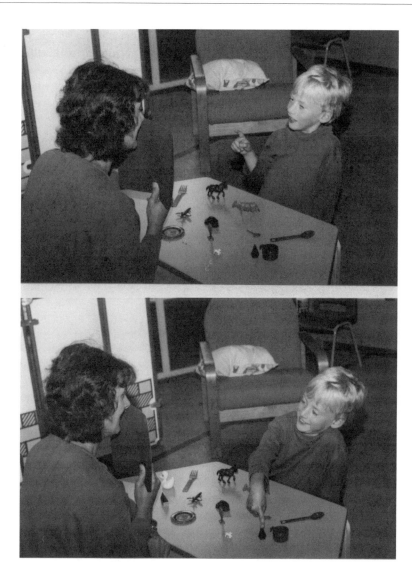

**Figure 11.7:** The McCormick toy test – 'Show me the ......'.

The ability to engage the child with the different tests in an age-appropriate test battery, should facilitate a reliable examination of hearing in almost all children. Accurate assessments should be possible for all ages, ranging from the teenager embarking on adulthood, down to the infant embarking on life. To the non-cognisant, physiological and electrophysiological tests often have greater scientific appeal, and they unquestionably have an important part to play in the paediatric test battery. However, the undertaking of behavioural tests requires the acquisition of different, reactive and flexible, child-friendly skills. Although they may appear deceptively simple, their value lies in their ability to both confirm and characterize even a very young child's hearing, and this subjective evaluation cannot be replaced.

# Chapter 12
# The management of deafness in childhood

PETER WATKIN AND ANNE DUFFY

## Multidisciplinary management – the cornerstone of effective habilitation

During the latter half of the 20th century, there was a gradual realization that the effective management of deaf children depended on their early identification. At long last this has become a real and practicable possibility and children are now being confirmed with deafness at younger and younger ages. However, while this is an important prerequisite for improving the effectiveness of intervention, it is only the first step in optimizing the quality of life for the deaf child. Diagnosing the impairment is but the beginning.

Evaluating the effect the deafness has on the child's performance of auditory tasks is necessary to facilitate participation in these activities. In particular, communication is affected. The world is an immeasurably complex environment in which to be born. We all spend a lifetime in a continuous spiral of questioning and learning. Effective communication is fundamental to gaining understanding and deafness has the potential of devastating this. Such difficulties cannot be redressed by conventional medical models of care. A seamless delivery of non-conflicting multidisciplinary input is required. This relationship is illustrated in Figure 12.1. At the very hub of the required model is the parent. Professor Court, in an eponymously named report into child health, lamented the fact that 'professions tend to gather a mystique to themselves which can be predatory to the proper role of the layman' (Court 1976).

This concern is particularly pertinent when increasingly esoteric hearing tests are used, and when subsequent management may appear to the incognisant to revolve around technology. Perversely, parental difficulties may be compounded by the best current practices. With identification

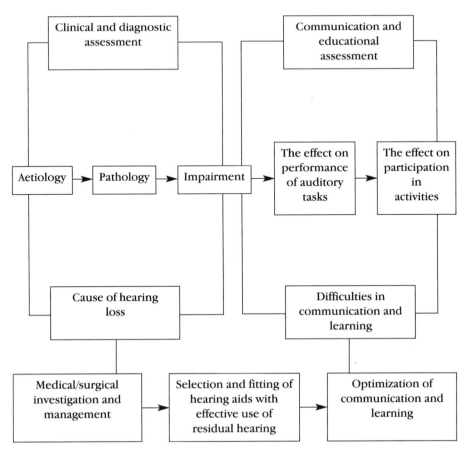

**Figure 12.1:** The multidisciplinary management of the deaf child (adapted from Baldwin and Watkin 1997).

possible before the effects have become fully evident, and interventions successfully facilitating auditory performance, small wonder that some families are uncertain that their child has special needs. Yet the family is central to the child's audiological care. For habilitation to be optimal, parents must be equal and valued members of the multidisciplinary team. Parental attitudes will, however, differ according to circumstance and should not be presumed. Deaf families may have no anxieties that their children are deaf. Naturally they resent the view of deafness as a medical condition to be investigated and treated, instead regarding it as part of the rich spectrum of humanness. They cherish and protect their communication, language and culture. Yet this does not negate the need for early and appropriate management of their children. For all parents, attitudes and aspirations must be individually assessed.

# Medical management – investigating the cause of the deafness

Even though in the conventional sense there is no prospect of a medical 'cure' for sensorineural deafness, every deaf child deserves medical investigation. A protocol of investigations is detailed in Table 12.1. While a causative exogenous factor may appear obvious, aetiologies may be multifactorial and these may only become evident with ongoing paediatric and otological examinations. The latter may now usefully include paediatric tests of vestibular function. Other specialist examinations should also now be routine. Vision is a vital sensory input for the hearing-impaired child and ophthalmological examination is necessary to exclude the many deafness–ocular syndromes, as well as the retinopathies of congenital infections and importantly the retinitis pigmentosa of Usher's syndrome. In early childhood, this diagnosis requires an electroretinogram. With the reduction in environmental insults, half the cases of childhood deafness are now attributable to genetic causes, and therefore the pedigree analysis and dysmorphology examination offered by clinical geneticists make an important diagnostic contribution. With the availability of molecular diagnosis for a wide range of deafness genes just around the corner, this input will surely become routine for every deaf child.

# Genetic counselling

Genetic counselling should be available to the parents of all affected children. At present it largely consists of counselling the family about the

**Table 12.1:** A protocol for investigating childhood deafness

---

1.  Clinical history including maternity and perinatal history, with specific inquiry into the presence of risk factors for congenital or acquired deafness. Also inquiry into family history of deafness or syndromic condition, with appropriate pedigree analysis
2.  Paediatric, dysmorphologic and otological physical examination
3.  Haematological investigations, including full blood picture, electrolytes and urea, thyroid function, TORCH antibodies and, if appropriate, chromosome analysis
4.  Urine examination for organic acids, amino acids, mucopolysaccharides, haematuria and viruria, if appropriate
5.  Electrocardiography to exclude a prolonged QT interval
6.  Radiology to exclude intracerebral calcification, and computerized tomography of the petrous bones when practicable
7.  Ophthalmological examination to exclude retinopathies, lens opacity and visual dysacuity
8.  Audiometric examination of first degree relatives, and genetic opinion

---

chance of recurrence. Clearly the timing and the information imparted must be sensitively individualized according to need. Additionally, despite the enormous strides in genetic knowledge, uncertainties remain. Although familial deafness usually follows simple Mendelian rules, conditions associated with deafness often demonstrate variation in severity (the expressivity of the genotype) and variation in the proportion of those with the gene mutation who actually have the condition (the penetrance of the genotype). Thus it may be possible to offer a precise recurrence chance of 50% for an autosomal dominant deafness traceable through one of the parents. However, the physical features may vary, as in Waardenburg syndrome type 1, where only around 20% have a hearing deficit (see Chapter 11).

Autosomal recessive deafness, with a recurrence chance of one in four, occurs when normally hearing parents are both carriers of the same deafness gene. This chance is clearer when the parents are consanguineous or when they already have two deaf children. However, for families with the first affected child, the chance of recurrence has been calculated empirically from the pedigree analyses of many such families and has been found to be around 10%. This is 100 times greater than the chance of any couple having a deaf baby. Other equally difficult problems may make counselling necessarily imprecise. Even in families where both parents have an inherited deafness, heterogeneity may make the mode of transmission uncertain. Most such parents are likely to be homozygous for an autosomal recessive gene but the chance of this being the same mutant gene is remarkably low. The often-held assumption that every child of such a marriage will be deaf is therefore far from correct.

It is apparent that the mode of inheritance and variability of expression and penetrance may not be clear even from a detailed pedigree analysis, and currently many recurrence chances remain empirically based. However, the routine availability of DNA testing, will, in the near future, remove much of this guesswork and an informed genetic opinion should always be made available.

## The provision of hearing aids for children

Children normally develop language and the ability to communicate through hearing other people speak. The majority of deaf children have enough residual hearing to allow oral/auditory communication if optimum amplification is available. It is therefore tremendously important for such children to use their residual hearing with early and effective amplification. Of course, this generalization cannot apply to all children. Spoken communication may not be the preference of the family, and the first language may be a manual system. In other children the severity of deafness does not allow access to enough of the speech signal to make spoken communication a realistic aim. Even then amplification should enable audition of the rhythms of speech and of environmental sounds. For these children cochlear implants may offer an alternative (Chapter 19); however, for the majority of deaf children, effective amplification with hearing aids is beneficial. This can only be achieved with appropriate fitting and consistent use.

## How do we select appropriate hearing aids for children?

The aim of hearing-aid fitting is to allow the hearing-impaired child to hear sound at levels which are both comfortable and safe. Ideally this must include access to his or her own speech, and to the speech of others. But how is this achieved in a child or even a very young baby? Although it cannot be a 'once and for all' process, there has to be an initial selection of hearing aids which offer the physical and electroacoustic characteristics required by the individual child.

## The selection of physical characteristics

When the first edition of this book was published, the only NHS hearing aid available was body-worn (BW) and of limited power. It was simply not possible to fit an aid that was child-friendly. However, with a rapidly increasing range of aids and earmoulds, this may now be achieved. BW aids may still be used for children when acoustic feedback limits the use of a behind-the-ear (BTE) instrument. This may occur when high power is required for a child with a profound hearing loss or when a child has an additional motor disability with poor head control. However, it is now usual to fit binaural BTE instruments even when the child has a profound deafness. Unilateral fitting is only undertaken when justifiable.

The size of the aid is important. With the increasing requirement to fit hearing aids in the first weeks of infancy, the use of miniature aids is not simply a matter of cosmetics. A comfortable fit is required for all ages. Children's hearing aids should also have facilities to make them compatible with other listening devices, such as type II radio aid systems. They also need to be tamper-proof, with secure battery compartments and volume covers. The recent availability of computer adjustment has also allowed some electroacoustic flexibility, which enables the settings of the aids to be tailored later, if the initial settings have been made on limited audiological data.

The earmould is an integral part of the child's amplification system, since well-fitting moulds prevent acoustic feedback. Fortunately, earmould technology has also progressed to allow this even for neonates. Both moulds and hearing aids are now available in a rainbow assortment of colours. Although seemingly trivial, anything encouraging aid usage is important and should not be undervalued. While it is self-evident that there is little point in wearing a cosmetically acceptable aid unless it is electroacoustically appropriate, the converse is equally true. To be consistently worn, the aid has to be physically appropriate and acceptable.

## The selection of electroacoustic characteristics

Hearing aids that give sufficient but not excessive gain over an appropriate frequency range are required; this involves using amplification targets that are suitable for children. While adult prescriptions use variations of the 'half gain' rule, the approach is fundamentally different in children. In an adult, hearing aids can be modified with the help of responses from the patient, but with children the fitting often has to be undertaken with limited audiological data. Additionally, the amplification requirements for those prelingually deaf, are quite different from those who have already acquired spoken language.

Paediatric methods are therefore based on a speech spectrum approach – aiming to provide amplified speech, which is audible and comfortable across a broad frequency range. But what speech is to be made audible? Although speech intensity delivered from a distance of one metre is usually around 60–70 dB SPL, the actual level varies considerably. It may be increased by some 20 dB SPL when a mother is holding her baby in her arms. Gender and age differences also occur. The child must also monitor his or her own voice and, on occasions, this may be very loud!

Hearing aids fitted to render speech audible can therefore never be ideal in all situations and a compromise is achieved by providing a gain and frequency response which aim to make 'average' speech audible. The compromise signal is a long-term average spectrum of speech (LTASS) being used at a conversational level and at a distance of one metre. Such a prescriptive strategy is the desired sensation level method (DSL 7, University of Western Ontario). As suggested by its name, the method aims to amplify average speech so that the different frequency components are heard at a 'desired sensation level' above the child's hearing threshold. This sensation level differs according to frequency. It takes into account the upward spread of masking, the greater sensation level required over the high frequencies, the reduced sensation level needed with increasing severity of deafness and the need to restore the natural ear-canal amplification, which is eliminated by inserting an earmould. The DSL method gives the real ear-aided-response values, which are required to amplify the LTASS to the desired sensation levels as a function of hearing threshold and audiometric frequency.

The desired real ear-aided targets are calculated in terms of dB SPL at the eardrum. A visual display of the different parameters, plotted in dB SPL on an SPL-O-Gram chart is illustrated in Figure 12.2. The method also calculates a desired maximum output in dB SPL for the hearing aid. Correct output limiting is crucially important if the hearing aid is to be tolerated.

Once the amplification requirements have been calculated, electroacoustic response shaping of a chosen hearing aid is required. Both the gain and maximum output of hearing aids are conventionally defined in terms of 2cc coupler measurements. However, the sound pressure level achieved by coupling the hearing aid to the ear is a function of the individual ear-canal characteristics. In an infant's small ear canal, sound levels may be increased by 20 dB. The child's real ear-to-coupler difference (RECD) must therefore be known. This can be simply obtained by measuring the same sound in both a 2cc coupler and with a probe tube microphone in the ear canal. When probe tube measurements prove too difficult, estimated RECD transformations by age and frequency may be employed. Although there is inter-subject variation, these estimates allow electroacoustically appropriate aids to be selected, even when probe tube measures are impracticable. If the increased sound level resulting from the reduced ear-canal size is disregarded then overamplification is inevitable.

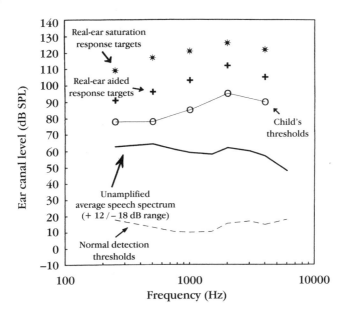

**Figure 12.2:** The SPL-O-Gram employed in the DSL method for fitting hearing aids (DSL® University of Western Ontario).

## The verification of amplification

Once aids have been selected and fitted, it is essential that benefit is assessed. Proper validation can only be undertaken over time by assessing the reduction of real-life disability. However, early verification is also necessary. This may be undertaken in two different ways.

### Probe tube microphone measurement systems

These systems have become widely available. It has been recommended that no facility should undertake paediatric hearing-aid fitting unless such a system is in regular use. It offers verification 'audiology by acronym'. The amplification provided by a hearing instrument at the eardrum of the patient is measured by means of a thin, flexible probe tube microphone placed in the ear canal. This amplification is termed the real ear-insertion response (REIR).

Several stages are required to measure the REIR. The system in place in a child is illustrated in Figure 12.3. Initially a signal of known SPL is emitted from a speaker and this is remeasured in the unoccluded ear canal. This quantifies the natural amplification of the external ear as the real ear-unaided response (REUR). The hearing aid is then placed in the ear and the real ear-aided response is measured (REAR). Subtraction of the two reveals the REIR. The REIR at a specific frequency is referred to as the real ear-insertion gain (REIG) and the insertion gain can be shaped to meet prescriptive targets. The great advantage of this verification methodology is that the amplification supplied independently at each eardrum can be relatively easily measured, allowing modification against calculated prescriptive targets. The method also enables the recording of multiple response characteristics to multiple signal levels. This is increasingly important for the verification of the latest non-linear instruments.

### Measurement of functional gain

This is the second method employed for amplification verification. Aided tests of speech perception offer the greatest validity. The speech perception tests described in Chapter 11 are undertaken with the child unaided and aided. Improvements are measured. To witness them is indeed gratifying for both parents and professionals, and they strongly reinforce the benefits of hearing-aid usage. However, even tests of speech feature perception way be beyond the capabilities of young, prelingually deaf children. Even when speech has been acquired, improvements may be subtle and difficult to assess. Thus a 50% unaided discrimination score on a single AB word list would have to improve by almost 25% to demonstrate a significant aided benefit. Similar large critical differences exist for other speech perception tests. Surrogate measures of functional gain are therefore usually used.

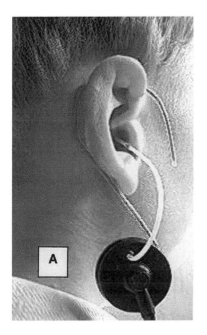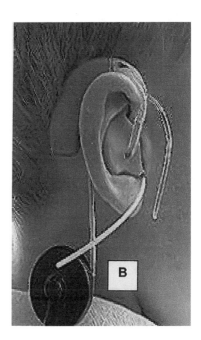

**Figure 12.3:** The measurement of (a) the real ear-unaided response (REUR) and (b) the real ear-aided response (REAR) using a probe tube microphone.

The use of sound-field threshold measurement is such a surrogate. Unaided sound-field thresholds are obtained using the behavioural conditioning techniques, described in Chapter 11. Warble tones, calibrated in dB SPL, are delivered through a speaker in a sound field. These stimuli prevent calibration inaccuracies resulting from the formation of standing waves. Behavioural thresholds are obtained with the child aided and unaided. Comparison of the two gives a measure of the functional gain across the frequency range. Comparison is also made with the LTASS (Figure 12.4).

Ideally, the amplified hearing should be above the LTASS, demonstrating the audibility of the different frequency components of conversational speech at a distance of one metre. Aid adjustments are possible. Such measures are of great benefit. Unlike probe tube measurements, they demonstrate to parents and professionals the actual level of aided hearing. They reinforce improvements achieved and also demonstrate inadequacies. Unfortunately there are limitations. As in all sound-field testing, it is difficult to audiometrically separate the ears. The cooperation required by the child may be excessive, test and retest reliability may be poor, information about frequency resolution is difficult to achieve and functional gain measures cannot verify all the benefits of non-linear amplification. While

Aided hearing thresholds

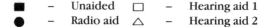

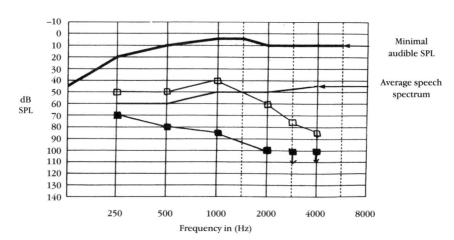

**Figure 12.4:** The functional gain measured by free field warble aones. Note that amplification above the long-term average speech spectrum (LTASS) is achieved up to 1 kHz, but at frequencies above this the LTASS is not audible to the child.

some of these reservations 'talk up' difficulties, others are well-founded and, as in so many aspects of audiology, there is an important place for both verification methods within a test battery approach.

## The introduction of habilitation for the newly diagnosed deaf child

The selection and fitting of appropriate hearing aids is, however, only a first step. Although there may be practical difficulties, these can be overcome. A much greater difficulty is the achievement of consistent hearing-aid use. The effective use of residual hearing depends on the use of amplification within an environment that provides both a good-quality signal and a good-quality listening experience. This can only be achieved through the introduction and ongoing implementation of appropriate habilitation strategies.

At the point of diagnosis, it is vital for the parents of the deaf child that all professionals work together in a way that is both supportive and informative. The reactions of parents when told that their child has a hearing impairment will vary according to a number of factors and according to the age and level of hearing of the child. Parents who have had no experience of deafness require simple and clear explanations of the prognosis, but those who are themselves deaf or have had experience of the deaf community may well wish to tackle the issues in ways that have been influenced by their own experience and knowledge.

Although in the UK the 'key worker' advising on early management may be a habilitatory audiologist, or occasionally another health professional, at this time it is nearly always a teacher of the deaf. Peripatetic teachers of the deaf have fulfilled a parental guidance role since the 1930s and it is now common practice for local education authorities (LEAs) to employ a teacher of the deaf to work with preschool children and their families as part of a discrete or generic support service.

The teacher should be involved from the point of diagnosis or hearing-aid issue. Large hospitals or cochlear implant centres also employ teachers of the deaf to work with their patients. The role of the teacher of the deaf in supporting the progress of the child can be most significant. He or she visits the family at home on a regular, often weekly, basis and can be instrumental in determining the approach taken by the family with regard to communication and future schooling.

Other professionals working with the family need to be aware of the statutory and local framework in which this advice will be given. The Department for Education has issued a Code of Practice for Children with Special Educational Needs (1994), which provides guidance in following the statutory requirements of the 1981 and 1993 Education Acts.

A five-stage process for the management of children with special educational needs is set out. These range from awareness of the child's needs at stages 1 to 3, an assessment at stage 4, and the issuing of a Statement of Special Educational Needs at stage 5. However, interpretation of the recommendations can vary between LEAs and educational management of the newly diagnosed deaf child is greatly dependent on local provision and policy.

Several models exist for providing this support and will vary significantly according to area. Thus, if a child is diagnosed in a large centre where the teacher of the deaf is present this teacher may support the family through hearing-aid fitting and will then contact the local support service, who will arrange home visits. Elsewhere, where diagnosis and hearing-aid fitting is undertaken by a district service, the local teacher of the deaf should be present from the outset. This teacher supports the family through hearing-aid fitting and at home, liaises regularly with the local audiological team, and involves other agencies such as social services.

Alternatively, a child may be diagnosed outside the district of residence, return home and await contact with the local teacher of the deaf. Contact may not be immediate if the local service is under-resourced. This is unsatisfactory and may result in the child making disappointing progress in the important days following diagnosis. In all cases, successful outcome following diagnosis depends to a large degree on the response made by the support service and the effectiveness of the early intervention.

The speech and language therapist may also be a member of the multi-disciplinary team providing early management. Although many parents and some professionals may perceive speech and language therapists as the experts on articulation and speech production, their remit is far broader. They have a comprehensive understanding of the development of early language and in many cases can help to piece together the full picture of the child's emerging communication skills. Some have specialist qualifications in working with deaf children, while others may be part of a generic therapy service. Some may be happy for the teacher of the deaf to take a lead role in the early stages of an intervention programme, while others, particularly those attached to diagnostic teams, become immediately involved.

Voluntary agencies also have an important role to play in supporting parental access to information. There is a requirement on diagnosing agencies to ensure that families are aware of how to contact the relevant organizations. Early contact with the National Deaf Children's Society, the Royal National Institute for Deaf People or the British Deaf Association can be invaluable, especially for parents who have no previous experience of deafness.

## The continuing role of the peripatetic home teacher

The School Curriculum and Assessment Authority views educational provision for the early years in terms of six main areas, all of which represent desirable outcomes for children's learning, and distinguishes that provision from medical or social services support. The six main areas are:

* personal and social development
* language and literacy
* mathematics
* knowledge and understanding of the world
* physical development
* creative development.

While it may seem impossible to consider planning in these terms for a newly diagnosed neonate, it should be borne in mind that educational provision should be clearly aiming to foster learning outcomes within the overall development of the growing child. The level of support offered should vary according to need, the development of the child and the requirements of the parents. Parents must be full partners in this early educational provision, with some services formally asking parents to take on board their responsibilities in this partnership. Parental views on what outcomes they wish their child to achieve must be sought. In any case, the parents have the right to demand of their peripatetic teacher that he or she is sympathetic to their home life, situation and culture. Fundamental to the teacher/parent partnership will be a common desire to support and extend the child's development of language.

## Approaches to communication

Language is fundamental to the learning process and the approach taken by parents and professionals is likely to have a long-lasting impact on a deaf child's education. All LEA services have a policy with regard to communication of deaf children. While this should be in written form, and accessible to parents, it can sometimes exist solely as a matter of practice, being steered by the teachers of the deaf involved. For many there still exists some uncertainty between the need to promote language development and the desire to elicit speech. The young deaf child can acquire a visual signed language, a spoken language or, over time, become bilingual. However it is the development of language, which is all important. Stephen Fry autobiographically expressed this importance: 'I am not actually sure that I am capable of thought, let alone feeling, except through language', and he quoted Oscar Wilde who wrote 'language ... is the parent, not the child, of thought' (Fry 1998).

Both communication practice and policy have developed and continue to evolve. The terminology used encompasses changes in practice. Recent definitions have been proposed.

### Monolingual approaches to communication

These are based on the use of English in all its forms – spoken, written and manually represented. They take as their premise the view that the mastery of English is of prime importance and that to learn to use English the child must be exposed to it and encouraged to develop it as a first or only language. There are four main monolingual approaches:

- *Natural aural*: children are presented with spoken English in a way that supports natural development of spoken language and makes full use of residual hearing.
- *Structured oral*: spoken language is taught systematically and includes structured sequences or steps aimed at the development of English through the use of residual hearing and the process of acquiring vocabulary and syntax, often supported by written language.
- *Maternal reflective*: this supports the development of spoken language through the types of interaction which are found between an immature and mature language user: the deaf child and the adult. This conversation acts as a base for reinforcement by written and spoken practice.
- *Sign-supported English/Signed English:* sign is used to support spoken English, which can be presented in any of the above ways. Signed English employs a manual representation of all words and grammatical structures while sign-supported English aims to provide a manual 'clue' for the spoken English which it supports.

**A sign bilingual approach to communication**

This approach uses British Sign Language (BSL) and English as two distinct languages. BSL, as the language of the deaf community, is given parity with English and with any home languages, and the development and success in both BSL and English, in all forms, is afforded value. There is a strong and growing argument that BSL supports the child not only in developing a fluent and strong language base, but also in creating a sense of value as a member of a minority group with its own culture and identity.

Views with regard to the communication approaches best used with deaf children have been subject to debate and dispute and are still shifting as new research is produced. What remains important is that parents are given informed and impartial advice on which they can base a decision about the future communication management of their child. As a general premise, a child who cannot hear his or her own voice when aided is unlikely to develop speech at a level that will support language and learning and so afford full access to education. The need to know how much useful, functional hearing the child has is therefore fundamental to the decision-making process. Yet this information may not be immediately available. Continuous assessment by the parents and those working with the child is essential to inform the decisions. Many parents will find this an almost impossible dilemma and will feel, following diagnosis, that they are returning home with a child who is a different one from the one they thought they knew. Any communication approach is therefore likely to provide them with further challenges and they will need ample opportunity to discuss and possibly research the alternatives themselves.

The peripatetic teacher needs to provide communication advice to parents based on knowledge of the child's audiological and environmental functioning coupled with a professional judgement backed by expertise. The many variables affecting a child's language development must be taken into account. The teacher must then support the parents through a decision which will ultimately have a tremendous effect on their child's personal, social and educational progress. Questions should then regularly be asked about why a child's language is developing as it is. Could it be bettered with better aiding or a different approach?

Decisions about whether or not to introduce sign as a method of communication have to be made. These must be based on more than a confirmed belief on the part of the teacher or service concerned and should be reviewed regularly. If necessary, signing classes should be available. These will be vital to enable both parents and other family members to keep ahead of the sign development of their child.

## Additional education support

Early programmes of management will offer, in addition to guidance on communication and language, audiological support and advice on the development of learning skills. This support may be offered to the family at home and within group settings. Audiological support will aim to provide parents with full information about all aspects of deafness as well as a clear explanation of their child's level of hearing. The teacher will help them to understand how hearing aids work and how to encourage their use with their child. He or she may provide ideas of useful toys and how to play with them, modelling appropriate ways to play in order to develop language and learning.

As the child grows older, there are benefits to both child and family in meeting other families with deaf children. Support groups can offer parents the chance to share experiences among themselves as well as offering a more structured programme of information giving, with deaf awareness training and access to a wider group of professionals. While parents learn and share, so too can the children, within a well-planned programme of play and activities. The peripatetic teacher may also link families and will introduce them to the LEA as they embark on their involvement with the Code of Practice for Children with Special Educational Needs.

# Assessment and school placement

The teacher of the deaf will work with the parents and other involved professionals to provide an ongoing assessment of progress. The teacher may also support children when they attend school, assessing progress and providing advice to teachers and support workers on the management of the deaf pupil in class. Ongoing assessment is thus an integral component of the educational role. In addition, deaf children require a statutory assessment, which serves to help the LEA to determine the additional and exceptional provision a child may require. A full, formal assessment will involve participation by health, social services and education representatives as well as seeking the views of the parents. At this stage an educational psychologist can provide more detailed information on the child's cognitive and developmental functioning, although the LEA is still required to seek the views of a specialist teacher of the deaf. For some children, their needs may be significant enough to warrant a Statement of Special Educational Needs, which outlines the needs and the provision that the LEA proposes to make to meet them.

For deaf infants, the Code of Practice states that 'If the LEA believes that a child in their area who is under the age of two may have special educational needs for which the LEA must determine the provision, they may make an assessment of their needs only if the parent consents to it, and must make such an assessment if the parents requests it'. At school and preschool level, a statement will be drawn up 'for children who require exceptional/additional support over and above that which is normally expected'. There will be a choice of placement, which will include the child's local mainstream nursery or school with support, a resourced mainstream nursery or school, a special school for deaf children or a special school for children with special educational needs other than deafness. Not all this provision will be available within the child's locality, and the removal of a child from his or her home environment will have many effects on the family. This may, in fact, be the first time that parents face the full, long-term implications of their child's deafness.

As children progress through school, their social and academic progress is monitored. Successful access to the full, whole school curriculum depends on peer group as well as child/adult interaction. For the child who is sign-dependent, access to school life, which depends on interpretation by a communication support worker, may be a very isolating experience. Where children have a Statement there is a statutory requirement for this to be reviewed annually. A meeting is usually held at the school and provides an opportunity for all, including the child, to report on progress made and to set targets for the coming year.

Where a Statement is not issued, pupils may be given an Individual Education Plan which outlines short-term targets and lists the support that will be needed. It is important that the relevant audiological details are available to all those working with the child in school, and the peripatetic teacher should be able to transfer this to set appropriate educational targets.

## Conclusion

From diagnosis to school placement the educational management of the deaf child is a complex and dynamic process. It relies heavily on trust, honesty and good liaison between all those involved with the child, on allowing parents to make informed decisions and on careful monitoring. There is no blueprint for the successful deaf child but no excuse for any child to achieve less than his or her full potential.

# Chapter 13
# Noise and hearing

Ross Coles

It is common knowledge that noise can damage hearing. This may result from a single exposure or very limited number of exposures to extremely high levels of impulse noise or blast, for example from being close to a large gun or an explosion, or very close to a smaller weapon. It is traditional to term this 'acoustic trauma'. More often though, damage to hearing by noise results from daily exposures to lower levels of noise, when the hearing loss gradually develops over months and years. The effect of this is called noise-induced hearing loss (NIHL). Of course, there are borderline levels and patterns of noise exposure, such as in recurrent firings of rifles, shotguns or pistols, but there is no need to distinguish precisely between the two as their effects on hearing are very similar.

## Harmful levels and durations of noise exposure

High-intensity noises capable of producing acoustic trauma are usually measured in terms of peak pressures, expressed as dB(peak). Their duration is of also some importance. While much damage can be done by noise of a very short duration (a few milliseconds), the same noise source occurring indoors in a small, enclosed space or near to reflective walls, ceilings or floors will have the same peak pressure but a longer duration due to reflections off nearby hard surfaces and this will make it seem louder. It may also cause more hearing loss. Although the evaluation of the auditory risk from such impulse noises is somewhat complex and uncertain, it can be concluded that exposure to noise with a peak pressure above 140 dB is liable to damage hearing. Above this level, irrespective of duration, preventative measures are required under the European Communities directive of 1986 and the UK Noise at Work regulations of 1989. A .22-inch rifle produces just under 140 dB (peak) at the firer's ear and is only a borderline hazard even when fired in an enclosed range. A 12-bore shotgun produces about 155 dB(peak) and a .410-inch shotgun about 4 dB less, while most military rifles produce about 160 dB(peak). Ear protection should always been worn with such rifles and shotguns, and most pistols. Heavier military weapons often produce much higher levels still.

Sound levels from more continuous types of noise, as often found in industry, are measured as decibels sound pressure level (dB SPL). Low frequencies and very high frequencies are less damaging to hearing and, incidentally, less annoying and they interfere less with speech. Consequently filters are often applied to the measuring equipment to take account of this. The filtering most commonly used is termed A-weighting, when the unit of noise level becomes dB(A). Noise levels down to about 80 dB(A), if experienced for many hours a day, for many days a year and for many years, will cause a small amount of damage to hearing in a small proportion of persons exposed. For regular exposures at 85 dB(A) there is risk of more damage and of a larger proportion of persons being affected: this is the 'first action level' under the Noise at Work regulations. People so exposed have to be advised about the potential risk and offered effective hearing protective devices, although their use is voluntary. The 'second action level' is 90 dB(A), and above this the use of hearing protection is mandatory.

Of course, noise levels are not usually constant in industry, nor are the daily durations of exposure. The variations in level and duration are taken account of by converting the actual noise exposures into a single figure, the 'daily personal exposure to noise' ($L_{EPd}$), or what used to be called the 'equivalent continuous 8-hour noise level' ($ECNL_{8hr}$). That is, the level of a constant noise continuing for 8 hours that has the same total energy as that experienced in the person's actual working day. The 85 and 90 dB(A) limits refer to $L_{EPd}$ or 8-hour ECNL values. The ECNL concept relates in turn to the equal energy concept, a useful working assumption but of limited actual validity. The concept is that noise exposures of different level and duration, which have the same total noise energy, involve the same risk to hearing. It also leads to a 3 dB trading relationship between SPL and duration of the noise. This means that a doubling or halving of the noise intensity, a 3 dB increase or decrease, has to be compensated for by a halving or doubling of the duration of exposure for it to have the same total energy and assumed risk to hearing. As the noise rises above 85 dB(A), so the permissible duration of 8 hours decreases. There eventually becomes a point where the distinction between a short-duration, high-level continuous noise exposure and an acoustic trauma becomes indistinct.

# Effects of noise on hearing

Prolonged exposure to high levels of noise puts an excessive biochemical load on the cochlea, which is very active in the process of transduction of acoustic signals from the environment into rapidly repeated nerve impulses in the auditory nerve. Waste products accumulate and the supply of oxygen and nutrients is depleted, with the result that the cells become fatigued, causing reduction of their function. If the noise exposure is not too high or prolonged, this process is reversible and may be measured as a temporary threshold shift (TTS) of hearing. It may also be noticed as a dullness of hearing after noise exposure and/or a ringing or other noise in the ears – tinnitus. But if the exposure is too great, then some permanent damage will result. With repeated such exposures, significant NIHL or permanent threshold shift (PTS) will gradually accumulate. With levels over about 100 dB(A), and in particular with impulses above 140 dB (peak), there is liable also to be direct mechanical injury to the hair cells. Because of this, the amount of damage done by impulse noise is more variable between individuals than with continuous noise, and that is why exposure to it is limited to 140 dB (peak) no matter how short the duration of each impulse or how few the number of impulses.

Research shows that quite a lot of hair cells can be destroyed before there is a measurable change in the audiogram. Nevertheless, this hidden damage does seem to matter, since a normal audiogram may be accompanied by such things as tinnitus, disturbance of frequency resolution and other forms of dysfunction such as abnormal otoacoustic emissions.

With most types of noise, the initial sign of noise damage in the pure-tone audiogram is usually a notch maximal at 3, 4 or 6 kHz. With further exposure, this notch gradually deepens and widens. After many years the upper limb of the notch may disappear, due either to added ageing effects or possibly to the effect of the noise itself, or some interaction between the two. Thus, while a high-frequency notch is the most characteristic feature of NIHL, its presence is not essential to the diagnosis. Indeed, after the age of about 65, it is probably more often absent than present. Figure 13.1 illustrates the gradual progression of hearing loss due to added effects of ageing in a case of NIHL. Note how the notch configuration gradually disappears, although there is still a bulge downwards and to the left around 4 kHz, which constitutes the remains of the noise-induced notch.

Some noises produce a slightly different audiometric pattern of damage. Low-frequency noise produced by turbulent airflow round a motorcyclist's helmet causes greatest PTS around 0.5 and 1 kHz. With high-intensity radio signals, often tones around 1 kHz, the main effect

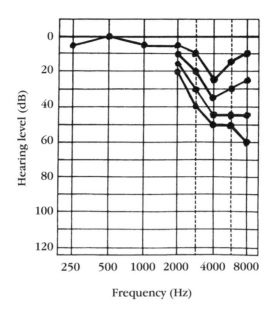

**Figure 13.1:** Hearing loss due to noise damage and its changing pattern with increasing age (40, 50, 60, 70 years).

seems to be around 1 and 2 kHz. Impulse noise, as from gun firing, produces a generally similar pattern to that of ordinary NIHL except that in some cases there appears to be greater involvement at and above 8 kHz.

The fundamental vibrating frequency of the human voice is at about 125 Hz in males and 225 Hz in females. However, there are many harmonics and the maximum energy of running speech is in the region of 300–500 Hz. Most of the information content of vowel sounds is between 250 and 2000 Hz. Consonants are even more important in terms of intelligibility of speech, and most of these are between frequencies of 1000 and 6000 Hz. Figure 13.2 shows these speech sounds roughly plotted on the audiogram.

One of the effects of NIHL can now be appreciated. The vowel sounds are heard at frequencies mostly below those affected by noise, and therefore NIHL has little effect on the apparent loudness of people's voices. On the other hand, the more informative and less intense consonant sounds are at higher frequencies, where the hearing has suffered much more damage. Failure to hear some of these sounds properly or at all leads to mis-hearing. This filtering effect of NIHL on hearing of speech leads to one of the common complaints of such people that: 'I can hear people speaking, but I miss parts of what they are saying.'

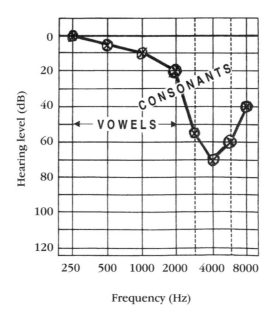

Figure 13.2: The filtering effect of noise damage on hearing of speech.

As already mentioned, loss of hair cells also causes more subtle changes in hearing, such as disturbances of coding of the acoustic vibrations into nerve impulses, in particular the coding of intensity, frequency and temporal sequence of sounds. This causes what might be called the distorting effect of NIHL. Perhaps the most important is impairment of frequency resolution, the ability to hear one sound in the presence of others, in particular hearing of speech in a background of noise or other voices. This leads to the other hearing complaint commonly made by people with NIHL: 'My hearing is not too bad in the quiet, but it's hopeless in a noise.'

## Prevention in industry

Of all forms of hearing disorder, that due to excessive noise exposure is both common and the most easily prevented. For such prevention, in industry, we have what is called a hearing conservation programme. There are five main components in this:

- identification and quantification of noise hazard
- engineering noise control
- hearing protection

- monitoring audiometry
- noise education.

## Assessment of hazard

Of course, one has first to have some indication as to when a noise may need to be measured and evaluated. A rough guide is that if two workers about 6 ft apart need a raised voice in order to be able to communicate with each other, then the noise level is likely to be at least 85 dB(A) and an acoustic investigation would be advisable.

Quantification of the noise hazard depends on acoustic evaluation using a sound level meter, an example of which is shown in Figure 13.3. This will usually measure the noise level both with and without A-weighting. In the past, a set of filters might have been added to enable measurement of the spectrum of the noise, i.e. its level in each of a range of frequency bands. However, this is less often needed nowadays, due to simpler methods of assessing the potential effectiveness of hearing protectors. Where the worker is exposed to noises having widely fluctuating level and frequency content, a more sophisticated meter with facility for measuring the total noise dose over specified periods of time will be needed. Likewise for high-level impulsive noises, a sound level meter with an impulse noise facility is needed.

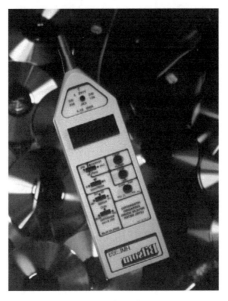

**Figure 13.3:** A typical industrial sound level meter (courtesy of SJK Scientifics, Southampton).

From the acoustic measurements, the $L_{EPd}$ can be calculated, taking account of exposure duration, intermittencies, rest breaks, overtime and so on. This is then compared with the legal requirements, and appropriate action is considered.

**Noise control**

The first principle of any medical management is, if possible, to prevent the condition in the first place, and the first principle of prevention is to remove the hazard. Much can be done to reduce sound levels in industry. First, there is choice of less noisy equipment. Nowadays, sound rating information is provided along with all the other technical information on new machinery. Older machines may become noisy with wear and tear, but careful maintenance and replacement of worn parts will often prevent or reduce rises in noise level. Vibrating surfaces can be damped, and isolated from other structures, which would otherwise be set into secondary vibration and thus produce yet more noise. Noisy equipment can be separated from workers, for example, by placing it outside or in a separate building, or it may be enclosed. Acoustic absorbent material may be placed on surfaces around the noisy equipment. Finally, the worker may be enclosed in a sound-treated control room.

Such acoustic engineering control should always be considered before resorting to hearing protection. But sometimes it is very costly, operationally inconvenient, not sufficiently effective or even impossible.

**Hearing protection**

Where the noise itself cannot reasonably be controlled, workers exposed to hazardous noise need to have their hearing protected. Various protective devices are available. They fall into the three main types, shown in Figure 13.4. Earmuffs are usually the most efficient and least dependent on careful fitting; and their use is easily monitored. But their headband has to be fairly tight, so they are uncomfortable and hot to wear for long periods. They may also give more protection than is actually needed, leading to an uncomfortable sense of isolation or to an unnecessary degree of communication difficulty. Earplugs are often preferable for noises below about 100 dB(A), but they have a wider degree of variation in effectiveness between one individual and another than do earmuffs, depending on how well they are actually fitted by the worker. They too can be uncomfortable.

A good halfway house is the canal cap. This is an earplug-like device, which fits onto the opening of the ear canal rather than penetrating into it, and is held there tightly by a headband. This is often the most comfortable

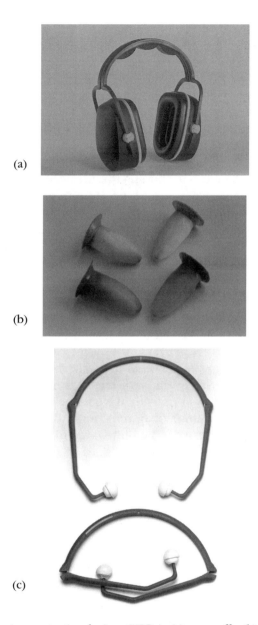

(a)

(b)

(c)

**Figure 13.4:** Hearing protective devices (HPDs). (a) ear muffs; (b) ear plugs; (c) canal caps (courtesy of SJK Scientifics, Southampton).

kind of hearing protector, and is also very convenient where the protector has to be used only intermittently – the device simply hangs round the neck when not in use.

Hearing protective devices (HPDs) have to be chosen with many wearability aspects in mind. It is best for the employer to offer a variety so that each worker can choose whichever suits him or her best; the adage that 'the best hearing protector is the one that is worn' is very relevant. Nevertheless, a major factor in choosing a protector is its effectiveness. In the past, one had to subtract the HPD's assumed attenuation (mean minus one standard deviation) at each octave frequency from the corresponding octave-band level of the noise, then apply A-weighting and finally combine the figures to see if the attenuated noise level in dB(A) was sufficiently low. Nowadays, simplified methods of doing this are available, such as the HML method. This uses the protector's high (H), medium (M) and low (L) frequency attenuation values and the A- and C-weighted sound level measurements (C-weighting is virtually linear or unweighted). An estimate of whether the HPD is good or acceptable is quickly obtained, and that device is then rejected if insufficiently protective or overprotective.

**Monitoring audiometry**

The only certain proof of effectiveness of a hearing conservation programme is to carry out a programme of monitoring audiometry of the noise-exposed workers. However, quite a lot of hair-cell damage can occur, reputedly up to 30% of the outer hair cells, before there are measurable threshold shifts. In any event, audiometry is not an accurate science, with test–retest differences at individual frequencies of up to 10 dB even in expert hands and with immediate retesting. Consequently, changes of hearing in one individual have to be quite large (e.g. over 10 dB between any two tests) before they can be identified as something that may be significant.

Then there remains the often difficult question as to what has caused the change in hearing thresholds. In this connection, one has to remember that the rate of accumulation of NIHL is really quite slow. For instance, using the National Physical Laboratory (1977) tables and assuming a fairly typical level of hazardous industrial noise of 95 dB(A), one finds that the average person after one, two, three, four and 10 years of exposure would develop NIHLs at 4 kHz of only 5, 7, 9, 10 and 15 dB. Thus, for monitoring the effectiveness of the programme as a whole, it is better to look at the statistical trends in substantial groups of people. But when in an individual case, perhaps in someone highly susceptible to noise damage, hearing loss having the clinical and audiometric appearance of noise damage is found to be developing, then that person should be warned and further preventative measures taken. These may involve making more effective use of their present HPD, a switch to one giving greater attenuation or removal from noise exposure.

## Education

Education of the worker and of those responsible for safety is very important. Noise levels in the 95 dB(A) region are potentially hazardous to the hearing of most people so exposed, and yet for many of them the noise will be very bearable, particularly as they gradually get used to it. They are also unlikely to notice any permanent effects on their hearing for many years. On the other hand, wearing a HPD is uncomfortable, leads to a sense of isolation and interferes somewhat with communication. Unless the programme is reinforced by explanation of why the protection is necessary in the first place and by supervision of its use, many of the workers will not use it properly or at all.

Before leaving the subject of prevention, there are some indications from recent research that it may be possible to prevent noise damage to the cochlea by other means. Prior exposure to lower levels of noise, of around 75 dB(A), may cause functional adjustments in the hair cells, which reduce their vulnerability to damage by a subsequent higher level of noise. There is also the possibility that ingestion of magnesium salts and certain other pharmacological agents may confer a reduction in susceptibility to noise damage. These are not practical means of prevention at present, but indicate future possibilities.

# Recreational noise

The main sources of recreational noise that may cause hearing loss are power tools, amplified music and shooting (see next section). What has been said above with respect to industrial noise applies also to recreational noise, but some additional comments are due. In general, less hearing loss seems to result and this is thought to be due to the relative infrequency of exposure and the beneficial effect of intermittency in the noise, a factor ignored in assessments based solely on the equal energy concept. What to do about these noises is also a more individual matter, and a useful personally applicable warning of potential hazard to hearing is the experience of sounds in the ears (tinnitus) and/or dullness of hearing lasting more than a few minutes after such noise exposure.

Most young people seem to use their personal stereos at sensible levels, but it is more difficult to limit sound exposure at discos and pop concerts. There are no regulations in the UK at present for limiting the music levels heard by those attending such events, the regulations only apply to noise levels at work. This is thought to be because of the difficulty in effective monitoring or enforcement, and because such noise seems to cause surprisingly little hearing loss. Many studies have struggled to show any effect at all, although it does seem to cause a somewhat increased incidence of tinnitus. Nevertheless, some limitation on very high music levels seems advisable, and those experiencing prominent temporary post-exposure symptoms would be better to use lower levels or seek less noisy venues.

### Impulse noise

The firing of virtually any weapon that uses an explosive propellant is a potential hazard to hearing, the main exceptions being the .22-inch rifle and starting pistols when fired in the open air. Air guns are acoustically safe too. Some firework rockets are fired from mortar-like tubes and may damage the hearing of those close to them, as may bangers if exploding close to the head or in enclosed places. With potentially noise-hazardous guns and fireworks, you should protect, move further away or avoid them altogether.

## Treatment

Once cochlear hair cells have been destroyed, there is as yet nothing that can stimulate them to regenerate. On the other hand, with damaged hair cells certain measures may enhance the chances of their recovery. In particular, anything that improves the supply of oxygen and removal of waste products in the cells could be beneficial. An acute acoustic trauma might well be helped by the same sort of measures as used in treatment of spontaneous sudden deafness. In the very long term, it is just conceivable that drugs may be found which would stimulate regeneration of hair cells, but the possibilities of that at present seem to reside either in non-mammalian species or in the vestibular hair cells of mammals.

At present, we have to accept that once the hair cells are damaged beyond repair, they do not regenerate. So treatment is directed towards hearing aids and other rehabilitational measures. In the past, it was difficult to obtain much benefit from a hearing aid in those cases where there was normal hearing at low frequencies and a moderate or severe hearing loss at high frequencies. But more modern developments in electronics – digital circuitry in particular – is improving matters. NIHL is often accompanied by tinnitus and sometimes this can be more troublesome than the hearing loss. Considerable improvements in treatment of tinnitus have also taken place (see Chapter 15).

## Compensation

Since NIHL is commonly of occupational origin, people suffering from it are often able to claim compensation. This may be from the state, through national or other insurance contributions related to their work. If they suffer an industrial disease or accident, then they are insured for that and can receive some financial recompense. Additionally or alternatively, people affected can sue their employers if the noise exposures or insufficiency of protective measures amount to negligence by the employer. The general guideline on what used to be needed was first set out in the UK by the government's advisory booklets 'Noise and the Worker' (1963, 1968, 1971). These were much elaborated in its Code of Practice in 1972, and the Noise at Work regulations (1989) have tightened up the matter still further and converted governmental advice into legal requirements.

The first compensation claims in UK were under common law, the worker suing his employer. The first to come to court was in 1967 in Exeter, but the claim failed. The first successful case was in 1971 in London. Since then there have been hundreds of thousands of claims, the vast majority of which have been settled out of court or under various settlement schemes. The government's compensation scheme for occupational deafness started in 1974, and has had a number of subsequent modifications and extensions. It is beyond the scope of the present chapter to elaborate on the compensation scheme, but people seeking further information should obtain DSS leaflet NI 207 'If you think your job has made you deaf', which is available from any national insurance office.

## Diagnosis

The diagnosis of NIHL depends first on whether there has been sufficient unprotected noise exposure to have caused the amount of hearing loss measured. However, there is such a wide variation in susceptibility to noise damage that mere exposure to a lot of noise does not automatically mean that all or even part of the hearing loss is necessarily due to that noise. With very intense, prolonged and repeated noise exposures, the chances of NIHL being present do of course increase, and very few people are totally resistant to noise damage. Nevertheless, in practical everyday terms, a diagnosis of presence of some NIHL cannot be made simply from a history of noise exposure.

After exclusion of other obvious causes of hearing loss, such as middle-ear disease and other causes of conductive hearing loss, and history of substantial alternative causes such as severe head injury, one then looks at the audiogram. Noise does not cause total deafness and there is plenty of epidemiological evidence available from which it is possible to define the extent of hearing loss that might arise from the estimated noise exposure plus ageing, and from ageing on its own, ranging from the most resistant person to the most susceptible person.

The audiometric configuration then needs to be examined. Most noises cause hearing losses maximal in the 3–6 kHz range, the main exceptions being where the frequency spectrum of the noise is concentrated in the lower frequencies. So in a case of NIHL, one should see either a notch in the audiogram at high frequencies, or at least a bulge downwards and to the left in the audiogram relative to the configuration most likely to result from ageing on its own. Notches tend to disappear after the age of about 65, probably mainly due to addition of ageing effects. But notches are not always present even in young persons with NIHL, as there may be some other cause for a pre-existing or added high-tone hearing loss or even a congenital absence of good hearing at high frequencies.

Comparison of the audiogram with what might be expected from ageing involves looking at normative data on presbyacusis, better described as age-related hearing loss (ARHL). The purpose of such comparison is not to contrast the amounts of hearing loss (unless grossly disparate), because one simply does not know to what degree the individual is susceptible to ARHL and to choose the average or any other statistic is entirely arbitrary. What is more important is the shape of the individual's audiogram as compared with that typical of ageing alone. But even here we have to be careful since the normative data only show the distribution of hearing losses in large populations as a function of age, sex and test frequency. In individuals, one finds many different configurations of ARHL. Some different patterns of this are shown in Figure 13.5. The different patterns have been attributed to different aetiologies or mechanisms of ARHL, but these associations are largely theoretical and unproven.

For most clinical purposes, and certainly for legal purpose, what matters is the 'probable' diagnosis, the legal criterion being on the 'balance of probabilities' or 'more likely than not'. ARHL having the type-B pattern shown in Figure 13.5 may occur, and addition of this to NIHL may obliterate any trace of a noise-induced notch or bulge. Such cases can be described as 'compatible with' a combination of NIHL and ARHL, or having 'possibility' of an element of NIHL. But often they fail to show sufficient audiometric evidence for a significant element of noise damage to be diagnosed at the required degree of probability. Keeping in mind that legal requirement of 'more likely than not' can be a great help in arriving at an opinion for or against NIHL.

## Noise-induced tinnitus

Any form of internal ear disorder is liable to be accompanied by tinnitus. Noise-induced damage is no exception. The prevalence of tinnitus depends strongly on the amount of high-tone hearing loss present. Of

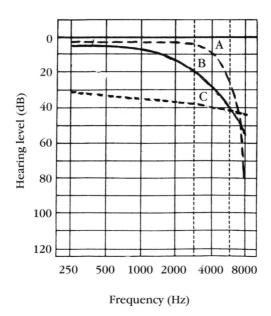

Figure 13.5: Some patterns of age-related hearing loss. A = the most common pattern in individuals, and the classical (averaged) pattern; B and C = other not uncommon patterns.

cases having sufficient hearing loss to qualify for compensation under typical governmental scales, about half would also have tinnitus. If it is of moderate or severe degree, additional compensation may be given. In common-law actions, tinnitus is usually compensated if deemed to be noise-induced and causing more than mild disturbance, but here it is irrespective of the amount of hearing loss. This is fairer, since you can have severe tinnitus with quite mild or no hearing loss at all, and vice versa.

Most commonly a noise-induced tinnitus has a pitch that is matched somewhere between 2 kHz and over 8 kHz, and has a descriptor suggestive of high-frequency content, such as whistle, whine, ring, screech or hiss. But sometimes the sound seems to be of a lower frequency. It can come on at any time during the period of noise exposure, from fairly early on to after many years, and quite frequently even years after the end of noise exposure. In the latter case, the link between the tinnitus and the noise damage is debatable, but as the critical factor seems to be the amount of hearing loss rather than its cause, it seems most unlikely that an underlying noise-induced hearing loss is irrelevant. Probably it is true to say that the tinnitus is at least due in part to the noise damage.

For legal purposes, diagnosis of noise-induced tinnitus is difficult. The problem is that as yet there is no objective test for presence of tinnitus, let alone one capable of measuring its severity. One has to assess the general demeanour of the patient and other evidence as to the honesty of his description of his tinnitus and the likelihood of it being noise-induced. In that connection, comparison of the volunteered pure-tone audiogram with the results of objective testing by cortical electric response audiometry can provide a useful check in a related area. In terms of amount of compensation, noise-induced tinnitus tends quite often to attract larger sums than the hearing loss. This is because of its sometimes devastating effects on a person's enjoyment of life, ability to work, earning capacity and so on.

# Chapter 14
# Non-organic hearing loss

Ross Coles

Hearing thresholds are sometimes incorrectly measured by pure-tone audiometry. This can be for a variety of reasons. That part of an apparent hearing loss that does not have an evident physical (organic) basis may be described as non-organic. Synonyms for non-organic hearing loss (NOHL) are spurious hearing loss and pseudohypacusis. NOHL may be on its own, i.e. where the hearing loss is wholly non-organic, or superimposed on a real hearing loss, i.e. partly non-organic. NOHL is most commonly seen either as the result of the patient's failure to respond properly to a hearing test in a way that could reasonably be expected of him or her, or as someone pretending to be more hard-of-hearing than is actually the case.

Classically, such cases are described as either psychogenic (synonyms functional or hysterical) or simulated (synonyms feigned or malingered). In fact, most of them have a mixed origin, with both psychogenic and simulated components in various proportions.

Purely psychogenic hearing loss is very rare, although much depends on its precise definition. Usually it is not difficult to find some potential advantage to the patient in having a hearing loss, which suggests an element of simulation. On the other hand, purely simulated NOHL certainly does occur quite frequently, either as a feigned or an exaggerated hearing loss. The most common motivation for NOHL in adults is in compensation claims for noise-induced hearing loss (NIHL) or traumatic hearing loss. In children, NOHL may simply be because they find it difficult to perform the test. In other cases, it may be a reaction to some stress, perhaps an attempt to gain attention or sympathy, or to provide an excuse for poor performance or disobedience. In yet others, there may be some underlying speech, language or educational problem, or a central auditory processing disorder.

NOHL can also be artefactual, particularly in children. The first kind of artefact, and one which is quite often missed, is when the patient is simply not capable of responding to the audiometric stimuli in the way that is required. The patient is thought to have been able to do the test properly and yet the results are not accurate. This may be due to inability to respond to the test properly, because the person is too young, too old, of insufficient intelligence, or too ill, tired or in pain. Other factors causing inaccurate results may be distraction by severe tinnitus or psychological distress, linguistic or hearing difficulties such that the test instructions were not understood, or inadequate instruction by the audiometrician.

Another artefactual cause of NOHL is where the ear canal is closed by pressure of the earphone and this is one to be particularly aware of. This tends to happen in elderly people with atrophic ear cartilage, in those with narrow ear canals and in those with thick tissue around the entrance to the ear canal, as found in some chubby children and in the post-traumatic condition of 'cauliflower ear'. Occlusion of the canal causes a conductive hearing loss affecting all frequencies, but most marked around 4 kHz, rather like the sound-attenuation properties of an earplug. Of course when bone-conduction tests are made, the conductive mechanism is bypassed and the bone-conduction thresholds are little affected by any occlusion of the ear canal. An apparent conductive hearing loss results. In the ears of the type described and in the presence of an unexplained conductive hearing loss, particularly if it is greatest at the higher frequencies or is at variance with tuning fork or impedance and reflex test results, the air-conduction thresholds should be remeasured with a small but firm tube, or stent, such as an acoustic impedance testing probe tip, placed into the ear canal to hold it open underneath the earphone.

Sometimes there can be an instrumental failure in the audiometer, which can lead to an apparent hearing loss. I recall one case where lengthy investigations were planned for an apparent total unilateral hearing loss and where explanation of the possible reasons for such a hearing loss had thoroughly alarmed the patient, but in fact the fault was simply a disconnected lead to one earphone. For this to have got past the audiometrician was of course a reflection on technique and lack of critical self-appraisal. Nevertheless, whenever there is an unexpected result that clashes with clinical observation, previous tests, tuning fork tests and so on, the first step should be to check or recheck the audiometer.

## Detection

An alert physician and audiometrician can detect many cases of NOHL by noticing discrepancies between various tests and observations. Most important is the comparison between the audiogram and informal observation of the patient's apparent ability to hear. To a considerable extent this is a matter of experience, and precise criteria cannot be given. Obviously there is something wrong if the patient can hear questions without lip-reading, e.g. while you are examining his or her ear or placing earphones on the ears, yet the audiogram shows a large hearing loss, such as over 60 dB averaged across the best two frequencies in the better-hearing ear. But where there is some apparent hearing difficulty and/or the measured hearing loss is rather less, then it becomes a matter of judgement and experience.

Comparison should be made with any other audiometric data that may be available. These may be tests carried out previously or elsewhere. Unexplained differences of more than about 10 dB averaged over several adjacent frequencies should raise the suspicion of NOHL. When more than one audiogram has been obtained on the same day, with the same instrument and by the same audiometrician, such variability should not be more than 5 dB.

Other types of audiometric tests may have been carried out. Commonly in NOHL the patient responds rather more acutely to bone-conduction than to air-conduction tests, giving an apparent conductive hearing loss. The conjunction of this with normal acoustic impedance and reflexes is strongly suspicious that something is wrong, or at least extremely unusual. Likewise in cases of severe hearing loss, you should not be able to obtain acoustic reflexes on stimulating the 'deaf' ear. If properly calibrated speech audiometry has been carried out, this will give an indication of the hearing ability for speech which should agree approximately with the pure-tone hearing loss. If the audiometric configuration is not flat, it is best to take the average across the two frequencies (out of 0.25, 0.5, 1, 2, 4 kHz) that show the best thresholds and compare that average with the speech threshold. Discrepancies in excess of 10 dB are suspicious. Increasingly in recent years, patients are being investigated by means of evoked otoacoustic emissions. By and large, these are unlikely to be present where the hearing thresholds exceed 25 dB at all frequencies in the 0.5–4 kHz range. Thus, if the audiogram appears to show greater hearing losses and yet such emissions can be evoked, the audiogram is probably incorrect.

A special case where there is an easy means of checking is in asymmetrical hearing loss. Clinical audiologists should be able to perform the Stenger test, and the patient need not know that he or she is being checked. From a two-channel audiometer the same frequency is presented simultaneously to each ear, at just above (more intense than) the apparent threshold of the better-hearing ear and just below the apparent threshold of the worse-hearing ear. If the measured hearing loss in the worse ear is true, he will not hear the sound presented to that ear, but will hear the sound presented to the better ear and so will respond. But if the hearing loss in the worse ear is non-organic, as quite often occurs in unilateral head- or ear-injury cases, he will hear the signal presented to the worse ear at quite a loud level, although not loud enough to admit to hearing it. But that sound will be loud enough to stop him hearing the much softer signal presented simultaneously to the better ear and so he fails to respond to the combined signal. That non-response indicates that he could in fact hear the sound delivered to the worse ear. The audiologist can then go on, by varying the levels between the two ears, to measure the real difference between them.

In compensation claimants for alleged NIHL, there is one other strong indication of possible NOHL. Particular suspicion is needed when the pattern of audiogram is rather flat, as distinct from the usual NIHL pattern of fairly normal hearing up to about 1 kHz and then a marked hearing loss with or without a notch at high frequencies. Recruitment of loudness – an abnormally rapid rate of growth of loudness – occurs where there is substantial cochlear hearing loss, such as at high frequencies in cases of NIHL. In cases of NIHL with a non-organic overlay, the effect of responding only to signals that are fairly loud is to reduce the apparent difference in thresholds between low and high frequencies, causing a relative flattening of the audiogram. Thus, excessive hearing loss at low frequencies is often an indicator of presence of a non-organic overlay in alleged NIHL cases. In these, it is advisable to have the hearing checked objectively (see below) if the hearing threshold level at 500 Hz exceeds about 25 dB.

This rule can be relaxed though, where compensation is only payable if the hearing losses exceed some larger figure, e.g. 50 dB averaged across 1, 2 and 3 kHz as in the British governmental scheme for compensation of 'occupational deafness' or of hearing loss acquired in military service. In fact, it seems likely that about half the cases appearing to qualify for such compensation have a substantial non-organic element in the audiograms they volunteer. I think it would be very cost-effective if all compensation cases apparently having that degree of hearing loss were routinely checked objectively.

## Objective audiometry

The purpose of objective tests is to obtain as accurate as possible a measurement of the true hearing thresholds in those cases where there is some indication of NOHL or a particular likelihood of it, and in a (objective) way which does not depend on the voluntary responses of the person being tested.

In adults, the best technique is cortical electric response audiometry (CERA). This is also known as evoked, or slow, vertex response audiometry. It gives a frequency-specific indication of the likely thresholds of hearing, usually accurate to about + or –10 dB at individual frequencies in the 0.5–3 kHz range. Above 3 kHz the tests become more difficult and less accurate. In any event, as the patient tires, becomes sleepy or becomes restless, the size and quality of the evoked responses in the brain waves (electroencephalogram) becomes reduced and so only a limited number of tests are possible. Quite often it is limited to about six in all, e.g. at three frequencies in each ear. Nevertheless, this is usually sufficient either to prove the presence of NOHL and indicate the probable true thresholds, or to corroborate the volunteered thresholds. It is less useful diagnostically though, because of the rather few frequencies that can be measured and their lesser accuracy at high frequencies (see also p. 112).

For children with NOHL, it is best to use CERA if the child is sufficiently old and quiet to collaborate by sitting quietly. But if sedation or anaesthesia is required, recourse will have to be made to auditory brainstem responses (ABR) (also called brainstem electric responses, BSER), which, unlike CERA, can be carried out under sedation or anaesthetic. They are much less frequency-specific however, although filtered clicks and derived responses can help somewhat in that respect.

## Management of NOHL

In the compensation context, it is usually sufficient simply to report the results. But occasional spurious results are obtained with CERA and so it is better to have some additional evidence of the presence of NOHL. Some clinicians inform the patient of their unsatisfactory responses to conventional pure-tone audiometry and then offer to retest, telling them that their present test results are unlike those of NIHL and would not qualify for compensation. Ideally, it is desirable to go on testing until a satisfactory pure-tone audiogram is obtained, i.e. one that agrees with the objective tests, but this cannot always be achieved and may also be too time-consuming.

In the case of children, I usually consider it best to inform the parents of the true state of affairs and, if possible, demonstrate to them that their child can in fact hear quite normally. This can often be done by means of speech audiometry, sometimes converting it into a sort of game with the child. I then tell the child that he or she can in fact hear quite well, but was not very good at the test. I advise the parents to treat the child as one who hears normally, but to be careful not to blame the child for his or her poor performance or for having 'pretended to be deaf'. In most cases, this is sufficient to rehabilitate the child. In some cases, subsequent audiometric tests continue to show poor responses, but in terms of everyday hearing the child can manage perfectly well. Just having an audiometric abnormality does not matter. If the child is wearing a (unnecessary) hearing aid, this is not removed, although the child is gradually weaned off it.

Nevertheless, in all but the artefactual cases, careful consideration needs to be given as to the possible cause of the child's behaviour, and this may entail multidisciplinary investigation and management.

## Non-organic tinnitus

In recent years, there has been an increasing number of cases of people claiming compensation for tinnitus, often as part of the effects of damage by noise, but in some cases arising from head injury or whiplash injury of the neck. This presents considerable problems, because there is no objective test to tell us whether or not the person really has tinnitus nor how severe it is. Moreover, severity of the tinnitus does not correlate with tinnitus loudness match measurements, so these are almost useless. Instead, its severity has to be assessed mainly from the patient's description of the effects of the tinnitus on him or her. So what can be done?

Rather little. There are only two tests which seem to help at all, and then only in a limited way. The first is to measure the pitch of the tinnitus, but even in a case of high-tone hearing loss due to noise, sometimes the tinnitus pitch is in a middle-range frequency, or occasionally even at a low frequency. Whether this is truly so and is due to the noise damage or whether it is simply an error of measurement is uncertain: tinnitus pitch matching is often very difficult for the patient, so rather little reliance can be placed on it. Nevertheless, a low-frequency tinnitus with a high-frequency hearing loss is at least unusual.

There is also the possibility of testing the person's 'auditory honesty'. In theory, if a person is going to exaggerate, he or she will probably do so not just about the tinnitus, but for the hearing difficulty as well. But of course the amount of hearing loss can be checked objectively by means of CERA. Then, if a claimant is shown to have some NOHL, it must throw considerable doubt on how truthfully he or she has described his or her tinnitus. Bearing in mind that tinnitus is a subjective phenomenon, highly dependent for its assessment on the honesty of the patient, it could be argued that the person should not be compensated for tinnitus if there is any substantial doubt about his or her honesty in any other aspect of the claim.

The problem with this test though is that the presence of NOHL in a compensation claimant is not automatically due to malingering or exaggeration. Some patients are just bad at audiometry. Others have not fully heard or understood the test instructions. Others are inattentive, or nervous and anxious, or may be over-breathing and thereby creating a physiological masking noise. And finally, those with severe tinnitus often find it difficult to perform audiometry due to the deleterious effect of the tinnitus on their ability to concentrate and thereby leading to spuriously high hearing thresholds and variable responses. Tinnitus may also interfere with the detection of test tones around the pitch of the tinnitus. In such cases, discrepancies between the audiogram and CERA tests might be ascribed to lack of honesty, whereas in fact it could be the very severity of the tinnitus that is causing the discrepancies.

In the end, it is simply up to the clinician to use his or her judgement as to whether the patient is being honest, whether his or her account of the tinnitus is an acceptable one or not, and to assess its severity from the patient's description of its effects.

# Chapter 15
# Tinnitus and hyperacusis: mechanisms and retraining therapy

JONATHAN HAZELL

In the past, patients complaining of tinnitus have not always elicited much sympathy from the professionals they consulted. For the most part, otolaryngologists, the specialists to whom most patients were referred, were concerned with the treatment of acute conditions. The common response to a complaint of tinnitus was 'there is no treatment' and 'you've got to learn to live with it'. As we will see, this approach has resulted not only in patients remaining untreated, but even in a worsening of their symptoms. At the turn of the century, psychiatrists tended to care for patients with severe tinnitus distress, and it could be said that the acquisition of tinnitus patients by otolaryngologists and audiologists in the 20th century was to some extent a retrograde step. With the development of multidisciplinary teams in otolaryngology and audiology, and with the new understanding of the mechanisms behind tinnitus and its distress, we are now in a position to offer real help to tinnitus and hyperacusis patients for the first time.

## The puzzles of tinnitus

Over the past 90 years most efforts to treat tinnitus have concentrated on the cochlea. This is partly because knowledge about hearing was restricted to the end-organ, and also because patients indicated so graphically that that was where sound was coming from. Enlightenment about tinnitus mechanisms only comes from a realization that perception of any sound occurs in the auditory cortex, after considerable processing in auditory pathways between ear and brain. The perceived location of sound depends on a complex rule book, built up in childhood, and based on the experience of our sound environment. All perceptions occur at a cortical level, but are then projected outside the individual to create a virtual reality of the world around us.

246

The first time that tinnitus is perceived, there are no rules for sound location within the head, and it is no surprise that the ear is chosen as the most likely place from which tinnitus should be emanating. Indeed 35% of patients first experiencing tinnitus think it is a sound coming from outside, and frequently scan the environment for a possible source.

Another simplistic view of tinnitus is that it relates to a part of the audiogram where there is a hearing loss, typically in the high frequencies. This has led to a naive explanation that tinnitus is caused by the same pathology as the hearing loss, i.e. hair-cell loss in the cochlea. It is assumed that since hair-cell damage cannot be repaired, neither can tinnitus be effectively treated. Unfortunately this line of thinking arises from a series of assumptions, which have led both patient management and clinical research consistently in the wrong direction.

In our clinical practice, we found that 30% of the patients with long-standing, troublesome tinnitus had normal audiograms. Furthermore, examination of a subgroup of these patients showed that there were no abnormalities of cochlear function as measured by otoacoustic emissions or distortion products. On the other hand, analysis of a database of 800 patients waiting for cochlear implants, who arguably have the worst cochlear damage of anyone, showed that 27% had never experienced any tinnitus at all. A further study was performed on 200 consecutive tinnitus patients attending our tinnitus clinic, which typically deals with the most severe cases referred after failed treatment elsewhere. Their audiograms were averaged and compared with normative data from the general population. There was no significant difference between tinnitus patients and the general population. These findings alone strongly suggest that something other than the cochlea is responsible for troublesome tinnitus.

## Neurophysiological model

Once treatment can be based on the underlying neurophysiological process, real progress can be made. Malaria, as its name indicates, was thought to be due to bad air. Little progress was made until the involvement of the mosquito was discovered, after which quite simple preventative treatments became effective. The important advance in tinnitus has been the analysis by Jastreboff (1990) of tinnitus and hyperacusis mechanisms and the part played in these mechanisms by the whole of the auditory system, and by the inter-connecting areas of the brain outside the auditory system (Figure 15.1). The account of this neurophysiological model is given quite simply, in a form that can be understood by patients, as part of tinnitus retraining therapy (TRT), called directive counselling. TRT is a therapy using teaching, behavioural and sound therapy techniques, based on the Jastreboff neurophysiological model, which has been shown to produce very significant improvements in 80% of long-term tinnitus cases within six months.

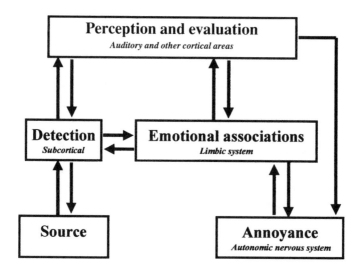

**Figure 15.1:** Jastreboff neurophysiological model of tinnitus.

## The auditory system

The outer, middle and inner ear are concerned with the collection of sound from our environment and with changing the physical sound waves into patterns of electrical activity in the auditory nerve. First, it should be realized that the individual sound locations are lost in this process, and are mixed together in a kind of 'sound soup'. Within the thousands of fibres of the auditory nerve, information is coded about the frequencies of sound that are present in our auditory environment, but without any knowledge of the location from which the sound originated. However, we do not perceive sound as a 'soup' made up of all the frequencies present, but rather a faithful reconstruction of the sound locations from which the different frequencies came. This complex task of reconstruction must be performed between ear and brain, in real time, and even in the absence of binaural hearing (although this definitely helps the process).

The connections between ear and brain are not simple cables, but complex neuronal networks capable of pattern recognition and selection, which are responsible for our selective hearing (Figure 15.2). Think of the ability we have to detect the sound of our first name in a nearby conversation or to wake from sleep at the sound of a creaking floorboard after we have a just slept through a thunderstorm. Clearly the auditory system has a complex mechanism of filters which can be set by our own individual experience of sound. These filters form part of our security system. Exposure to warning signals, or in the animal world the sound of predators, results in a conditioned response that automatically activates survival by 'fight or flight' mechanisms. The auditory system is particularly important in this regard, as these subcortical filters are monitoring our environment 24 hours a day. Sometimes aversive conditioned responses can be generated to seemingly harmless parts of our environment, such as spiders, lifts, aeroplanes or high buildings. Each of these conditioned reflex responses results in a varying degree of emotional reaction combined with an enhancement of autonomic activity shown by a change in the arousal state. The emotional response frequently involves fear, while the autonomic activity results in alterations of bodily functions such as heart rate, breathing, muscle tension and sweating. A very small response or reaction might only involve a feeling of unease or irritation; a full response might result in a strong phobic or panic reaction.

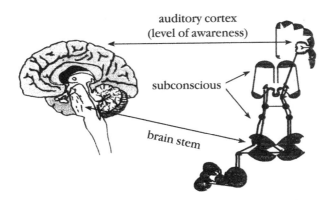

**Figure 15.2:** Auditory pathways.

# The source of tinnitus

In 1953, Heller and Bergman performed a classic experiment. They took 80 normally hearing young adults and placed them one by one in a sound-proof room for five minutes. They were told to listen carefully, and did so anticipating a test of their hearing. In fact they experienced five minutes of complete silence. On questioning, 94% described hissing, ringing, pulsing or a sound in their ears or head during this period. The description of sounds was identical to that experienced by another group with hearing loss who had tinnitus. Clearly the ability to detect sound generated within the auditory system or by the body is almost universal, provided that the environment is silent enough.

All the elements within the neuronal networks making up the auditory system are electrically active during life. In a normal environment, with a sound being generated and the auditory system responding, the background electrical activity diminishes. If the system ceases to receive information, because the environment becomes unnaturally quiet or because there is a hearing impairment, the background activity increases in an effort to turn up the volume or increase the gain. This explains why tinnitus can be heard by anyone in a quiet environment provided that they listen carefully enough. It also explains why increasing hearing loss may be associated with tinnitus, although the relationship is a weak one.

## The conditioned aversive response

There is a difference between those experiencing tinnitus in the Heller and Bergman experiment and those who have suffered for 10 or more years from a cacophony of noise in their ears or head that has destroyed their quality of life. The answer lies in understanding the way in which the brain reacts to any sound (whether it comes from inside or outside the head). If the sound represents a threat, an intrusion or even some kind of change in the environment, then our selective hearing mechanisms will tune subcortical filters on to it. If the sound is categorized or evaluated as a threat, intrusion or change in our sound environment that is unwelcome, an aversive reaction and conditioned response will be set up against it.

In exactly the same way as our security system works, each time the signal representing tinnitus is detected by the subcortical filters, a reaction involving the limbic and autonomic nervous systems will be produced. Therefore each time the environment is quiet enough, and there are no other distractions, tinnitus will be heard and will cause varying degrees of distress. Whether or not there is distress from the tinnitus depends on whether there is an aversive conditioned response. As our research has shown, the characteristics of the tinnitus sound are irrelevant. It does not even matter how loud the tinnitus is. Tinnitus distress depends on the understanding of what tinnitus means, what is the conventional wisdom, what the patient has been told and what the cultural background happens to be. In northern India, tinnitus is believed to be the gods speaking to you and is considered a blessing. Any experience of tinnitus without an unpleasant reaction does not become a clinical problem, and statistics show us that this is extremely common and clinically unimportant. Those who come seeking help with problem tinnitus all have a degree of aversive conditioned response, which may range from very mild alterations of autonomic activity to a powerful phobic reaction with continuous anxiety and panic states.

Once the conditioned response is established in the subconscious part of the brain it cannot be interfered with just by thinking. It is impossible to change a reaction to the motor horn as we cross the road, just by wishing to. Moreover, the responses from the limbic and autonomic systems create a vicious circle connected to detection of the tinnitus signal, which can automatically strengthen the response as well as tuning the filters more directly on to the tinnitus. Tuning of the filters, rather like a radio tuning on to a distant station, results in an increased perception of the tinnitus, provoking stronger conscious feelings of dislike and increasing concerns about the future outcome of tinnitus. The source of tinnitus remains unchanged.

## Hyperacusis

The neurophysiological model successfully predicts a similar mechanism for hyperacusis. External sounds often cause mild annoyance for a variety of reasons. Many people naturally seek silent places where they know they will be free from external pressures and stresses. Others may take to wearing earplugs to avoid environmental sound, particularly at night. This search for silence results in an increase in auditory gain, whereby subcortical filters 'open' in an attempt to gain auditory information. As a result, normal environmental sounds are enhanced and the resulting perceptions are overloud. This is the mechanism of hyperacusis. It is important to differentiate this from auditory recruitment, which is always associated with hearing loss and is caused by a reduction in dynamic range, usually as a result of hair-cell loss in the cochlea.

While hyperacusis indicates an increased sensitivity to all sounds in the environment, some patients also develop phonophobia. Here there is a specific aversion to certain sounds, but not others. For instance, doors shutting, dogs barking or the sounds of cutlery may be very upsetting, while loud music is well tolerated. There is often a fear that sounds will damage the hearing or cause an increase in tinnitus or hyperacusis. In practice, hyperacusis and phonophobia tend to be present together in varying degrees.

Some 40% of our tinnitus patients have a degree of hyperacusis, and in many cases a history of hyperacusis and sensitivity to external sounds for a long time before the onset of tinnitus. This indicates that the whole auditory system was in a sensitized state, ideal for the detection of internally generated signals – the 'music of the brain'. In each case of hyperacusis, particularly when phonophobia is also present, an aversive conditioned response is generated to the external sound, in exactly the same way as it is in tinnitus distress.

## Tinnitus retraining therapy

This treatment has developed, and is still developing, from our understanding of the Jastreboff model. It should be remembered that TRT is not the only way to treat tinnitus, but at this moment it is the most effective, with published results of 80% effectiveness over a six-month period. Elements of TRT are present in the approaches used by many healthcare professionals treating tinnitus and all are helpful. However, high levels of success can only be expected if all the elements are incorporated.

### What is the goal of TRT and how does it work?

The goal of TRT is to produce a complete removal or habituation of any reaction or conditioned response to tinnitus or external sounds; this means any reaction involving the limbic and autonomic nervous system in the subconscious, that results from conditioning by tinnitus or by an external signal. The problems created by tinnitus and hyperacusis only exist as long as they are producing unpleasant reactions. These may frequently interfere with sleep (increased autonomic arousal), concentration, quiet recreational activity, etc. In fact, once a complete removal or habituation of the reaction has been achieved, subconscious filters are no longer directed to focus on the signal and its perception weakens. This process takes a long time, commonly 18 months for habituation of the reaction. Following habituation of the reaction, habituation of perception occurs spontaneously, with a gradual reduction in tinnitus awareness.

TRT works by combining a number of different approaches. First, there is teaching, directive counselling and a 'demystification' process. It is impossible to believe that tinnitus perception can be a natural phenomenon, or can be altered, without a full knowledge of the auditory system. The patient (and the doctor) must learn the mechanism of the auditory system, its interaction with the limbic and autonomic nervous system, and the importance of subcortical or subawareness filters which are involved in our selective hearing process. This knowledge is essential in the process of reclassifying tinnitus (or external sound, in the case of hyperacusis). Following the acceptance and understanding of these mechanisms, it is possible by behavioural retraining to gradually reduce unpleasant and aversive reactions to the sounds. This last element in the training resembles phobic desensitization techniques. As treatments are aimed at the removal of aversive reactions to tinnitus, the trigger factors or underlying pathology that may have resulted in an emergence of tinnitus in the first place are irrelevant.

**Specifics of TRT**

In each case, it is essential to emphasize the importance of avoiding silence. Specific counselling about the use of sound reinforcement will always be needed. This is not simply a matter of instructing patients to leave their television on. Many patients will be aversive to environmental sounds, and it can be difficult to choose a sound-enrichment source that is not intrusive, distressing or likely to generate an aversive reaction itself. Natural sounds are best, and where, because of security or bad weather, it is not possible to leave the window open, alternatives should be sought. Commercial devices that generate the sound of gentle rain or wind or the sea, or tape or CD recordings of these may also be used. A large domestic or ceiling fan can generate the sound of air movement. Sound enrichment should not be loud and intrusive, but it should continue throughout sleep, as the filters are active during this period. Sleep disturbance is common in tinnitus patients, partly due to inadequate sound enrichment and a tendency to be disturbed by any environmental sound that occurs during the night, while the subcortical filters are enhanced by silence.

Where white noise generators are required they must be fitted to both ears, as long as there is serviceable hearing, and not just to the ear indicated by the patient. Tinnitus and hyperacusis are disorders of central auditory processing, not of the ear. It is better to fit one patient properly than two patients with a single instrument each, where a serious imbalance of auditory input may result.

Where hearing aids are needed (category 3, see below), they must be fitted with attention to the highest possible standards of auditory rehabilitation, and sometimes without regard to cost, when appropriate amplification dictates specialized hearing aids. Wherever possible, binaural amplification must be used to ensure symmetry within the auditory system.

Demystification and directive counselling are essential parts of TRT in all patients. No benefit will be gained simply by fitting instruments and sending the patient on his or her way. Each patient must understand how the auditory system works, and the mechanism of tinnitus and hyperacusis, according to the Jastreboff model. Instructing the patient requires the use of simple stories or parables to illustrate the complex brain mechanisms involved. Doing this with regard to the patient's unique and individual experience of tinnitus or hyperacusis requires skilled and special training. In the absence of this, professionals must at least avoid any negative counselling, which might strengthen the aversive reaction to the tinnitus or external sound. The most important messages to get across are: (a) that the problem is an aversive conditioned response to a sound; (b) that the loudness of tinnitus or external sound depends on the disposition of changeable filters in the auditory subcortex; and (c) that retraining therapy can permanently fix these problems.

### The Jastreboff categories

In the development of TRT, it proved helpful to divide patients into categories according to the kind of treatment they need. These categories have nothing at all to do with medical or surgical diagnosis. The categories of patients and their consequent treatments are based on the impact of tinnitus or hyperacusis on their life, the patient's perception of hearing loss, the presence of hyperacusis and phonophobia, and the presence of 'kindling' or winding-up effects (sounds or events that trigger the enhanced perception of tinnitus). It depends on which of these symptoms are dominant.

- *Category 1: tinnitus only.* Here tinnitus is the predominant symptom without significant hyperacusis or hearing loss. Treatment involves the regular daily use of noise generators set at just below the 'mixing point' of loudness (when the external sound blends into the tinnitus), repeated appropriate directive counselling and advice about sound enrichment.
- *Category 2: tinnitus with hearing loss.* Tinnitus is the most important symptom, but there is a hearing loss, which is significant to the patient, who may already be wearing hearing aids. Hyperacusis is absent. Treatment is undertaken with appropriate binaural amplification and counselling about sound enrichment. Care is taken to avoid asymmetry of auditory stimulation. Hearing aid provision must be of the highest possible quality.
- *Category 3: hyperacusis.* Hyperacusis is the predominant symptom, with or without tinnitus. There should be no prolonged exacerbation of symptoms by environmental sound (see category 4). Treatment is with demystification and teaching, and the use of white noise generators applied binaurally. The intensity of the white noise may be varied to suit different environmental sound situations.
- *Category 4: hyperacusis with 'kindling' effect.* Severe hyperacusis is present and moderate levels of environmental noise make symptoms worse for periods longer than 24 hours. Phonophobia is nearly always present and needs to be dealt with by appropriate counselling. There is a severe disorder of the subcortical filters, and desensitization with white noise generators must be introduced with extreme care. Binaural instruments are set just above threshold and gradually increased to a comfortable listening level over a period of many weeks. Patients should be screened for Lyme disease.

- *Category zero: tinnitus or hyperacusis of low severity.* Here the symptoms have only a small impact on the patient's life and the strength of reaction is weak. These patients can be effectively treated by one or two sessions of directive counselling with demystification and instruction about sound enrichment. Follow-up is essential to ensure that categorization has been appropriate.

## Assessment of the patient

Proper assessment of the patient is a vital part of TRT, and the questions asked should be relevant to the model. Time should be spent inquiring about the effect of tinnitus on the patient's life and the activities that have been prevented by it or by hyperacusis. An assessment of habituation of reaction can be made by recording the change in the percentage of waking hours during which irritation, annoyance or distress is experienced. Habituation of perception can be measured as a change in the percentage of waking hours during which the patient is aware of tinnitus. For proper categorization of patients it is essential to measure the pure-tone audiograms and loudness discomfort levels at each frequency. These are the only measurements which are essential for TRT, but minimal suppression levels for tinnitus are also useful. Loudness discomfort levels consistently quieter than 100 dB nHL are generally found in hyperacusis. Other tests and investigations will be indicated by the general audiological or otological picture.

Emergence of tinnitus is frequently triggered by emotion or stress. Inquire about contemporary experiences of unrelated illness, accidents, bereavement, work stress, etc., which are frequently responsible for a state of the 'red alert' with consequent alterations of auditory filters. Take a careful history about the sound environment in which the patient lives. Information about other aversions, dislikes or phobias can sometimes be helpful in getting an overall picture of the patient.

## Follow-up

Serial appointments, ongoing assessment and repeated directive counselling are necessary for most patients, particularly those who are the most distressed and have the strongest aversive reactions to their tinnitus or external sounds. However, in a general audiological practice patients may fall into different categories. It is essential to organize the tinnitus and hyperacusis patients into a special clinic because TRT takes time to apply and do well. It is best to set aside a period each week, or at least each month, specifically for tinnitus and hyperacusis patients, during which time experience and expertise in their management can develop.

Remember to make regular measurements of the percentage awareness and annoyance or distress to assess the degree of habituation of perception and reaction. A 40% change in awareness and annoyance, together with the ability to perform at least one activity previously prevented, constitutes a significant improvement leading to a successful outcome. With TRT performed properly, 80% of patients should reach this goal within six months to one year, while the remaining 20% will take longer.

## Syndromic tinnitus

So far, the tinnitus and hyperacusis we have discussed has been non-syndromic tinnitus. That is to say, the symptoms were not associated with any other medical or surgical conditions. In about 5–20% of cases, according to the practice and referral patterns of the specialist, tinnitus will be part of a medical condition containing other symptoms or signs (a syndrome). In dealing with tinnitus and hyperacusis patients it is essential to bear in mind all the possible conditions of which tinnitus is a symptom, and make sure that these are excluded by careful history taking and appropriate investigation and tests. The most common conditions encountered in audiological practice are Ménière's syndrome and, rarely, acoustic neuroma. Tinnitus is 20 000 times more common than acoustic neuroma, so it is unhelpful to alarm patients unnecessarily. Where investigations for a unilateral hearing loss are indicated, patients should be counselled with sensitivity. If a magnetic resonance imaging (MRI) scan is needed, earplugs should be worn during the scan, which can be noisy.

## Other treatments for tinnitus

Because patients with tinnitus and hyperacusis can be so desperate for a 'quick fix', it is not surprising to find that almost everything has been tried somewhere. Medical and surgical treatment aimed at the cochlea indicates a lack of understanding of the mechanisms involved in tinnitus and hyperacusis. Likewise, potentially harmful treatments such as using lasers, hyperbaric oxygen and intravenous infusion are to be avoided. The drugs most commonly prescribed are tranquillizers and antidepressants. These may produce temporary changes in limbic and autonomic function, but no permanent benefit. Antidepressants may sometimes be separately indicated. Herbal remedies, vitamins and ginko biloba enjoy anecdotal support, but are unproven in proper trials. Relaxation techniques and acupuncture have a strong effect in reducing autonomic overactivity and may temporarily help tinnitus. Long-term effects are most likely when combined with a TRT programme.

Successful surgical treatment of middle ear conductive deafness often improves tinnitus, as can surgery for Ménière's syndrome. Destructive surgery for tinnitus alone must be avoided at all costs. It is based on the belief that tinnitus is an ear disorder, and nearly always makes things worse. In profound deafness, where hearing aids can no longer be of help, several studies have shown that cochlear implants can help tinnitus as well as deafness. Before any surgery it is important that the patient should be counselled about temporary increases in tinnitus, which are common at first because the ear may often be blocked with a dressing and the patient stressed by the trauma of surgery. Failure to do this may result in the emergence of tinnitus, which the patient wrongly associates with surgical failure, initiating a strong aversive reaction to the tinnitus, which can lead to its persistence.

## Summary

The outlook for well-established, distressing tinnitus and hyperacusis has dramatically improved following the publication of the Jastreboff neurophysiological model, and the development of tinnitus retraining therapy (TRT) on which is based.

## Further reading

The Tinnitus and Hyperacusis Website (Hazell) http://www.tinnitus.org
Proceedings of the Sixth International Tinnitus Seminar, Cambridge, UK, September 5–9 1999. Immediate Proceedings Ltd. Tel 44 –(0) 1379 586628.

# Chapter 16
# Psychological aspects of acquired hearing loss

Laurence McKenna

## Hearing loss and psychological state

### The popular image of hearing impaired people

Sensory restrictions are an almost universal part of human existence and almost everyone experiences some problems with listening, especially in demanding auditory situations. In spite of the widespread nature of hearing difficulties the popular image of people with hearing impairment is not flattering. Hearing loss is associated with old age and, as a consequence, with frailty of body and mind. In word association, deaf is likely to be followed by dumb and to have connotations of stupidity. Hearing-impaired people are commonly regarded as suffering from psychological disturbances such as depression or paranoia. It has also been observed that people who use hearing aids are regarded less favourably by others than people without a hearing aid.

There are certainly good reasons for supposing that hearing loss might lead to psychological disturbance. Acquired hearing impairment involves losses of one kind or another. Depression may come about when a person experiences a sense of loss, or of helplessness, and the perception that his or her actions do not influence events. Anxiety may arise when a person anticipates loss or believes that things will go wrong in some way. Intuitively, one might expect to find high rates of both depression and anxiety and possibly other psychological disturbances among people who experience hearing impairment.

Given the popular images of deaf people as weak, stupid, possibly mad or at least disagreeably suspicious, and given the apparent relevance of emotional disturbances such as depression to the experience of being hearing impaired, the psychological circumstances of hearing-impaired people demand serious attention.

258

**Hearing loss and emotional state**

There are many descriptions of the negative emotional consequences of hearing loss. Early reports came from the observations of psychiatrists involved in the care of deafened people. Often they described their hearing-impaired patients as neurotic or paranoid. It must be remembered, however, that these descriptions came from general impressions formed by psychiatrists rather than from formal studies and may therefore have been biased. Attempts have also been made to record the psychological impact of simulated hearing loss in experimental subjects. While negative emotional consequences have been described, it is difficult to draw conclusions from these studies. They have been restricted by the difficulty in achieving meaningful levels of simulated hearing loss and by their temporary and artificial nature.

Another approach has been to examine the prevalence of psychological disorder among hearing-impaired people. Some studies have pointed to a high prevalence of emotional disorder among hearing-impaired people attending hospital clinics. Only a small number of these studies have sought to assess deafened people according to accepted psychiatric guidelines as laid out in the *Diagnostic and Statistical Manual* (DSM) of the American Psychiatric Association. When this has been done the psychological symptoms of people with hearing loss have not always met the criteria for a psychiatric classification. More usually, studies in this area have employed questionnaires that identify psychiatric cases and that are commonly used to quantify particular forms of psychological disturbance. They have reported elevated levels of psychopathology and maladjustment, including depression, neurotic symptoms, anxiety and social isolation in hearing-impaired populations. A study by McKenna, Hallam and Hinchcliffe (1991) reported that 27% of people attending a neuro-otology clinic with a main complaint of hearing loss were suffering from significant psychological disturbance. This is considerably higher than the prevalence of psychological disturbance among the general population (approximately 5% of whom have significant psychopathology). It is, however, lower than the prevalence rates reported to be associated with other audiological symptoms, such as tinnitus and vertigo.

An improvement in psychological wellbeing has also been observed in deafened people who have had some restoration of hearing. The experience of cochlear implant patients is important in this respect. Improvements in questionnaire measures of emotional wellbeing have been observed along with reports of positive changes in their self-confidence and a reduction in their sense of reliance on others.

The link between hearing loss and mental health has also been studied by examining the extent of hearing impairment in patients who are known to have a psychiatric disorder. The results of this approach have suggested that a hearing loss increases the chance that a patient will have a diagnosis of schizophrenia, and that hearing loss is one of a number of premorbid factors that distinguishes patients with paranoid psychosis from those with affective psychoses. However, the studies involved in this work did not properly take into account other factors, such as general health, age and noise exposure. These factors could have explained the differences observed. There is, however, the potential for a hearing loss to lead to misclassification in psychiatric cases and it is important for this to be taken into account in the diagnostic process.

While other studies have also suggested that hearing loss is associated with emotional disturbance, the empirical picture is mixed, and some studies report conflicting results. When other health problems have been taken into consideration the correlations between hearing loss and anxiety and depression are weaker. The presence of multiple symptoms, for example, hearing loss with tinnitus, leads to a greater likelihood that a person will suffer from significant psychological distress. The high co-morbidity between hearing loss and tinnitus is particularly relevant in this respect: many hearing-impaired people may experience significant psychological distress as a consequence of the combined effects of that loss and tinnitus.

### Hearing loss and cognitive functioning

A possible relationship between hearing loss and cognitive dysfunction has received some research attention. Both hearing loss and brain disorders that lead to cognitive impairment are common in the elderly, and a number of studies have noted a strong association between the presence of hearing loss and of confusion or dementia. Some researchers have considered the correlation between hearing loss and dementia to be too strong to be explained simply by the advanced age of the people studied. This observation has led to the suggestion that deficits of sight and hearing may play a part in the production of cognitive impairment, by reducing the person's contact with the outside world. However, much of the work involved did not include the collection of audiometric data. Research that has taken account of audiometric information has found that the association between hearing loss and dementia is lost when the age of the people studied is taken into account. This weakens the strength of the argument that hearing loss might have a role in causing dementia.

Complaints of difficulty in concentrating are common even among younger hearing-impaired people when they are seen in a clinical setting. It has usually been assumed that difficulties in concentration stem from fatigue, due to the effort of listening and lip-reading, or from emotional distress. However, recently, subtle difficulties in information processing have been observed in hearing-impaired people that are not easily explained in terms of fatigue or emotion. It has been observed in at least one study that the degree of difficulty in information processing was related to the duration of hearing loss. The implication is that hearing loss may lead to changes in the way the brain processes information. This does not mean that hearing-impaired people have a general intellectual deficit, only that they are less able to process certain types of verbal information. The evidence to date also suggests that not all hearing-impaired people show evidence of such changes.

## Complexities in the relationship between hearing loss and psychological state

The complexity of the relationship between hearing loss and psychological disturbance is further highlighted by the fact that many people, particularly older people, do not complain about their hearing loss. It is often the case that older people tolerate a greater degree of impairment before taking action than do younger people, and regard a hearing aid as of little use to them. It has been noted that some people deny that they have a hearing problem even when confronted by audiometric evidence of a hearing loss. The link between audiological thresholds and psychological disturbance is also unclear. If hearing loss is associated with psychological disturbance then it might be expected that there would be a relationship between the extent of the hearing loss and the extent of the psychological problems. Many research studies, however, have found that this is not the case, although one study (Thomas and Gilhome-Herbst 1980) suggested that this may be so in people with severe hearing loss and poor speech discrimination.

At first sight, therefore, the evidence about the relationship between hearing loss and psychological wellbeing seems mixed. In part this may be because of an overly simple approach to assessing psychological status. Many studies have used an approach that classifies people as either psychiatrically disturbed or not. This runs the risk of neglecting those people who experience emotional distress that falls short of being classified as disturbed. For example, it seems reasonable to suppose that acquired hearing impairment, because it involves loss, might lead to a grief reaction. Clearly, not everyone experiencing grief about hearing loss will react in ways that would allow them to be classified as psychiatrically dysfunctional. One recent study used a different approach to the study of hearing loss. The researchers (Kerr and Cowie 1997) used a questionnaire to discover the subjective experiences of people with acquired hearing loss. As a result of their analysis of the responses to the questionnaire they emphasized the multidimensional nature of the experience of hearing loss, and described its effects in terms of six factors. Only one of these factors referred to the communication problems that one might expect to be associated with hearing loss. One factor was concerned with social restrictions such as employment difficulties and strained family relationships. Another factor referred to poor interactions on the part of others: deafened people perceive others as using strategies that undermine the confidence of a hearing-impaired person. For example, hearing people may use gestures rather than speech when communicating with hearing-impaired people or ignore them in conversation. The other factors emphasized the psychological dimensions of the experience. One of these factors was concerned with the distress associated with interactions. It referred to the emotional distress of anticipating and trying to avoid communication breakdown as well as the aftermath of that breakdown. It also referred to a sense of social isolation. The next factor highlighted a sense of loss and bereavement as a result of hearing loss and the feeling that hearing people do not understand what it is like to be deafened. The final factor was concerned with positive experiences associated with hearing loss, such as the value of social support and of gaining greater inner philosophical resources. In common with other studies, Kerr and Cowie (1997) found that audiological factors alone did not predict how much impact a hearing loss would have on a person's life.

The finding that hearing loss might be associated with some positive consequences may seem surprising. However, this has been noted by other workers in the field. Positive consequences such as not having to listen to unpleasant noises, a sense of success in overcoming difficulties and an affinity with other hearing-impaired people have been recorded by researchers examining the psychosocial aspects of hearing loss. The effects of hearing loss are therefore not always those that one might intuitively predict. It is also worth noting that not all cochlear implant users report a positive psychological outcome, even when they acknowledge that the implant provides obvious acoustic benefit. It is sometimes the case that the 'restoration of hearing' provided by the implant does not lead to all the changes in life that the person hoped for. For example, the author is aware of one young implant user who lost his hearing in his early teenage years, with a range of social and psychological consequences. He considered that one of the most important of these consequences was his inability to get a girlfriend. Following cochlear implantation he performed very well in speech perception tests. However, he became agitated and depressed. He had hoped that the implant would improve his confidence with women, and when it did not, he had a sense of despair.

## The World Health Organization model

The complexity of the relationship between hearing loss and emotional wellbeing can be accounted for by the fact that hearing loss does not occur in a vacuum but rather in the 'rich tapestry of life'. Two people with the same level of hearing loss may have quite different life experiences. The effect that their hearing loss may have on their daily lives and emotional wellbeing may differ substantially. The World Health Organization (WHO) (1980) classification of impairment, disability and handicap has been used when seeking to explain the lack of a clear relationship between the extent of hearing loss and the level of psychological disturbance.

Stephens and Hetu (1991) provided definitions of impairment, disability and handicap within an audiological context. They defined impairment as the defective function that may be measured using psychoacoustical techniques. They suggested that this is independent of psychosocial factors. They defined disability as the *auditory* problem experienced and complained of by the individual. They refer to handicap as the *non-auditory* problems that result from hearing impairment and disability. This will be determined by the social and cultural context within which the hearing impairment occurs. Because handicap refers to the disadvantage that the individual experiences there will not be a direct relationship between impairment, disability and handicap. Put very crudely, a hearing loss is likely to interfere with a concert violinist's ability to fulfil his role more than it will interfere with an artist's ability to make paintings; the handicap in one case is likely to be greater than in the other.

The WHO (1980) model has, however, been challenged in other areas of healthcare. The psychologist Marie Johnson (1996) summarized a number of difficulties when the traditional model is applied to physical disorders and suggested amendments to it. The WHO (1980) model assumes that different health professionals would rate a person's behaviour similarly. Johnson pointed out that nurses consistently rated patients as more disabled than did physiotherapists and occupational therapists. She sought to explain this observation in terms of differences in the patient's behaviour elicited by different professionals. Social circumstances also influence the level of disability observed. Some psychological models used in the study of people with chronic disease postulate that people cope with their own mental concept of the problem rather than with the problem itself. Studies have also indicated that patients' perceptions of the control they have over their disability influences the outcome of rehabilitation, whatever the original level of disability.

**The theory of planned behaviour: a psychological model**

It cannot be assumed that all disabled people have an equal and full intention to perform everyday tasks. For example, past failures to perform tasks may lead a person to give up even when there has been a recovery from impairment. Johnson (1996) argued that levels of disability are influenced by a combination of a person's intention to behave in a certain way and their perceived control over being able to do so. She placed considerable emphasis on the theory of planned behaviour in this context. This theory suggests that a person's intention to perform a task is determined by a combination of their attitude to the behaviour, subjective norm for the behaviour and perceived control over the behaviour. In a hearing rehabilitation context, the behaviour in question might be speaking with others. An attitude associated with this might be 'when I speak to people I mishear and feel embarrassed and I dislike embarrassment'. The subjective norm might be 'my spouse wishes to do the talking for me and I am happy to go along with this' and an example of perceived control over the behaviour could be 'I am not confident that I can hear what people say'. Applying the theory of planned behaviour to the WHO (1980) model, Johnson proposed that physical impairment influences mental representations which, in turn, determine behavioural intentions and the behaviour itself. In summary, the suggestion is that disability, like handicap, is a form of behaviour that is subject to manipulation in the same way as any other behaviour.

The point that social factors influence the level of disability has long been recognized. Stephens and Hetu (1991) pointed out that the disability caused by a hearing loss depends not only on the extent of the impairment but also on factors such as lifestyle, employment and social situation. In a wider context, the social model of disability emphasizes social barriers as the determinants of disability, for example, a wheelchair user is disabled when confronted by a flight of steps rather than a ramp. Johnson's argument, however, goes beyond this by highlighting not only social determinants of disability but also cognitive or mental ones.

While the notion that hearing-impaired people face social barriers is now considered self-evident, from a clinical point of view it is also apparent that they encounter psychological obstacles. Few would challenge the idea that the way a person complains about hearing loss can be emotionally determined and that reduced motivation, or anxiety about failure, may lead a person to abandon the goals of rehabilitation, so maintaining levels of disability and handicap. It is also widely accepted that emotional factors can interfere with a person's ability to carry out tasks such as lip-reading and the use of non-verbal information, so influencing levels of disability. It might be argued that this simply represents feedback loops in the traditional WHO model of impairment, disability and handicap, and is not a new structure. To the author's knowledge, Johnson's ideas have not been directly tested in the field of hearing impairment. There is, however, evidence indicating that the effects of acquired hearing loss go beyond difficulties in communication; there are strands of support for the idea that psychological factors influence hearing disability directly. One piece of research from the field of cochlear implants is informative in this context. An assessment was carried out of a group of implant users' retrospective perception of changes in their psychological status. The assessment indicated that almost all of the group studied believed that their lives were close to ideal prior to the onset of hearing loss, and that this was radically changed by their hearing loss. It seems implausible that so many people in the group would have had near-perfect lives before losing their hearing, and it seems more likely that there has been a cognitive manoeuvre or a change in people's mental maps of their psychological status. The effect is to increase the perception of the loss experienced; this in turn may have acted as a determinant of the subsequent disability behaviour.

**A new WHO model**

A new classification of impairments, disability and handicap is being developed by the WHO (1997). The proposed new classification again refers to three levels of disablement: losses or abnormalities of bodily function and structure (previously referred to as impairments), limitations of activities (previously disabilities) and restriction in participation (previously handicaps). The proposed new classification is set within the context of the social model of disability. It suggests that disablement occurs within and by means of 'contextual factors'. Two sorts of contextual factors are identified: social and environmental factors, and personal factors. Social and environmental factors include physical conditions such as climate and terrain, as well as aspects of the social environment, including social attitudes, laws, policies and social and political institutions. Personal factors include gender, age, other health conditions, coping styles, social background, education, occupation, past and current experience, overall behaviour pattern, character style and other factors that influence the way in which disablement is experienced by the individual. This new classification is broad enough to incorporate the ideas put forward by Johnson. However, Johnson's model more clearly delineates the role of psychological factors.

It can therefore be seen that, in addition to the depression and sense of isolation from which a deafened person may suffer, there are a number of other less obvious areas in which hearing loss may interact with an individual's psychological state. These include:

- the individual's own image of a deafened person, derived from social stereotypes and his or her own encounters with hearing impaired people and relatives
- the fact that deafness has the power to make people less socially capable
- the fact that deafness may make the processing of verbal information harder and so slow up the normal flow of social interaction
- people's differing tolerance of, and compensation for, their disability
- the fact that a person's handicap from deafness can be related to his or her own attitude to the disability.

In addition, all the above factors are influenced by the age, social circumstances and education of the deafened person.

## Treatment

From a psychological point of view much of the emphasis within a clinical setting has been on providing a psychotherapeutic or counselling response to the emotional consequences of hearing loss.

### Loss and bereavement

The element of loss in acquired hearing impairment suggests that some knowledge of the bereavement process may be important in understanding and helping the hearing-impaired person. Freud suggested that the process of adjustment to loss is an active one that he referred to as 'grief work'. It has been widely believed that grief reactions proceed through stages.

Different authors have labelled the processes involved differently, but there seems to be a considerable degree of overlap in the descriptions. One classic model suggests that the process begins with a period of denial, followed by anger and then bargaining in which the person adheres to the advice given to him or her in the hope that the problem will go away. It is thought that when these strategies do not lead to the removal of the problem there follows a period of depression. Only after this comes an acceptance of the loss; this involves a change in the person's identity and a redefinition of 'self' to incorporate the loss. The evidence, however, suggests that while grief does involve a variety of emotions it does not strictly follow through the stages traditionally suggested. It is now accepted that a person can experience a variety of emotions but can then return to emotions experienced earlier in the process: for example, after bargaining the person might return to anger.

There is an enormous variation in the degree of distress and in the time taken by different people to adjust to similar losses. This is thought to be related to different styles of coping, but another important variable is the circumstances in which the loss has taken place. For a hearing loss, this may include factors such as whether the loss was sudden or gradual and whether other distressing symptoms such as tinnitus or vertigo are present. It is still widely assumed that it is beneficial for thoughts and feelings to be confronted. However, more recent research suggests that suppression of thoughts and feelings may be just as helpful as confrontation with them as a means of adjusting to a grief reaction. There is a general psychotherapeutic maxim of not forcing a person to confront an issue and this would seem to be just as relevant when counselling a hearing-impaired person as when counselling anyone else.

### Behavioural treatments

The WHO (1980) model and its replacement use a behavioural perspective in the assessment and treatment of hearing loss and of other disabilities. Johnson also suggested that a focus be placed on disability behaviour rather than just on emotional responses to disability. With a behavioural approach, emphasis is placed on considering each patient as unique and in need of a tailor-made set of rehabilitation strategies. The therapist must identify both the forms of behaviour that need to be changed and the factors that control them. It should to be remembered that the patient experiences the loss of hearing in his or her own environment. Identifying the controlling factors involves observing those circumstances in which the relevant behaviour takes place and also observing the consequences of that behaviour.

A behavioural approach to audiological rehabilitation has been described by McKenna (1987). The approach suggested follows the principles of goal planning, a system widely used in mental health rehabilitation and with learning-disabled people. It involves the use of clear behavioural language in the description of the patient's needs and of the things that each person involved in the rehabilitation will do. Abstract concepts are avoided and goals are described in terms of what the person says or does. For example, rather than having a vague objective for a patient, such as 'better communication', specific goals may be stated, such as 'he needs to wear his hearing aids for six hours a day' or 'he needs to tell people how to talk to him'. These goals are then broken down into achievable steps and each person's role in achieving the steps is described. An emphasis is placed on abilities rather than disabilities and positive language is used, e.g. 'the patient needs to practise relaxation techniques' rather than 'he cannot relax'. Goal planning does not impose any theoretical framework nor dictate what therapies should be used in the rehabilitation. Rather, it is a framework for organizing the rehabilitation process. It is a means of stating what should be achieved but does not dictate the method of intervention.

A study by Andersson et al. (1995) described a behavioural approach to the management of hearing loss in a group of elderly people. This focused on the use of hearing tactics, i.e. the methods used by hearing-impaired people to solve the everyday problems that result from hearing loss. The treatment involved setting individualized treatment goals and achieving these through the use of behavioural tasks. It included the use of video recording, the rehearsal of tactics, and teaching of relaxation and coping skills. The results indicated that subjects treated in this way were better able to cope with their hearing loss. The authors concluded that disability resulting from hearing impairment could be regarded as a behavioural problem and that this behaviour can be the central focus of rehabilitation. They suggested that cognitive, and especially motivational, factors are of the utmost importance in how hearing disability is viewed.

### Cognitive therapy

Cognitive factors can be changed through the use of cognitive therapy. This is a form of psychotherapy that focuses on discovering people's thought processes and changing these when they are unrealistically negative or unhelpful. It is based on the cognitive model of Beck (1995) and forms the basis for the practice of many clinical psychologists in the UK. The model proposes that people's thoughts influence their emotional state and that negative thoughts are not only a feature of emotional disturbance but that they maintain the disorder. Negative beliefs relate to the person, the world and the future. They are maintained by cognitive distortions such as 'all or nothing thinking' or the selective acceptance of information that confirms the person's ideas and rejection of information that contradicts them. Cognitive distortions are, in turn, thought to occur as a consequence of a poor emotional state.

Cognitive therapy is pragmatic in style and is usually brief, ranging from as few as six to about 20 sessions, over a course of months rather than years. Part of the therapeutic effort is in elucidating the person's thoughts about his circumstances. People are often unaware of the content of their thoughts until they pay specific attention to them and they are usually much more aware of the emotions that their thoughts produce. Thoughts often have an automatic quality and take the form of a 'running commentary' or 'dialogue' and are frequently in a shorthand form. Automatic thoughts are not necessarily the result of reasoning or reflection on a situation, but often arise spontaneously. They tend to be specific and can be plausible, in spite of evidence that contradicts them. They do not necessarily arise as a result of external events but can be provoked by ruminations or memories. Techniques such as questioning and diary keeping help to reveal the content of automatic thoughts.

Another part of the therapy involves assessing the accuracy of automatic thoughts through the use of techniques such as questioning (rather than persuasion) or behavioural experiments. The discovery of negative distortions in a person's automatic thoughts can lead to these thoughts being reformulated and a consequent improvement in the associated emotion. In addition to awareness of their day-to-day thoughts, the person can be helped to become aware of deeper 'core' beliefs that are formed through early learning experiences. These are more difficult to articulate and may take some effort to access. These core beliefs are generalized in nature and ultimately have a determining influence on how the person thinks about all events. Most people maintain relatively positive core beliefs most of the time, but at times of emotional distress negative ones can emerge and become dominant. When they have a negative content, core beliefs are commonly concerned with the idea that the person is 'not good enough' in terms of either being inadequate or unloveable in some way. Intermediate beliefs in the form of attitudes, rules and assumptions lie between the core beliefs and the day-to-day automatic thoughts. Intermediate beliefs help the person to cope with any painful ideas that may be inherent in the core beliefs. Initially, therapy usually focuses on identifying and changing automatic thoughts to produce symptom relief. Subsequently, intermediate and core beliefs become the focus of the treatment.

In the context of audiological rehabilitation, cognitive therapy extends the discussion to include what the person *thinks* about his hearing loss or the rehabilitation. For example, a woman in her late sixties with a moderate hearing impairment was unwilling to wear her hearing aids or to use hearing tactics and felt very anxious at the prospect of social encounters. Questioning within a cognitive therapy context revealed that the automatic thought that underlay her anxiety about socializing was that others would mistake her hearing impairment for stupidity. This reflected an 'all or nothing' style of thinking in which she saw any slip in her social performance as tantamount to total failure. Her reluctance to wear her hearing aids had a similar automatic thought behind it: that other people would identify her as deaf and so classify her as stupid. The automatic thought behind her reluctance to use hearing tactics was that others would think her unpleasant or too assertive for doing so.

These ideas were tackled in cognitive therapy by having her evaluate her performance and the reactions of others in social situations to date. To help her get a clearer perspective on the issue she was also asked to consider how she might advise another person with a hearing loss who was facing similar situations. This was followed up by having her attempt a relatively safe social encounter wearing her aids with people she trusted; this was an experiment to test out her automatic thoughts. These strategies brought about some reduction in her anxiety.

The patient was a writer and in the course of the therapy she complained that she had not submitted any work for publication for years, and had left many scripts unfinished. Her automatic thought behind her avoidance was that her scripts might be rejected. She believed that she could not bear the emotional pain of this. Further questioning revealed that she had been an awkward and clumsy child who often made mistakes and that her elder sister would not let her play with her because she was too young. She therefore spent much time alone as a child. She developed strong core beliefs that she is ultimately someone who others would reject and that she would end up 'an old maid' alone, unless she succeeded at everything that she did. These deeper beliefs formed the setting for her automatic thoughts about her hearing loss and her work as a writer, and became the focus of the cognitive therapy. A change in her core belief that she was not good enough led to a further reduction in her anxiety and to lasting behavioural change.

## Conclusions

Reactions to hearing loss are determined in a complex way and are multidimensional in nature. People's responses to hearing loss or to the restoration of hearing are not always easily predictable. They depend on cognitive, behavioural and social influences as well as the changes in their ability to hear. The stereotypical images of hearing-impaired people do little justice to the actual experience of having a hearing loss. An approach to rehabilitation that focuses only on an attempt to alter the input of sounds to the ear runs the risk of ignoring fundamental aspects of the experience and therefore faces the prospect of only limited success. It is therefore perhaps not surprising that there is a large variation in hearing-impaired people's acceptance and use of hearing aids. The management of acquired hearing loss needs to go beyond the provision of hearing aids and should include the manipulation of many factors, including psychological ones. This was recognized almost 20 years ago when Goldstein and Stephens (1981) recommended that aural rehabilitation should address psychological factors. Our understanding of the issues involved has improved since then and the argument for the involvement of clinical psychologists in rehabilitation of hearing-impaired people has become all the more persuasive.

## Summary

- Responses to hearing loss depend on cognitive, behavioural and social influences.
- Disability can be regarded as behaviour, subject to the same laws as any other behaviours.
- Success in rehabilitation may depend on changing psychological factors as well as acoustic ones.
- Responses to hearing loss can be the focus of psychological therapy.
- Psychological therapy can also seek to change the behaviour that represents hearing disability.

## Further reading

McKenna L, Andersson G (1998) Hearing disorders. In: Bellack A, Hersen, M (eds) Comprehensive Clinical Psychology, Vol 9: Applications in diverse populations. Oxford: Elsevier.

# Chapter 17
# Deafness and mental health

PETER HINDLEY AND NICK KITSON

Deaf children and adults are at greater risk of developing mental health problems than their hearing counterparts. This is primarily the consequence of being deaf in a hearing-oriented society and, in this sense, the vast majority of these mental health problems are preventable.

*This chapter is primarily concerned with people with severe to profound bilateral sensorineural deafness, hereon called deaf people.* It has a number of objectives. First, it describes a cultural model of deafness. Second, it identifies the main factors that lead to deaf people being more vulnerable to mental health problems. It goes on to identify factors and interventions that can enhance deaf people's resilience. This part of the chapter will be of particular relevance to audiology and otolaryngology professionals, whose views and advice often have a powerful impact on the parents of deaf children. Finally, the chapter describes how deafness and the consequences of deafness affect the presentation of mental health problems in children and adults, and how therapeutic approaches can be adapted when working with deaf children and adults.

## A cultural model of deafness

The majority of deaf children will grow up to use some form of sign language and many will feel more at ease with deaf rather than hearing peers (Gregory, Bishop and Sheldon 1995). The vast majority will, of necessity, spend their working lives in primarily hearing environments but will choose to spend their social lives with other deaf people. The worlds of deaf and hearing people intersect but are separate. Deaf people learn to live within and across these separate worlds. Over the past 40 years, a model of deafness has grown, which sees deaf people as a linguistic and cultural group rather than a disabled group. Like all cultural groups, deaf people are not homogeneous but the use of sign language is often seen as the central defining feature of deaf culture, alongside an experience of the world in primarily visual terms. Traditionally, attending a school for deaf children and membership of deaf organizations such as deaf clubs have been seen as other key experiences (Meadow-Orlans and Erting 2000). However, over the past 30 years increasing numbers of deaf children have attended mainstream schools. Membership of deaf clubs has declined to be replaced by more informal associations supported by modern telecommunications devices such as text telephones, faxes, videophones and e-mail.

Deaf culture is unique in that the transmission of beliefs is primarily horizontal rather than vertical. Approximately 90–95% of deaf children are born into hearing families. Most of these families have no prior experience of deafness. Their beliefs about language use and educational placement will be partly shaped by their own experience. For many, local professionals and local service provision will determine whether or not their child acquires spoken or signed language first and whether or not they attend a mainstream school or a school for deaf children. Their child's experience of being deaf and their beliefs and attitudes will be shaped by these experiences. Their child's contact with deaf culture will be through deaf peers and deaf adults from outside the family.

## Sign language

Sign languages are the naturally occurring languages of deaf communities. Sign language is not international, each national deaf community having its own sign language; in Britain this is British Sign Language or BSL. Each national sign language will have its own dialects and regional variations. Sign languages are visuospatial languages, which use a combination of hand shape and movement, facial expression, eye gaze and body movement to convey semantic and syntactic information. All sign languages are theoretically capable of communicating ideas as complex and subtle as ideas conveyed by spoken language. The extent to which this happens depends in great part on the educational opportunities and experiences available to deaf children and adults.

Each sign language has its own grammatical structure, although most use a specified sign space and placement within this sign space as a central grammatical structure. The syntaxes of most sign languages are completely distinct from those of their native spoken languages. In the case of BSL, where English uses noun–verb–object structures, BSL uses topic–comment structures, more akin to Navajo or Yoruba. When sign language is written down, usually in word-for-sign order, it can resemble psychiatrically disordered spoken language. In fact, this reflects the different underlying grammatical structures. Most sign languages use some form of finger-spelling (i.e. different handshapes used to represent different letters of the alphabet) to convey words, and especially names, in the native spoken language. The vast majority across the world use one-handed finger-spelling, BSL and Auslan (Australian Sign Language) are among the few that use two-handed finger-spelling. For further information about BSL and other sign languages see Kyle and Woll (1985).

## Vulnerability and resilience factors

This brief account of a cultural view of deafness will provide the framework to discuss vulnerability and resilience factors for deaf children and adults. The first context we consider is the family environment in which children grow up.

Two related sets of factors will have a powerful impact on deaf children's psychological development and mental health. The first is the family's response to having a deaf child. By family we mean parents, siblings, members of the extended family and especially grandparents. The response of parents to being told that their child is deaf has been likened to a bereavement, in the sense that the parents have lost the idealized child they had wished for. Although there are elements of loss, it may be equally useful to think about this experience using a stress/adaptation model. In this model, the nature of the stressor, the extent to which families have been able to prepare for the stressful event and the resources – both intrapersonal and social – available to members of the family, will all have an influence on the way in which the family adapts.

Clinicians who are the first to inform parents that their child is deaf can play a significant part in supporting effective adaptation. A number of practical steps can help parents. First, ensuring that parents have plenty of time to absorb information and ask questions and offering early follow-up appointments to allow parents to ask the questions they thought of after the first appointment had finished. Second, trying, as far as possible, to ensure that both parents attend together or, in the case of lone parents, that they have a relative or close friend with them at these initial appointments. Third, offering balanced written information about all the options open to their child from the outset, so that parents can go away and begin to understand the nature of the problems they face. It is often very difficult for parents to remember fully all that has been said under conditions of stress. The National Deaf Children's Society (see p. 287) provides useful information packs that describe all the options open to deaf children. Luterman (1987) provides a thoughtful and sensitive account of the management of this period.

There is evidence (Greenberg and Calderon 1984) that early introduction of sign language, combined with parental counselling about the needs of their deaf child, has a positive impact on children's social and emotional development and parents' sense of wellbeing. Such an approach will support parents in processing the emotions and the desire for information that such news can provoke in many parents. The processing of this information and these emotions can be a major challenge for many parents. Our experience is that parents who either angrily reject the possibility of their child being deaf or deny that their child is deaf have the most worrying prognosis. The extent to which parents are able to process these thoughts and feelings is influenced by the degree of social support they can access. Parents who have limited social networks and parents whose extended family impose their own views of the child's diagnosis and needs, or support a state of denial, are again more vulnerable. Finally, it is worth noting that there is tendency for the social networks of some parents of deaf children to become professionalized, with a corresponding reduction in natural social networks as friends and family withdraw (Quittner, Gleuckauf and Jackson 1990).

The outcome of this process of adaptation is positive for most parents of deaf children. However, some will remain in persistent denial or angry rejection and others will maintain a sense of persistent grief. Although there is no research in this area, our clinical experience, and our knowledge of the effects of maternal depression on child mental health, suggest that these feelings will have a detrimental effect on the development of an attachment relationship between the deaf child and his or her parents. Disordered attachment can persist into adulthood and is a significant risk factor for a range of child and adult mental health problems. Early identification and intervention for such families is likely to have a significant preventive effect. Two forms of intervention can be of benefit. Those parents who appear stuck in either angry rejection or denial may benefit from sensitive discussion of these feelings. Once the parents are able to recognize the difficulty, referral to a local clinical psychology or counselling service may help parents to move on. Second, contact with other parents of deaf children who have been through similar experiences may help parents to reflect on how their thoughts and feelings are affecting their child. The National Deaf Children's Society has developed residential weekends for families, which are highly effective in creating an environment in which these conversations between parents can occur.

## Access to the developmental environment

Given that most deaf children are born into hearing families, most with no prior knowledge of deafness, differences in communication and language need are likely to be the rule rather than the exception. It appears that as long as the fundamental relationship between the child and the parents is sound, these differences do not act as a barrier to the earliest stages of attachment formation. However, from the child's second year onwards, verbal communication (whether in spoken or signed language) becomes increasingly important in supporting the child's development. Thus parents who use visual means of communication with their deaf child are far more likely to achieve mature attachment relationships in which the parents and the child can separate by agreement and without undue distress by the time child is four years old.

Other aspects of psychological development are intimately linked to language development. To give two examples, the development of an understanding of emotions and emotional experience and the development of consequential thinking are highly dependent on language development. In most hearing children, these capacities will be well-established by the time they first enter school (at five years in the UK), but most deaf children will experience considerable delays, some continuing into adolescence and adulthood. Equally the development of abstract operational thinking, occurring from late childhood onwards for most hearing children, is frequently delayed and sometimes even fails to develop in deaf children. The fact that these developmental delays are rarely seen in deaf children of deaf parents who use sign language suggests that early and continuing effective communication are key factors for deaf children's healthy development.

Deaf children face similar difficulties face in their interactions with their peers. Longitudinal studies of the development of deaf children's peer relationship (see Hindley and Brown 1994 for a review) show that deaf children in mainstream settings experience increasing difficulty in accessing meaningful peer groups as they progress through school. This becomes particularly important at the transition to adolescence, when conversation about shared interests replaces physical play. Deaf children begin to feel increasingly isolated from, and at times rejected by, their hearing peers. This is further compounded by the high levels of teasing and bullying of deaf students which occur in many schools.

### Other vulnerability factors

There are two other main areas of vulnerability for deaf children. First, there is considerable evidence that deaf children are at greater risk of all forms of abuse than hearing children (Sullivan, Brookhouser and Scanlan 2000). This is both within and outside the family. The factors relating to early family relationships outlined above, disrupted attachments and angry rejection, are similar to abuse risk factors seen in hearing children and may contribute to higher rates of abuse within families. Second, problems of communication make it less likely that deaf children will be believed if they disclose abuse or that successful criminal proceedings will be brought. These two factors make deaf children attractive targets for paedophiles. Finally, residential schools, without effective child protection procedures, are arenas within which abuse by both peers and staff and other adults can take place.

The other main area of vulnerability is with respect to central nervous system (CNS) abnormalities. Deaf children are at greater risk of CNS abnormalities, either because of acquired aetiologies such as intrauterine cytomegalovirus (CMV) or anoxic brain damage, or because of congenital anomalies, such as CHARGE (see Chapter 11) syndrome, where CNS abnormalities form part of the syndrome.

## Preventative interventions

Preventative interventions can be considered at primary and secondary levels. Tertiary prevention will be considered later. At a primary level the early provision of sign language to all deaf infants, from as soon after diagnosis as possible, is the single intervention that is most likely to prevent additional child mental health problems. The effectiveness of deaf language aide projects (Vaccari and Marschark 1997) shows that such provision is both practical and practicable. The evidence from Scandinavia, with over 20 years of experience of introducing native sign languages to deaf children and their parents, shows that rates of psychiatric disorder among deaf children in these countries are no greater than among hearing children (Sinkkonen 1994).

At a secondary level a range of educational interventions have been described to enhance deaf children's social and emotional development (see Hindley 1997 for review). The most well-tried approach is Greenberg and Kusche's (1993) social and emotional curriculum, Promoting Alternative Thinking Strategies or PATHS. This was initially developed in the USA specifically for deaf children and has now been adapted for use in the UK (Reed 1999). It is also used extensively in countries such as Holland. It promotes self-control, emotional understanding, reflective thinking skills and social problem solving. The efficacy of PATHS has now been demonstrated in a variety of countries and educational settings – both mainstream and segregated – and has proved to be usable in a variety of settings and educational philosophies – oral and signing. Promoting the development of these social and emotional skills in deaf children will be beneficial in both childhood and adulthood in preventing a range of behavioural, emotional and personality difficulties. PATHS will also enhance the efficacy of a range of self-protection programmes designed to help deaf children who experience abuse (see Sullivan et al. 2000). However, these programmes cannot disguise the need for protection agencies to provide appropriate resources when investigating allegations of abuse involving deaf children (Kennedy 1992), nor the responsibility of all, but especially residential schools, to ensure that their pupils are adequately protected.

# Child psychiatry and deaf children and their families

Deaf children experience the same range of psychiatric disorders as their hearing peers, but two factors can prevent identification and accurate assessment of these problems. First, difficulties in communication. Many child psychiatric disorders, particularly emotional disorders, depend on the children communicating their distress and people in their environment accurately identifying this distress. Deaf children may not have sufficient vocabulary to express feelings of sadness, self-blame or anxiety. Equally, parents and teachers may not have sufficient signing skill to identify these feelings when children try to express them. The second factor is misattribution of all additional problems to the child's deafness. Thus behavioural problems can be explained because 'all deaf children have behavioural problems', or perhaps, more worryingly, autism can be explained as being part of the communication problems that deaf children experience. Both factors can have an impact on mental health clinicians with limited experience of working with deaf children and can lead to a sense of panic that prevents the clinician from using their basic skills.

The presentation of mental health problems in deaf children does not appear to differ fundamentally from hearing children, but the factors that account for their increased vulnerability to mental health problems are different (see above). It is important to bear these factors in mind when assessing deaf children and their families and when planning and delivering treatment.

### Assessment

As with hearing children, the assessment of deaf children with mental health problems needs to consider the child in context. That is the child and family or carers, the child in school and the child and his or her friendships and peer relationships. Preschool children are best seen with their families, with an individual interview with the child less often needed. The older the child the more essential an individual interview becomes and some teenagers may choose to be seen without their parents. Interviews with families need to assess the form and quality of communication within the family; in some families there may be no meaningful communication between the deaf child and his or her parents and siblings. The family interview also provides a means of assessing relationships. It is vital to gain an understanding of how the child sees him or herself and how parents and siblings see each other. For many parents the process and the moment of the diagnosis of deafness remain enduring memories and for some, profoundly affect their relationship with their child. For some parents, being parents of a deaf child has become a major part of their view of themselves as parents. Gathering an understanding of these aspects of relationships within families plays an important part in shaping a treatment plan.

It is our impression that schools play a larger part in the lives of deaf children and adults than of their hearing peers. This may be partly because their teachers are often the adults in their lives with the best communication skills. Equally, if they are in a deaf school or hearing impaired unit, their deaf peers may be their only friends. Information from school is essential. This can be gathered either by report or by a standardized questionnaire (e.g. the Strengths and Difficulties Questionnaire, Goodman 1996) or by direct observation. Direct observation, in both classroom and playground, often yields the most useful information.

A considerable proportion of deaf children, approximately 15%, will have additional disabilities, therefore physical examination is frequently indicated. A high index of suspicion for epilepsy should be maintained: ictal and peri-ictal phenomena can mimic behavioural and emotional disorders and predispose children to such problems. Equally, anticonvulsants have beneficial and adverse psychotropic properties.

**Management and treatment**

Clinically, the largest group of children referred to our specialist service is children with conduct disorders. However, the majority of these children also have emotional problems and/or disorders ranging from lowered self-esteem to major depression coincident with conduct disorder. Following assessment, the majority appear to benefit from a multi-modal approach to treatment. For preschool and early school-aged children, a parent management approach (such as the Parent–Child Game) combined with enhancement of communication and work aimed at encouraging a positive view of deafness appears the most effective approach.

For older children the need for individual work becomes greater. Some deaf children and young people appear to engage more easily with a deaf professional, certainly ease and flexibility of communication is of prime importance when working with teenagers. Depending on the underlying psychopathology, some children whose difficulties relate primarily to early trauma respond to psychodynamic approaches. In other children, where impulse control and irritability are underlying mechanisms, cognitive behavioural approaches are more effective. Both these approaches can be successfully adapted for use with deaf children. Some children with aggressive conduct disorders, particularly where there is evidence of brain disorder, benefit from psychotropics such as carbamazepine or sodium valproate. The major neuroleptics (e.g. chlorpromazine) are very rarely indicated in these circumstances.

Emotional disorders present in similar ways to hearing children. Depression with loss of interest, irritability and sadness. All of these symptoms are often more changeable than in adults. Subtle emotional distress is often not picked up: a quiet, depressed child sitting at the back of the classroom is less likely to gain attention than an angry, disruptive child. The main means of treating depression in children and adolescents is by psychotherapy and family therapy. Children and adolescents appear to respond more variably and generally less well to antidepressants than do adults. Deaf children experience obsessive-compulsive disorder and other anxiety disorders and again psychotherapies are the main means of treatment.

The assessment and treatment of the major psychoses are similar in children and adults, and are covered below. It is worth noting that deaf children frequently have complex networks of professionals surrounding them. Major difficulties in relationships in families with children with psychotic disorder are sometimes played out within these professional networks, often to the detriment of the child or young person's wellbeing. It can be very difficult for the parents of a deaf child, who may already have difficulty in accepting deafness, to accept the diagnosis of a major psychiatric illness. Parents will need time to think through the implications and work through their emotions.

Finally, there appears to be an increased risk of deaf children presenting with autism and other pervasive developmental disorders. Our service has assessed 30 such young people and children, and a study in the USA (Jure, Rapin and Tuchman 1991) found an overall prevalence of 4% in a clinical population of deaf children compared with a prevalence of 0.4% in hearing children. This is likely to be due to co-morbidity. The majority of deaf children with autism appear to benefit from the use of sign language, which enhances their communication and their social functioning.

# Adult psychiatry

## Assessment

### Language

Communication between doctor and patient is, for psychiatrists, the major part of the examination, not merely history taking. The psychiatrist for deaf people could be significantly handicapped by lack of shared, comprehensive, fluent communication. Individual deaf people vary their use of language widely, shifting code to match the needs of others. Psychiatrists must be able or enabled to assess the normal and abnormal form and meaning of this use of language.

On the face of it, informants or interpreters can enable an accurate history to be taken, but are they reliable and who but the patient can relate the subjective experience of events? All mental health workers, except those who themselves are fluent in sign language, will be handicapped in examining a mental state. The majority of this assessment relies on direct observation of the patient's behaviour, attitudes and emotions associated with the content of the interview. The assumed emotion, attitudes and roles of others or past self that is part of storytelling in sign must be distinguished from the current mental state. This is important for both diagnosis and psychotherapy.

### Attitude

Attitude and assumptions are also a handicap. Mental health workers in both generic and deaf services have been found to rate 'deaf' cases as needing more supervision and medication. Experienced psychiatrists have been found to make negative prognostic assumptions. As for deaf children, abnormal behaviour may be attributed to the patient's deafness. Frustrated communication or irritability secondary to CNS abnormalities may be mistaken for evidence of mental illness.

### Phenomena

It is generally agreed that the standard classifications of mental disorders such as the WHO *International Classification of Disorder*, ICD-10 (WHO 1992) and the American Psychiatric Association's *Diagnostic and Statistical Manual*, DSM IV (APA 1994) are appropriate to deaf people. Similarly the phenomenology is generally the same or a signed equivalent. However, there are some differences between phenomena observed in hearing and deaf people.

Deaf patients may suffer concrete, absolute right or wrong, thinking, have difficulty sequencing time and have difficulty with 'who', 'why', 'where', 'when', 'what' and 'how' questions. The one way around this can be the use of multiple-choice questions, but with the risk of suggesting answers. Additionally, the direction of actions related by the deaf person may be unclear, as pronouns for subject and object in sentences are usually redundant in sign language. Either the patient may sign with inadequate context and direction due to poor development of language or illness, or the interviewer may have difficulty perceiving the subtle sophistication of directionality in sign.

Deaf patients not suffering mental illness may appear to suffer tangential thinking. Topic changes can be rapid and without context, or subtle context changes and cues can be missed by all except the most skilled signers. It is not uncommon for deaf people (and hearing people signing to them) to talk rapidly and anxiously to avoid the reception mode of conversation, which usually feels more difficult.

Clinical experience suggests that delayed personality development and an agitated appearance may mask depressive illness in some deaf people. The somatic symptoms of depressive illness, where present, may be particularly useful as well as being indicators of a response to antidepressants. A family history of affective disorder, good premorbid function prior to otherwise unexplained behavioural change, lack of reactivity to circumstance and phasic episodes are also potential indicators of underlying affective illness.

The words in deaf people's writing not uncommonly take the order of the signs as used in sign language. Such writings have been found to suggest thought disorder, presenting as fragmented and confused. If writings are to be used in diagnosis then they need to be compared with the same patient's premorbid writings. The signs of formal thought disorder, a cardinal feature of major mental illnesses such as schizophrenia or bipolar affective disorder, seen in sign language are broadly equivalent to those seen in spoken language, with some subtle differences (Kitson and Thacker 1999). However, one common feature of sign language, the repetition of a sign for emphasis, may be mistaken for perseveration.

*Epidemiology*

The majority of those referred to deaf mental health services are not found to be mentally ill. Behavioural problems and developmental disorders associated with deafness predominate.

Schizophrenia appears to be no more or less common in deaf people than the 1% found in the overall population. Additionally, the rates of schizophrenia in the parents and siblings of deaf schizophrenia sufferers were found to be similar to those of hearing sufferers. Rates of schizophrenia in a community survey and studies of referrals to deaf mental health services are no more than would have be expected.

Most authors have reported less depressive illness or its presentation as an agitated state in deaf people. A reported absence of guilt in presentations was argued to be due to a lack of superego with a resultant 'lock' on rage. Similarly, it has been argued that low rates of depressive illness have been attributed to delayed personality development in deaf people, suggesting that hearing is required for normal development of human relations, including a conscience. Even Freud commented, 'the ego ... wears an auditory lobe'.

With the increasing sophistication of mental health outpatient clinics and domiciliary services for deaf people, major depression has been found to be increasingly common. For example, in London, diagnoses of major depression have more than quadrupled over a three-year period. This was associated with a referral rate increase of three times, approximately half of the patients being assessed in their homes, the consolidation of deaf people as mental health workers in the service and the employment of a psychotherapist. The frequency of depression in community psychiatric research in the deaf population also supports the idea that the low rates were an artefact of poor services.

Bipolar affective disorder has been described as rare. One author reported only one deaf person with at least one truly depressive phase followed by a manic phase in 15 years. In contrast, the London deaf service, which covers a general population base of up to 20 million, has diagnosed four cases, each with at least one truly manic and one truly depressed phase, and two further cases with diagnoses of mania only from new referrals over a two-year period. An additional six patients with unipolar mania were on the long-term case load in 1994.

## Physical examinations and investigation

Usher's syndrome or retinitis pigmentosa, usually an autosomal recessive disorder of early childhood deafness associated with later onset progressive blindness through pigment deposits on the retina, has been associated with a fivefold increase in the likelihood of schizophrenic-like psychosis. The most common complication of maternal rubella is sensorineural deafness. Thirty-seven per cent of people with deafness due to rubella have additional impairments, compared with approximately 25% of deaf people (Sever, South and Shaver 1985). Rubella is associated with the late development of eye disease, epilepsy, diabetes, thyroid disease or, rarely, progressive rubella panencephalitis, all of which can have psychiatric presentations. Additionally, new behaviour disorders can be directly caused. Pendred's syndrome, an autosomal recessive genetic disorder, also associates congenital deafness with thyroid disease. Both hypothyroidism and hyperthyroidism are associated with psychiatric disorders, which respond to the treatment of the thyroid disorder.

## Assessment and management of specific disorders

### Schizophrenia

Schizophrenia is the commonest major mental illness with a lifetime prevalence of approximately 1%. It can be severely disabling, but prompt diagnosis and early intervention with multimodal treatments (see below) can significantly limit the extent of the disability. The assessment of schizophrenia in deaf people poses a number of problems. First, that some of the symptoms seen in hearing people suffering from schizophrenia, such as poor insight, labile affect, vagueness and inability to see through a course of action, are seen in some deaf people without schizophrenia. Second, that other symptoms, such as delusional perception and hallucinations, require relatively sophisticated language skills that not all deaf people with mental health problems possess. Asking about such unusual experiences can also challenge the language skills of hearing mental health professionals. Third, that apparent delusional beliefs can in fact arise from naivety as a consequence of limited experience. Fourth, that idiosyncratic signs or unusual regional dialects may be mistaken for neologisms seen in schizophrenia. Finally, that unusual experiences, such as auditory hallucinations, may be discounted because professionals do not believe that deaf people can experience such phenomena. In fact, auditory hallucinations are not uncommon in deaf people with schizophrenia, although visual hallucinations, uncommon in hearing people, are commonly reported. Prolonged assessments and detailed observations by skilled staff are often essential to making an accurate diagnosis of psychotic disorders in deaf people. Kitson and Thacker (2000) provide a more detailed account of the above.

The management of schizophrenia depends on three principles. First, rapid treatment with antipsychotics. The newer antipsychotics, such as olanzepine or risperidone, have better side-effect profiles and are better tolerated than older medications. This is particularly important for those deaf people with CNS abnormalities, who are often more likely to experience side-effects, and deaf people with limited communication skills, who may not be able to inform professionals that they are experiencing side effects. Second, social management. A combination of a semi-structured environment, with low levels of hostility from and overinvolvement with carers appears to reduce the likelihood of relapse. Third, a range of cognitive behavioural techniques have been developed to help patients learn how to manage unpleasant auditory hallucinations and challenge delusional beliefs.

## Emotional disorders

Historically, emotional disorders such as depression and anxiety have been thought to be less common in deaf people than in hearing people. However, community surveys of children and adults show that deaf people do develop such disorders. As with major depression, as mental health services for deaf people in the UK have become more sophisticated, the numbers of people with such disorders presenting to the services have increased. In contrast, the number of young people presenting with eating disorders, such as anorexia nervosa, seems relatively low, with only three patients with such problems referred to the service. However, an American study of deaf college students (Hills, Rappold and Rendon 1991) suggested that the prevalence of symptoms of eating disorders, such as binge eating and body image distortions, in a non-clinical population were the same as that in an equivalent hearing population.

The management of emotional disorders depends on accurate assessment. As noted above, the symptoms of these disorders can be subtle and require sophisticated lanaguage skills in the assessor. Management is normally with a combination of psychotherapy and drug treatment. Biological symptoms such as loss of appetite and sleep disturbance are often indicative of a good response to antidepressants. Modern antidepressants such as fluoxetine are equally efficacious as older tricyclics and are much safer in overdose. Suicide risk always needs to be assessed in depressed patients. Both psychodynamic and cognitive behavioural psychotherapy are effective in managing emotional disorders. The choice of psychotherapy will, in part, depend on the individual patient's personal motivation and understanding of his or her own problems and in part on the mental health professional's assessment.

## Behaviour disorders

Psychiatrists for adults rarely use the terms 'behaviour' or 'conduct' disorder. Those with disturbances of behaviour referred to adult services tend to have behaviours that can be understood in the context of the patient's personal development, are long-standing and can be predicted to be resistant to treatment. They are considered part of the patient's personality and labelled as 'personality disorders'. The diagnosis of personality types or disorders is notoriously unreliable.

Until recently it had been generally agreed by psychiatrists for deaf people that deaf people exhibit concrete thinking, rigidity, decreased empathy, projection of responsibility on to others, lack of insight or self-reproach, unrealistic views of their ability, increased demands and impulsivity with poor control of rage (Altshuler 1971). The implication was that these behaviours were generally characteristic of deaf people and their culture. For example, 'Egocentric and rigid behaviours, products of deaf enculturation, can be mistaken for personality disorders' (Misiaszek et al. 1985). Mental health workers who work with hearing people will recognize that such behaviours are not at all exclusive to deaf people. Contact with deaf people who did not have mental disorder appears not to have been common among mental health workers for deaf people. Had there been more contact it is unlikely that such statements would have been written.

One cross-national study in America and Yugoslavia (Altshuler et al. 1976) found greater impulsivity in 'normal' deaf people as well as patients. Sarlin and Altshuler (1978) found a delay in the development of the relationship between cognition and affect, which provides a potential model for impulsivity. When confronted with a challenge there is inability to trust the environment and a lack of practice at sequential responses through lack of imaginative play. The result is an inability to think out a sequential plan and therefore an immediate response to their feelings by impulsivity actions. They found similar patterns of behaviour in deprived children to those in deaf children, one presumably through neglect, the other through the problems imposed by deafness in a hearing family. An alternative or more likely concurrent model is that of organic brain damage, resulting in irritability. Chess and Fernandez (1981) found rubella children with only deafness as a sequela to suffer impulsivity, which resolved by age 13–14. Notably more of those rubella children with deafness and additional sequelae where impulsive, and it did not resolve. Altshuler (1986) compares deafness with other deprived groups and cogently argues it is lack of audition, in other words the deprivation of deaf people in a hearing world, that leads to impulsivity. The world of deaf people is changing with recognition of sign language in schools and in later life, and the introduction of preventative programmes such as PATHS in childhood. Anecdotally, it seems that along with these changes there is a general reduction in impulsivity in deaf patients.

Research into the prevalence of behaviour disorders in deaf people has mostly been conducted in children. It shows that such disorders are at least twice as common as in their hearing counterparts (Hindley et al. 1994), but they are not the norm. Basilier (1964) first highlighted the prevalence of behaviour disturbances in young deaf people, emphasizing impulsive and aggressive behaviour. He also emphasized a better prognosis than for hearing people, a point that is generally agreed on by psychiatrists for deaf people. Deaf people presenting to psychiatric services with such behaviours often have personal histories and current behaviour that would result in the label of personality disorder, yet many have a much better prognosis.

There is little evidence that deaf people are more or less prone to any particular personality disorder. Paranoid personality has been said to be common, though it appears this is due to lack of clarity between early childhood deafness and later acquired deafness. In the latter case, there is a greater sway of opinion, though even there its justification is questionable. Vernon and Andrews (1990) suggest any increased prevalence of paranoid personality traits is reality-based in deaf people, as well as suggesting 'schizoid' personality is more frequent in rubella and low birth weight causes. Grinker, Werble and Dye (1977) claimed 'borderline' personality is not seen in a deaf client group. The authors have had experience of successfully treating deaf patients who fit the diagnostic criteria for borderline personality disorder. Farrugia (1992) suggests that the diagnosis of borderline personality disorder is probably less common in the deaf population, due to reduced access to mental health services. Farrugia also suggests that borderline personality disorders might be more common in deaf people due to frustrated relationships with parental figures in early life.

From clinical experience it appears that behaviour disorders are becoming less of a problem in deaf patients. It may be that Gerber (1983) was right in noting that due to communication difficulties 'behaviour disturbances are observed more often than problems of interpersonal concerns or neurotic symptoms'. Now that society's reaction to deaf people has improved and mental health services are staffed by deaf people, maybe we are better able to see the neurotic problems previously hidden by behaviour disturbance and poor communication. Those deaf people presenting with behaviour disturbance often respond to a combination of an appropriate communication environment and specific therapies such a behaviour therapy or cognitive behavioural therapy. Those individuals presenting with significant emotional difficulties in association with behavioural disturbance may also benefit from psychodynamic psychotherapy.

Our understanding of the mental health of deaf people is still in its infancy, but it is definitely growing. One message is clear, to avoid error and unintentional adverse labelling of deaf people, it is vital that deaf people themselves are involved in furthering that understanding and delivering services to deaf people.

National Deaf Children's Society, 15 Dufferin Street, London EC1Y 8PD

# Chapter 18
# Hearing aids

MIKE MARTIN

For people who have a hearing loss, and whose hearing condition requires no further medical or surgical treatment, a hearing aid becomes the primary means by which they can minimize the handicap caused by the loss.

The provision of a hearing aid may appear at first sight to be a relatively simple matter. When people first think of a hearing aid their first thought is usually about the device itself. They tend to think about its size, its performance and the benefits that the technology might bring. However, what people often do not realize is that, like many other devices, a hearing aid is only going to be of benefit to the wearer if a number of other factors are in place. These factors are listed below in order of importance in the successful fitting of a hearing aid:

1 the attitude of the user to wearing a hearing aid
2 the attitude of the person fitting the aid
3 the type and degree of hearing loss
4 the care with which the hearing aid is fitted
5 the physical comfort of the aid when fitted
6 the giving of factual information as to the benefits and limitations of using a hearing aid
7 the use of a trial period of the aid
8 the aftercare available to the wearer to help maximize its use
9 the knowledge of other devices and systems that support or complement the use of the aid
10 maintenance and repair.

A short discussion of these factors may help the reader appreciate that while the technology used in the hearing aid is a very important element of its beneficial use, the successful use of the aid depends on a lot more besides. The final factor is the individual who is going to wear the aid and, as in every other sphere of life, people vary enormously. The relevance of the factors for any individual will therefore also vary.

## Attitude of the user

It is a fact that nobody wants to wear a hearing aid. Very often it is friends and relatives who make the potential user come forward for an aid. It is also well documented that most people who come for a hearing aid for the first time have had their hearing loss for a good number of years. This is compounded by the fact that the majority of people with hearing losses are over the age of 60 (see Chapter 2) and the average age of people coming for their first hearing aid is over 70. Consequently they have formed attitudes towards wearing a hearing aid that may have been largely influenced by years of misinformation, by the stigma that still exists towards having a hearing loss, and even by the attitudes of their GP and other health advisors.

However, many people do not get the opportunity to try a hearing aid because of the misunderstanding by GPs and other professionals of the value of an aid, particularly in relation to who will benefit from an aid and who will not. Consequently the potential hearing aid user will either not be referred or may even be actively advised against the use of an aid.

It is therefore very important that any person coming for a hearing aid for the first time has an attitude that is at least biased towards giving the aid a fair trial. If a person has a negative attitude towards trying an aid then it is better not to proceed with the fitting until that person can be educated into a frame of mind that will allow him or her to give the aid a realistic trial. Some clinics and dispensers will not try to take the fitting process any further than a first interview if they consider there is too negative an attitude towards using an aid.

## Attitude of the hearing aid dispenser

It may seem odd to consider the attitude of the dispenser in the fitting process, when clearly it should be one of wanting to fit an aid that will benefit the user the most. However, there are a number of approaches to fitting an aid, the main two being holistic and analytic. The holistic approach will take into account the needs and lifestyle of the potential wearer. The analytic approach is to concentrate on the technicalities of the hearing loss and the hearing aid and treat the ear rather than the person.

Two other important considerations are whether the dispenser is working within a hearing aid delivery system that is integrated with rehabilitation and aftercare, and whether this system (private or public) limits the time available for fitting an aid.

## Type and degree of hearing loss

### Type of loss

The main considerations here are whether the loss is conductive or sensorineural, and the shape of the audiogram. There has been a long-held belief in some quarters that people with sensorineural losses will not benefit from the use of hearing aids. This is not the case, although there are more problems to overcome than with conductive hearing loss as can be seen below.

People with conductive losses benefit greatly from the use of amplification, as they do not incur any significant degree of loss of speech recognition, i.e. the ability to be able to recognize the words they hear (see the section on speech audiometry in Chapter 5). They also do not have any significant reduction of dynamic range of loudness perception. Where conductive losses involve any discharge into the ear canal, care has to be taken to provide earmoulds that provide adequate ventilation and to ensure that the user understands what must be done to keep the ear in good condition.

People with sensorineural hearing losses may, however, have serious problems with speech recognition and reduced dynamic ranges for loudness perception. These people will be able to hear what is being said but will not be able to understand the words because of the effect of the sensorineural hearing loss, i.e. their speech recognition ability is poor. The variability from individual to individual in their ability to recognize speech may be quite significant, even though they may have the same type and degree of hearing loss. This leads to problems in identifying the needs of individuals when one person benefits greatly from one particular aid and another person, with apparently the same degree and type of loss, does not.

The shape of the pure-tone audiogram reflects the sensitivity of the ear at threshold across the audible frequency range. Consequently it provides valuable information, at a basic level, of the degree of loss and an initial guide to the fitting of an aid. It does not, however, indicate what the perception of loudness is likely to be as sound goes from very quiet to very loud, nor does it quantify the speech recognition abilities of the individual. The provision on the audiogram of loudness discomfort levels is essential for hearing aid fitting purposes as it indicates the dynamic range of the ear across the frequency range.

*Degree of loss*

The degree of loss relates to the gain and maximum acoustic output of the aid required. Consequently the type of aid that can be used becomes more limited as the hearing loss increases.

However, with the range of hearing aid performance available today, the type of aid becomes a limiting factor only in the more severe hearing loss ranges.

It should be remembered that with today's aids it is possible to make all but the truly totally deaf hear something. However, the ability to hear something says little about a person's ability to recognize speech and make use of what they hear.

In the fitting process, the above factors have to be taken into account. However, even when the acoustic performance of the hearing aid is carefully selected to match the individual's hearing, users often complain that they can hear but cannot understand what is being said. This is not the fault of an appropriate hearing aid but the limitation of the individual's ability to recognize speech due to their sensorineural hearing loss. The problem of speech recognition is also made worse by the presence of any background noise.

**Care with which the aid is fitted**

This may again appear to be an obvious factor and it could be assumed that all hearing aids are fitted with the same degree of care. Unfortunately this is not the case, because of different attitudes and practices of dispensers and the amount of time that is available for fitting the aid. This means many first-time users are put off using their aids. This is often because of some simple error on the part of the dispenser, e.g. aid in the wrong ear, aid too loud for comfort, etc. The fact that a first-time user has problems should not be surprising and steps should be taken by the dispenser to identify the problem and see how it might best be resolved.

**The physical comfort of the aid when fitted**

Hearing aids today are very small and light and the major problem from the comfort point of view is the way the aid or the earmould fit into the ear. Ideally the user should be unaware of the mould in the ear. For people who are allergic to the acrylic material normally used for the earmould, special materials are available on request to help overcome most problems. The various types of earmould are described on pages 305–7.

## Provision of factual information

There is a strong tendency for the new user of a hearing aid to be given the impression that the aid will solve all of their hearing problems. This is obviously the aim of any good fitting, but realistically it is not going to be the case. It is therefore very important that the new user is told truthfully what the advantages of wearing the aid are and when the aid will be of more limited use, even when it is best to switch it off. The advice should be given in an encouraging but realistic manner. The user should be encouraged to report back with any problems and not to just put up with them.

It is important that a hearing person should accompany the person being fitted with an aid, so that he or she can pick up any information the hearing-impaired person misses. In any event, the amount of information is probably too great for any one person to absorb in the stressful situation of a first fitting. The need for clear, written factual information to be available at the first fitting is therefore very important.

## Trial/learning period

Even if all the right things are done during the initial fitting of the aid, it is still a new experience for the first-time wearer. Consequently the user does not know what he or she is going to hear, or not hear, and may well find problems that are quite unexpected, even with advance warning.

The fitting of an aid, particularly for the first time, has to be seen as part of an iterative process, where the best efforts are made to provide an aid that is suitable at the first fitting. However, the fitting of an aid is a complex matter with many uncertainties due to the subjective nature of the process. To obtain user satisfaction it is important to have a trial period when the user can determine, in the real-life situations that are important to him or her, whether the aid is giving benefit. The term trial period is widely used but it should be seen as a learning period for both the user and the dispenser.

The user should be encouraged to wear the aid and report problems. There should be an easy means whereby the user can return with the aid for further adjustments to deal with any problems encountered. There may be misunderstanding of the situations where the aid will be of benefit and where it will not. Problems are likely to be situation-specific. It is interesting to note the approach taken by Stuart Gatehouse (1999) in the Glasgow Hearing Aid Benefit (GHAB) Profile, which takes into account the range of factors that affect a person with a hearing loss. Table 18.1 shows how the questions in the profile are structured to take into account the variables associated with the handicap. It shows that it is not sufficient to ask if hearing aid users have a problem, it is important to know the degree

**Table 18.1:** A question from the Glasgow Hearing Aid Benefit profile illustrating how the effect of deafness and the use of a hearing aid may vary depending on the question that is asked of the individual

| Does this situation happen in your life? | Listening to the television with other family or friends when the volume is adjusted to suit other people | | In this situation how much does your hearing aid help you? | In this situation, with your hearing aid, how much difficulty do you now have? | For this situation, how satisfied are you with your hearing aid? |
|---|---|---|---|---|---|
| 0 No   1 Yes | | | | | |
| | How much difficulty do you have in this situation? | How much does any difficulty in the situation worry, annoy or upset you? | In this situation, what proportion of the time do you wear your hearing aid? | | |
| | 0 N/A | 0 N/A | 0 N/A | 0 N/A | 0 N/A |
| | 1 No difficulty | 1 Not at all | 1 Never/Not at all | 1 Hearing aid no use at all | 1 Not satisfied at all |
| | 2 Only slight difficulty | 2 Only a little | 2 About a quarter of the time | 2 Hearing aid some help | 2 A little satisfied |
| | 3 Moderate difficulty | 3 A moderate amount | 3 About half of the time | 3 Hearing aid quite helpful | 3 Reasonably satisfied |
| | 4 Great difficulty | 4 Quite a lot | 4 About three quarters of the time | 4 Hearing aid a great help | 4 Very satisfied |
| | 5 Cannot manage at all | 5 Very much indeed | 5 All of the time | 5 Hearing is perfect with aid | 5 Delighted with aid |

(The column "In this situation, with your hearing aid, how much difficulty do you now have?" scale reads: 0 N/A, 1 No difficulty, 2 Only slight difficulty, 3 Moderate difficulty, 4 Great difficulty, 5 Cannot manage at all)

of the problem, whether it actually causes any concern and whether intervention has any effect. It also records the amount of time that the hearing aid produces benefit.

Neither the user nor the dispenser should feel that the presence of problems reflects lack of expertise, care or goodwill; it is the nature of hearing-aid fitting that problems will occur and have to be addressed. It is also important that there is recognition from both parties that some problems cannot be resolved.

Obviously the wearer of the new aid must wear it during the trial period, particularly in the situations that were causing difficulty without the aid. This is not to say that he or she should wear it all the time, rather it should be worn in a controlled and careful manner. A period of one month should be sufficient to determine if there are any problems in the use of the aid and for steps to be taken to resolve or minimize these problems.

### Aftercare

As indicated above, the fitting of an aid is not a one-off event. It is therefore essential that there should be a good line of continuing communication between the dispenser and the hearing aid user. The benefits obtained from the hearing aid will also depend on the user's general ability to communicate. The development of lip-reading skills and 'hearing tactics' will considerably increase the benefit obtained from the aid. Knowledge of the assistive devices indicated below will also increase the use and benefit of the aid.

### Assistive devices

There are a number of situations where the user will have difficulty in hearing, no matter how good the hearing aid is. A range of devices can complement and supplement the use of an aid and all users should be aware of the potential of such devices. A description of the most widely used devices is given later in the chapter.

### Maintenance and repair

Hearing aids are virtually maintenance-free except that they need batteries to power them. The user should be aware of the type of battery required and keep an adequate supply to hand. He or she should also know how long the batteries should be expected to last. The zinc-air cells that are now provided with hearing aids have a limited life once the tab that allows the air in is removed. Consequently, someone who only uses his or her aid infrequently may be surprised that the battery is flat after a period of unuse.

Earmoulds, or the sound outlet from in-the-ear (ITE) aids, require regular attention to prevent them becoming blocked with wax. Earmoulds for behind-the-ear (BTE) aids need to be retubed from time to time as the tubing becomes hard and can crack. Users and carers should be encouraged to acquire the skills needed to undertake these tasks.

When an aid becomes faulty, and it is inevitable that it will, there should be a clear and recognized means for the user to have it repaired quickly. Once a user has become accustomed to wearing the aid it is not acceptable for him or her to be without it for any period of time.

## Hearing aid delivery services

There are a number of ways that an adult can obtain a hearing aid and these are illustrated in Figure 18.1. The following descriptions apply to the UK, but it should be remembered that hearing aid delivery systems vary considerably from country to country.

In general, hearing aid delivery systems can be divided into those that require the potential user to go to a medical practitioner/hospital clinic first and those that allow the person to go directly to the hearing aid dispenser. In most countries, the hearing aid dispenser is licensed by a regulatory body, which in the UK is the Hearing Aid Council. The role of the Hearing Aid Council is to register dispensers, to regulate their examinations and, when appropriate, to take disciplinary action. It is a criminal offence to dispense hearing aids by way of retail trade if not licensed to do so.

The procedure for obtaining a NHS aid in the UK is for the patient to go to his or her GP, who then refers him or her, if considered appropriate, to an ENT/audiology outpatient clinic. After diagnosis and treatment as necessary, the patient is passed to the hearing aid clinic that then dispenses the required NHS hearing aid. All treatment and provision of the aid, including after care, batteries and repairs, are free of charge to the patient.

In some areas it is possible for a GP to refer a patient directly to a hearing-aid clinic based in the hospital, a system known as direct referral. This service is based on the fact that a large proportion of hearing-aid users are over 60 and have no treatable hearing loss. This is coupled with the training of the staff in direct referral clinics to be able to recognize a set of conditions that require ENT referrals.

In the private sector, the client goes directly to the registered hearing aid dispenser and pays for all equipment and services – there is no cross-subsidy available from the NHS. The private hearing aid dispenser also has criteria laid down by the Hearing Aid Council, indicating when the client must be referred to a medical practitioner.

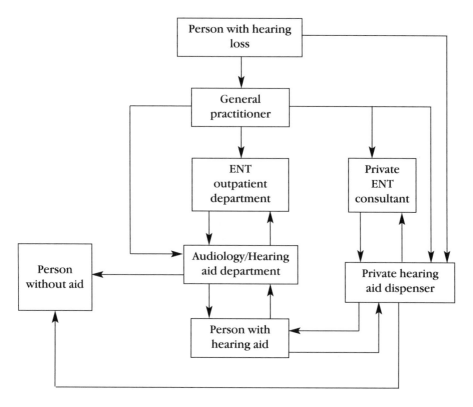

**Figure 18.1:** A general model of the hearing aid delivery system in the UK. A hearing impaired person may obtain a hearing aid by going through the NHS system or by the private sector.

### Hearing aid delivery services for children

The provision of hearing aids for children is much more varied than for adults and requires a more flexible and interactive service. Hearing aids can now be fitted to children from the age of a few weeks or months old. The recommendation for a hearing aid will be made by the clinic to which the child is referred, having been diagnosed as having a hearing loss. This is very often a paedo-audiological clinic or it may be the ENT/audiology department in a hospital. There is a need for regular follow-up appointments for children, particularly very young ones: new moulds are needed as the external ear grows and the aid(s) must be checked to make sure that it is functioning and that the child is benefiting from its use. The involvement of parents in this process is very important, as they need to know how to look after the aid and support the child's communication development.

The range of hearing aids for children that is provided free of charge in the UK is larger than the range for adults; clinics dealing with children provide a range of private-sector hearing aids in addition to the standard NHS ones, where appropriate. These aids may include ITE aids, programmable aids, etc. There is also a need to provide aids that are compatible with classroom equipment, such as radio (FM) systems where an electrical input is required. The provision of these aids is made out of the budget given to the NHS fitting department and is at no cost to the parents/guardian of the child.

However, if a private-sector aid is provided, the cost of maintenance has to be met by the family once the child leaves full-time education. It may also be difficult to continue with the maintenance or replacement of the aid if the child moves from one area to another, where the policy for providing private-sector aids is different.

## Hearing aids

The functional parts of a hearing aid are shown in Figure 18.2 and the specific types of aid are described below. Functionally, the hearing aid is an audio frequency amplifying device usually worn in or behind the ear. Developments in technology have led to these devices being made in very small packages. The introduction of digital technology has led to the availability of more sophisticated aids, which can be remotely controlled by the user and can provide digital signal processing of speech signals. When considering a digital aid, care should be taken as to what the digital processes are – the word digital does not imply any particular function apart from the fact that the amplifier and associated circuitry uses a digital processor rather than an analogue one.

The wide range of aids now available should be seen as a set of devices from which the most appropriate one has to be selected to give the hearing-impaired individual the opportunity to maximize his or her hearing. It is obvious that not every person requires the most sophisticated of devices and that the aid should be chosen to match the specific need.

### Hearing aid controls

Many hearing aids today have only a limited range of user controls. ITE aids usually have a volume control with a combined on/off switch. For BTE aids the on/off switch may be separate from the volume control and where an induction pick-up coil is incorporated in the aid a control marked O-M-T is used. O is for off, T is for the induction pick-up coil input and M for microphone input (see Figure 18.3). On some BTE aids there is a provision to connect an external device such as an additional microphone or a

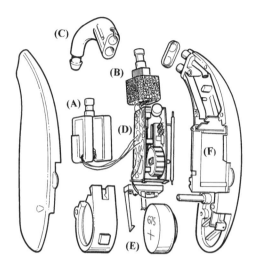

**Figure 18.2:** The functional parts of a typical behind-the-ear hearing aid. The same parts are found in all hearing aids but constructed differently to meet the requirements of the particular configuration of aid. (A) Earphone/receiver, (B) microphone, (C) hook to connect tubing of earmould to aid, (D) amplifier with volume control, (E) battery and battery compartment, (F) casing of aid.

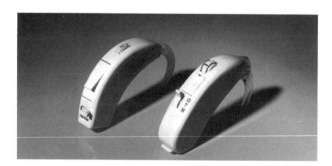

**Figure 18.3:** Behind-the-ear aid with user control. O = off, T = telephone/induction pick up coil position, M = microphone.

radio receiver, via contacts near the base of the aid. The external device requires a 'boot'-shaped plug to fit on to the bottom of the aid to make the connection. This connection may be indicated with an 'E' or O symbol. However, some digital aids do not have any controls at all, all changes being made by the software.

Some hearing aids have user controls for altering the frequency response. These will be marked N, H and L. N is the normal and widest frequency response, while H is for high emphasis and L is for low emphasis.

Figure 18.5(b) shows the relative responses of such a tone control. For aids with separate keypad controllers the same legends are used.

A wide range of fitting controls is also available on many BTE aids and these are hidden behind covers. Aids that have to be set up using software and a PC also tend to use the same legends for the user controls, but the software fitting controls may have very different legends in different products.

## Types of hearing aid

Hearing aids can be grouped in a number of ways, e.g. by the way they are worn, by their performance and by the technology involved. The first consideration for the user is normally how the aid is to be worn.

Hearing aids available today are worn on the head behind the ear (BTE), in the bowl of the ear (ITE), in the ear canal (canal aids), completely in the canal (CIC aids) close to the eardrum or in the form of spectacles. Aids worn on the body (body-worn aids, BW) are also available. All aids are air-conduction devices, but BW and spectacle aids can also be provided as bone-conduction instruments. Figure 18.4 shows the various types of aid. Below is a brief description of the essential elements of each type.

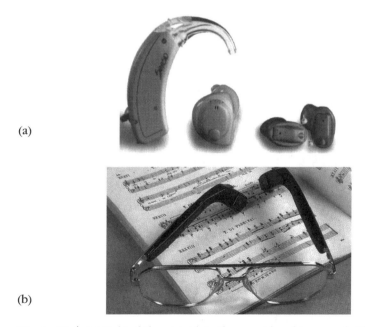

(a)

(b)

**Figure 18.4:** (a) Behind-the-ear aid, in-the-ear aid and two canal aids. Picture courtesy of Widex. (b) Bone-conduction spectacle aid with an independent bone-conduction aid on each side. Picture courtesy of Coselgi.

### Behind-the-ear (BTE) aids

The complete aid is housed in a package worn behind the ear. Sound is conducted from the hook of the aid into the ear, via the earmould, by means of a plastic tube. The aids vary greatly in size and performance as well as the user facilities they offer. They are capable of providing sufficient acoustic output to meet the needs of a very wide range of hearing losses.

### In-the-ear (ITE) aids

ITE aids have all their components housed in a shell that is small enough to fit into the bowl of the ear. With most of these aids the components are mounted on a face plate that fits into a shell whose shape is taken from an impression of the individual's ear. These aids are known as 'custom-made'.

ITE aids that are made in a fixed form and require an earmould are called 'modular aids'.

Due to their small size, these aids are limited in their acoustic output and therefore are most suited to mild to moderate/severe hearing losses. There is usually only a volume control on the aid, but some aids also have induction pick-up coils.

### In-the-canal (ITC) aids

These aids are smaller versions of the ITE aids and are worn with the major part of the aid in the ear canal, not filling the bowl of the ear. Due to their even smaller size they are most suited to mild to moderate losses.

### Completely-in-the-canal (CIC) aids

Here the aid is small enough to be worn close to the eardrum and has a stem protruding from the aid to allow for its withdrawal from the ear canal. The even smaller size limits the acoustic output, but this is offset by the closeness to the eardrum. Consequently the same range of hearing losses can be fitted as for the ITC aids.

### Spectacle aids

Spectacle aids come in a variety of forms that include both air- and bone-conduction aids. They are capable of providing high degrees of amplification and acoustic output as well as providing a very inconspicuous means of wearing one or two hearing aids. However, the number of companies providing spectacle aids is limited.

Air conduction spectacle aids may come built into the spectacle arm or as add-on devices to be fitted to the back of spectacle frames. The same configuration may be also achieved with a BTE aid and a special adapter that is fitted to the back of the spectacle arm.

Bone-conduction spectacle aids require strong spectacle arms to provide enough pressure for the bone vibrator to press very firmly against the head.

In addition, spectacle aids provide the means for using a CROS aid. CROS stands for contralateral routing of signals, and is used for people who have one good ear, often with normal hearing, and one ear with a profound loss. A microphone is placed on the deaf side of the head and the signal is run around the head through the spectacle frame to the good ear. The sound from the deaf side is fed into the good ear through an open mould that does not obstruct the ear. The person then hears sounds coming from the deaf side as slightly different from those coming from the good side and can hear sounds on the deaf side that they previously could not. The CROS aid effectively fills in the acoustic shadow caused by the head being between the source of sound and the good ear. The same arrangement can be formed by using two BTE aids joined by a lead running behind the head. In this arrangement, one aid contains a microphone and the other the amplifier and earphone. A further alternative, called a wireless CROS aid, is where the lead running around the head is replaced by a very small radio transmitter coupled to the microphone on the deaf side, which transmits to a receiver on the hearing side.

### Body-worn (BW) hearing aids

BW aids offer the potential for the highest acoustic outputs but are cosmetically unappealing. The use of a button earphone connected by a lead (cord) to the body of the aid worn on the chest, makes their use difficult compared with head worn aids. However their performance in terms of the frequency range of the maximum acoustic output can make them the only form of aid that meets the requirements of a small proportion of profoundly deaf people.

## Hearing aid performance

The purpose of all hearing aids is to amplify speech and other sounds so that they are audible to a hearing-impaired person. Hearing aids are audio-frequency amplifiers whose main characteristics can be described by a small number of objective parameters: gain or amplification, frequency response and power output. The main difference between a hearing aid and, say, a hi-fi amplifier is that the range of frequencies amplified is much smaller. In particular the dynamic range of the level of sounds is much smaller, often by design, to meet the needs of the reduced dynamic range of the listener.

The performance of a hearing aid can be measured objectively in a number of standardized ways. The performance can also be measured subjectively on an individual. The relationship between the objective and subjective performances is not necessarily highly correlated. The reason for this is that the objective method of measurement must be made using measuring devices that are, at best, average replicas of the acoustic characteristics of the human outer ear and ear canal. Most objective measurements do not take into account the presence of the head and torso of the wearer. In addition, they do not take into account the perceptual properties of the ear to which the aid is fitted – this has to be attempted in the fitting process. However, these objective measurements provide a uniform and reliable method of obtaining and exchanging information on the acoustic performance of an aid.

## Objective measurement

The main characteristics that are measured objectively are as follows:

- the frequency response of the aid – the range of frequencies over which the aid provides amplification
- the maximum acoustic output of the aid – the highest level of sound that the aid will produce given sufficient input
- the gain or amplification that the aid provides and the manner in which this is controlled.

The frequency response of an aid is measured by presenting the microphone of the aid with a known constant sound pressure level (SPL), usually 60 dB SPL. The output of the aid is then measured in an appropriate acoustic ear simulator and the plot of this output against frequency gives the frequency response. Figure 18.5(a) shows such a curve and in addition shows what happens as the level of the input is increased from 60 to 90 dB. This multiple plot is called a family of curves and shows that the aid performs differently at different input levels. Where the input and output levels change by the same amount is called the linear portion of the input/output characteristic of the aid. It is normally accepted that the frequency response of the aid is taken in the linear portion of the input/output characteristic.

The frequency range over which the hearing aid is deemed to operate is called the bandwidth of the aid. The effect of tone controls on the bandwidth and consequently the tone of the aid are shown in Figure 18.5(b)

The gain of an aid can easily be determined by subtracting the input level from the output level. In the example in Figure 18.5(a), at 500 Hz this is 50 dB, i.e. output 100 dB SPL – input 50 dB SPL = gain 50 dB.

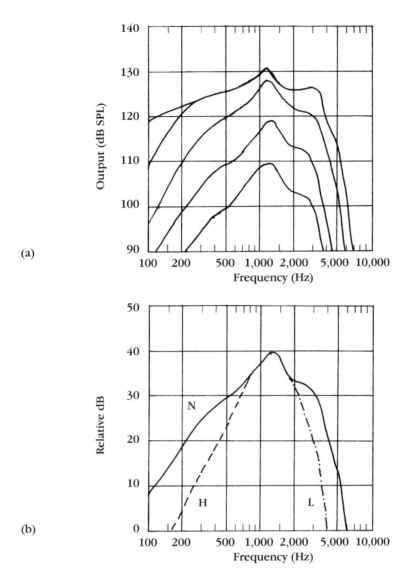

**Figure 18.5:** (a) Family of frequency response curves. Constant input sound pressure level over the whole frequency range. Lowest curve input 50 dB SPL increasing in 10 dB steps up to 90 dB SPL. (b) The effect of a tone control marked N (full frequency range), H (high tone emphasis), L (low-frequency emphasis).

The maximum acoustic output of the aid is usually taken, for practical purposes, as being the output sound pressure level (OSPL) that occurs for an input of 90 dB, called $OSPL_{90}$. It should be noted that the frequency response of the maximum output is a flat curve compared with that on the linear part of the input/output characteristic at lower input SPLs, e.g. in Figure 18.5(a) at input levels of 70 dB and below.

Because the dynamic range of the ear is restricted in cases of sensorineural hearing loss, both the maximum output of the aid and the dynamic range of the output need to be controlled to prevent the aid from being uncomfortably loud to the wearer. The control of output is achieved in two ways: first, by peak clipping, which occurs in most hearing aids when the input signal is so great that it saturates the aid; and second, by automatic gain control (AGC) or compression. The effect of peak clipping is to instantaneously limit the signal to some predetermined output level. Above that level the signal does not increase and the signal is then in a non-linear portion of the input/output characteristic of the aid. This then leads to distortion of the output signal. The level at which peak clipping takes place can be adjusted on many aids and provides a means of limiting the likely effect of loud sounds causing discomfort to the wearer.

With compression, circuits in the amplifier control the level of the signal and can both limit the output and alter the way the signal is amplified as the input signal varies in level. Compression circuits take a finite time to operate and these time constants can be varied to achieve different effects. The value of a compression circuit is that it prevents distortion occurring with high-level signals and should be set to keep the signal within the comfortable listening range of the wearer.

## Subjective performance

As has been stated above, there is not a good correlation, on an individual basis, between the objective measurements of performance and the subjective impression of the hearing aid user. There is usually a reasonable statistical correlation on a group basis, but this is often only of limited help to the person fitting an aid on an individual. Consequently fitting procedures need to take into account the individual perceptual properties of the hearing aid user.

A number of so-called prescription methods exist for the initial setting-up of the hearing aid. These should be seen, in the author's opinion, as a starting point for the fitting and not as defining the optimum settings. Hence the use of the word 'prescription' is perhaps unwise.

The basis for most of the formulae that predict the gain required uses the well-established fact that hearing aid users do not require the same gain as their hearing loss. In other words, a person with a 50 db hearing loss does not require 50 dB of gain but only approximately half this value. With regard to maximum output, it has been shown that the increase required is only about a third of the level of the increase in hearing loss.

The preferred method today for measuring the performance of an aid on a person is by means of real ear testing. This involves measuring the output of the aid in the ear canal of the individual while he or she is wearing it.

The value of this measurement is that it cuts through all the uncertainties that surround the objective measurements and measures the amount of sound going into the individual's ear. It is then possible to set up the aid to give optimum amplification to ensure that the widest range of sounds is heard comfortably. What this does not give is a measurement of the ability of a person to recognize speech. This has to be done separately using some form of speech audiometry.

## Earmoulds

The earmould should be considered an integral part of the hearing aid as it can substantially affect both the acoustic performance of the aid and the comfort of wearing it.

Earmoulds are made from an impression taken of the outer ear and ear canal using a self-setting compound that is syringed into the ear. The quality of the impression determines the quality of the earmould and therefore it has to be taken with great care. To prevent the impression material going further down the ear canal than is required, a tamp is placed in the canal before the material is syringed in. Once the impression material has hardened it is withdrawn from the ear, trimmed as necessary and then sent to an earmould laboratory where it is used to produce an acrylic mould in a similar manner to that used to produce dentures. The earmould laboratory is instructed about the type of mould required, the type of material and any special features, such as vents. Figure 18.6 shows a range of typical earmoulds.

The fit of the earmould determines both the comfort of the fitting and the degree of amplification that can be achieved. A poor-fitting earmould is very often identified by the fact that the aid whistles due to sound leaking past the earmould and being picked up by the microphone. A further problem with the fit of the aid is that many users, particularly those who are very elderly, have problems inserting and positioning the earmould correctly. It is important that users are fully aware of how to insert the mould correctly and that they acquire this skill. Inability to insert the mould is one of the major reasons for aids whistling and failing to provide sufficient amplification.

A vent is a second tube in the mould that provides a controlled acoustic leakage and a means of balancing the pressure between the earmould and the eardrum. Balancing the pressure often relieves a blocked-up sensation

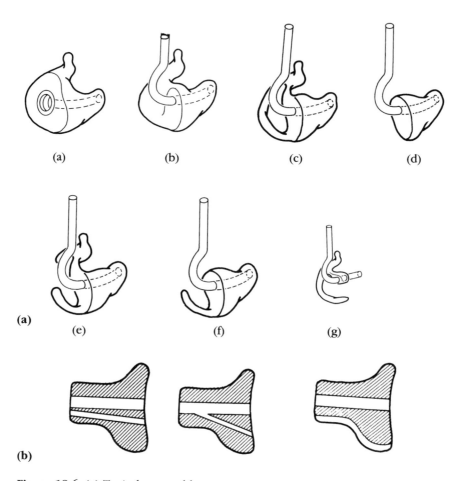

**Figure 18.6: (a)** Typical earmoulds.
**(a)** Solid mould for use with bodyworn hearing aid, (b) solid mould for use with BTE aid, (c) skeleton mould, (d) ear tip, (e) half skeleton mould, (f) quarter skeleton mould, (g) open mould.
**(b)** Forms of earmould vent.

that wearers sometimes experience and also reduces the amount of low-frequency sound being fed into the ear. The effects of leakage are seen in Figure 18.7, where the amount of low-frequency amplification from the aid is reduced below 1 kHz depending on the diameter of the vent. As this effect occurs at the output of the hearing aid it also reduces the maximum output of the aid, which can be very helpful in reducing loudness discomfort from low-frequency sounds. This is particularly helpful to people with high-frequency losses and good low-frequency hearing.

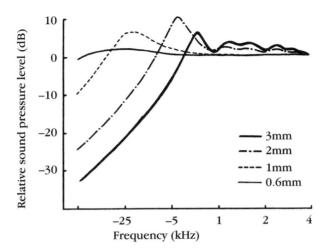

**Figure 18.7:** The effect of increasing the size of the bore of a vent in an earmould. The curves show the difference between a tightly sealed earmould and the introduction of vents of varying sizes. The larger the vent the more low frequencies are reduced.

The extreme of a vented earmould is an open mould that is no more than a tube held into the ear canal. This leaves the ear open and therefore sound is allowed to reach the eardrum in a normal manner. This approach is often used with CROS aid fittings.

# Assistive devices

While the hearing aid is the primary means of benefit for hearing-impaired people, there are many situations where the acoustic situation prevents the hearing aid from providing optimum benefit. Also for those who are profoundly deaf and cannot benefit from amplification there is an urgent need to provide an awareness of sound or to provide alternative communication.

In the above situations there are a range of devices known as assistive listening devices (ALDs) or assistive devices when they are not used for listening to speech.

### Assistive listening devices

When hearing-aid users are at a distance from someone speaking and when there is a background noise they often have great difficulty hearing what is being said. These situations occur in everyday life, for example at meetings, in church, at the theatre, etc., and often prevent hearing-aid users from attending such events. The problem can also occur at very much shorter distances, such as when people are listening to the television and even at small meetings. The solution is well-known in broadcasting and recording circles, where microphones are placed very close to the person speaking in order to optimize the pick-up of the speech and minimize any background noise present.

It is not always practical for a hearing aid user to be wired up to a microphone or to be close to the person speaking at all times. However, the principle of placing the mouth of the person speaking close to the microphone is one that still holds for hearing-aid users. To overcome this problem a number of approaches have been adopted.

One of the oldest and most widely used forms of assistive listening device is that of the induction loop system. The principle is very simple, as indicated in Figure 18.8, and can be used in a variety of ways, as shown. The most important point in all uses of the induction loop system is that of having the magnetic field strength at the correct level of 100 mA/m as

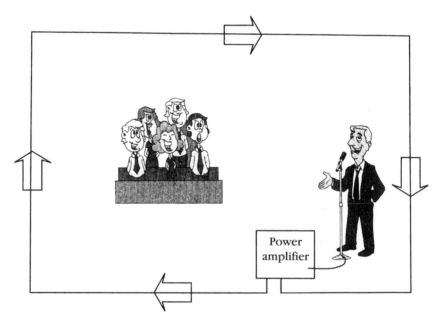

**Figure 18.8:** Induction loop system. A wire forming a loop is run around the area in which hearing-aid users wish to listen to the speaker. This area can be as small as a desk or as large as a football pitch, depending on the power of the amplifier. The signal being driven round the loop is an electric current that corresponds to the speaker's voice. The loop produces a magnetic field that fills the area of the loop and is picked up by the coil selected by the T position on the aid, effectively bringing the speaker's voice directly to the ear of the hearing aid listener. This ensures that the effects of background noise and distance are minimized.

specified in IEC 60118-4. The reason why many loops do not work well is because they do not meet this standard.

The induction loop principle is also applied to the telephone, where inductive couplers are placed in the earphone of the phone to provide a magnetic field for hearing-aid wearers with the appropriate 'T' position on their hearing aid.

The use of radio microphones, where the microphone is connected to a small radio transmitter, is widely used with hearing-impaired children, particularly where they are being educated in normal schools. The signal from the transmitter is picked up by a small receiver, which may feed into the electrical input on a hearing aid or into a loop amplifier. Adults can also use these systems, often called FM systems, in a similar manner.

A range of listening devices are available for listening to the television, which allow the hearing-impaired person to listen at his or her required level without having the sound too loud for anyone else in the room (Figure 18.9).

---

**1 HEADPHONES**
Headphones or miniature earphones can be plugged directly into many TV sets. These can be tried in Hi-fi stores and some TV dealers and are usually best suited to those with less severe losses.

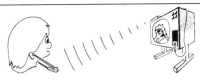

---

**2 LISTENING AIDS**
These aids comprise a small control unit connected to the TV set through which you can adjust the level of sound. Normally you listen through an earphone on the end of a long lead.

---

**3 INDUCTION LOOP SYSTEM**
'Sound' is sent to you in the form of a magnetic field and you can stay 'tuned in' so long as you remain within the area of the 'loop'. If your hearing aid has a switch marked 'T', or if you have a suitable receiving unit the loop system is very effective.

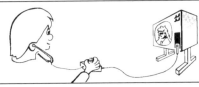

---

**4 INFRA-RED**
With this system, signals are sent to you as 'infra-red light'. A transmitter unit is attached to the TV set and you listen through a special receiving unit which responds to the infra-red transmissions.

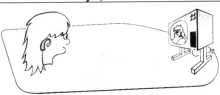

---

**Figure 18.9:** TV listening devices.

## Other assistive devices

Where a person is profoundly or totally deaf, means have to be found to provide an alternative form of indicating the presence of sound. For warning and alerting signals, such as doorbells, fire alarms and alarm clocks, the acoustic signal is replaced by a flashing light or a vibratory signal and a range of such devices are available from specialist suppliers.

For communication over the telephone, the use of text phones is a long-established method. These are keyboards that have a built-in display and a modem to send text data over the normal telephone lines. The person at the other end needs to have a compatible device. Today, a range of text phones are available and personal computers can be configured to provide the same function. Telephone relay services have been introduced to enable hearing people to communicate with deaf people who have text phones. This involves a service centre that acts as a relay, whereby a hearing person's speech is transcribed into text and the deaf person's text is spoken to the hearing person. If the deaf person has intelligible speech over the telephone then he or she can speak directly to the hearing person, as in Figure 18.10.

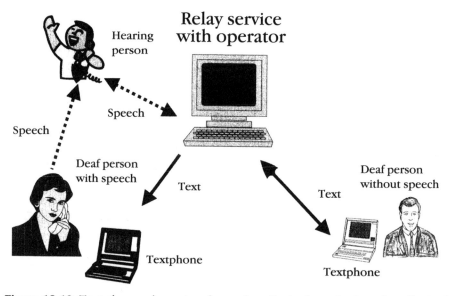

**Figure 18.10:** Text phone relay system for profoundly deaf people. A profoundly deaf person whose speech is intelligible over the telephone can speak directly to a hearing person using the phone normally. The hearing person's speech is transcribed into text by the operator in the relay centre and appears on the screen of the deaf person's textphone. A profoundly deaf person whose speech cannot be understood over the telephone types what he or she wants to say on the text phone and the operator relays that text verbally to the hearing person. The hearing person's speech is then transcribed into text by the operator and appears on the deaf person's screen.

# Chapter 19
# Cochlear implants

## Huw Cooper

In recent years, cochlear implants have joined the mainstream of modern audiology and ENT practice, and are now widely accepted as a safe and effective management for profound deafness. The report by Summerfield and Marshall (1995) gave clear, well-documented evidence of the benefits and cost-effectiveness of multi-channel implants in adults as well as valuable indications about the way that the already well-developed implant programme in the UK should mature and develop over future years, based on predicted demands. The National Institutes of Health Consensus Conference (1995) also gave recommendations about possible expansions and restrictions of implantation.

Perhaps the most exciting aspect of the development of cochlear implantation since the last edition of this book has been the accumulation of increasing evidence of the benefits of implants in very young children. It may be that the controversy concerning this work will never go away. All those involved in paediatric implantation should continue to take heed of some of the concerns expressed by some 'culturally' deaf people, while carefully collecting the data to show the great potential benefits.

Meanwhile, many hundreds of deafened adults continue to come forward for cochlear implants each year and many thousands around the world are long-term users of implants, in many cases with transformed lives. An inevitable consequence of the growth in numbers of implant users worldwide is that the proportion of time spent by cochlear implant teams and other professionals on maintenance and ongoing support of implant users, as opposed to assessing new cases, is increasing all the time. This fact is one that urges careful thought about development of services to meet the needs of this growing population in a cost-effective manner.

# Implant design

### Electrodes

Multi-channel intracochlear devices are now used almost universally and most surgeons are now much more confident at drilling into the cochlea when ossification prevents easy insertion. Designs of the implanted receiver/stimulator package and electrodes vary slightly between the main commercially available systems but the essential elements remain the same (Figure 19.1).

Multi-channel devices use a flexible array with up to 22 intracochlear electrodes spaced along thir length. In the most widely used system (Nucleus), the array is essentially straight in its resting state, with 22 intra-cochlear platinum/iridium band electrodes and 10 extra-cochlear 'stiffening rings'. The array is sufficiently flexible so that it easily finds its way around the turns of the cochlea and no special tools are required. A leading competitor (Advanced Bionics) uses a curved array with radially spaced pairs of electrodes. The rationale behind this so-called 'modiolus hugging' design, which originated in early work at the University of California at San Francisco, is to reduce the distance between the electrodes and the spiral ganglion cells to be stimulated, and so reduce current requirements and increase selectivity of stimulation. However, the design necessitates the use of an inserting tool and not all surgeons are

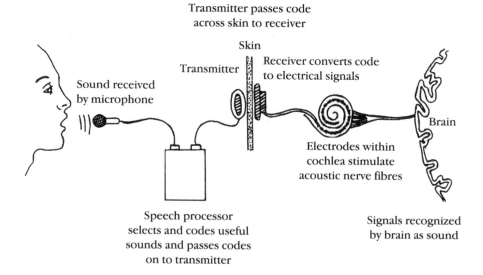

**Figure 19.1:** Principles of the cochlear implant device.

comfortable with the shape of the array. Recently, the manufacturers of that device have been evaluating an electrode positioner, which effectively wedges the electrode array within the cochlea with the intention of optimizing its position in proximity to the modiolus. At the time of writing, only preliminary results with this method are available, and there may be concerns about the possible trauma such an insertion might cause. Other variants in design, such as the Digisonic multi-array implant, which comprises three arrays each with four electrodes, and the MedEL and Nucleus 'split' electrodes, open up possibilities for implantation in cochleas obstructed by new bone growth and are potentially useful in these rare cases (Richardson, Clarke and Hawthorne 1998).

**Brainstem implants**

Patients with bilateral acoustic neuromata, such as in neurofibromatosis type 2, have in the past often been left bilaterally profoundly deaf following tumour removal accompanied by surgical damage to the auditory nerve. Experience with the auditory brainstem implant (ABI) has now grown such that the results, although still somewhat variable and unpredictable, in many cases justify the complex surgery it entails. The ABI consists of a receiver–stimulator package similar to the conventional intracochlear device, with a flat, silicone electrode carrier plate with 21 electrodes arranged in three rows instead of the usual thin electrode array. This plate is placed on the cochlear nucleus directly. The speech signal is processed as in the normal implant by the externally worn speech processor and transmitted from the transmitter to the internal device; a careful process of pitch ranking is required to ensure that stimulation is as tonotopic as can be achieved. Careful intraoperative monitoring of other neurological functions is also practised as the stimulation in the brainstem area could potentially affect other structures with undesirable effects, such as pain, bodily movement, etc. With these safety measures, some patients can achieve limited open-set speech understanding and most obtain awareness of sound at least (Laszig et al. 1995).

**Speech processing**

Development and investigation of different speech-processing strategies for cochlear implants has occupied much research time and effort in recent years, as it has been shown that the way in which the speech signal is processed and delivered to the electrodes can make significant differences to performance. A full explanation of the principles underlying different speech-processing strategies is beyond the scope of this chapter, but can be found elsewhere (e.g. Tyler 1992).

The first purpose of the speech processor is to ensure that stimulation is delivered via the implant at an appropriate and comfortable level to each stimulating electrode. These levels are established during 'programming' (see below). A second purpose is to encode the incoming speech sounds according to the speech-processing strategy being implemented.

Earlier designs of implant made use of 'feature extraction', in which those features of speech thought to be most important for speech understanding were detected and 'extracted' from the incoming speech signal, coded and delivered to the stimulating electrodes. For example, the 'F0F1F2' strategy, which was implemented in previous designs of the Nucleus implant system, detected the formant frequency (F0) and first and second formants of speech (F1 and F2). This determined, respectively, the rate of stimulation and location of the electrodes that were stimulated at any moment. This method, although intuitively a good one, had its limitations and was superseded by the 'speak' strategy, which rather than deliberately extracting speech features, continuously picks out those frequency bands containing the most energy and stimulates the particular electrodes allocated to those bands, at a constant rate. The result is a representation of the spectral pattern of the speech signal in the pattern of stimulation across the electrode array. More recently, the 'advanced combination encoder' (ACE) strategy has allowed much greater flexibility in terms of both the rate of stimulation (including the potential to increase the rate of stimulation from 250 Hz up to 1200 Hz) and the number of channels activated at any one time. It is hoped that this could lead to benefits in performance, and initial results are good, but as ACE is a relatively new approach more time is needed for evaluation.

Another method that has been implemented widely since the original demonstrations of its effectiveness by Blake Wilson and colleagues at the Research Triangle Institute (Wilson 1997) is continuous interleaved sampling (CIS), and most implant systems are able to deliver this strategy in one form or another. In CIS, instead of the stimulation 'roving' across the electrodes as in 'speak', all the electrodes are continuously stimulated in rapid cycles with high-rate pulsatile stimuli. Interaction between channels is reduced by 'temporally interleaving' the stimulation. The stimulus level in each channel is determined by the input level to its particular frequency band, so that the spectral pattern of the speech signal is represented (as in 'speak'). Enhanced speech-recognition performance has been demonstrated in some patients using CIS (Wilson et al. 1991), and work aimed at establishing which parameters of the speech processing (for example speed of stimulation) can be altered to further improve performance continues. Until recently it has not been possible to implement all the various speech-processing strategies in a single device, so true intra-subject comparisons have not been possible. One exception is the recent work coordinated by Advanced Bionics Ltd, using the 'Clarion' implant system. These studies measured performance using either CIS or an alternative analogue speech-processing system (simultaneous analogue stimulation or SAS). The results do not provide evidence of a universal advantage for one strategy over another, but show that there is considerable inter-subject variability. Also, they seem to suggest that in general, patients achieve the best performance with the speech strategy they subjectively preferred.

The most recent version of the system made by Cochlear also opens up the possibility of intra-subject comparison as the body-worn 'Sprint' speech processor can deliver the 'speak' strategy as well as CIS and ACE under the heading 'custom sound'. It can also be set up with four different programs so that patients can compare strategies easily and performance can be compared within the same subject. Hopefully some interesting results concerning the effects of varying parameters in CIS and ACE and patient preferences will emerge from studies currently in progress.

### Ear-level speech processors

Until recently, all multi-channel cochlear implants have necessitated a body-worn speech processor, and for the vast majority of patients this has been an acceptable compromise in view of the benefits to hearing they have achieved. Inevitably, implant designers have worked towards smaller equipment and ear-level processors (e.g. the 'Esprit' system from Cochlear and the ear-level processor, which was launched by Med-El in 1999) are now available and gaining wide use, and have obvious advantages for many patients. The benefits of a very small processor are offset somewhat by its limitations in speech-processing flexibility and the loss of some other functions (e.g. visual sound-level display, telemetry), but there is no doubt that for a very large number of patients an ear-level device is going to be hugely attractive. One can anticipate all implant manufacturers producing their own ear-level versions in the near future as part of a continuing move towards miniaturization.

## The implant team

There are many factors to consider when contemplating a cochlear implant as a possible treatment for a deaf patient and most teams have successfully developed a multidisciplinary approach, including audiologists, speech and hearing therapists, psychologists and otolaryngologists. With children, teachers of the deaf have a leading role to play in the assessment and habilitation process, and in some paediatric teams the ENT nurse has developed a valuable role in counselling children and families about the hospital stay. In both adults and children, various other professionals can become involved in particular cases as needed, for example, psychiatrists and social workers for the deaf.

## Patient selection

It is to be hoped that those involved in the provision of cochlear implants adhere to the philosophy that an implant is one of a range of possible treatments for deaf patients. Assessment should therefore be aimed towards selecting the best treatment for each patient rather than selecting the patient for the treatment. A significant number of people referred for consideration for an implant would not benefit from one but can be helped in other ways, including (most frequently) enhanced conventional amplification, and these other options should be explored carefully in each case.

In adults, postlingually deafened patients with little or no useful hearing are the main 'traditional' candidates for cochlear implantation. Little evidence of the usefulness of implants in prelingually or congenitally deaf adults has emerged and such individuals are unlikely to come forward for consideration. Data concerning those intrinsic factors in adults that are probably related to outcomes with an implant have been accumulated as the number of implanted patients has increased, but there remains a high degree of variability in results and performance. It has become clearer over time that the outcome of a cochlear implant results from a complex interaction of a quite large number of otherwise unrelated variables, making accurate prediction of results difficult.

Duration of deafness has consistently been found to be a variable with one of the strongest associations with performance, with shorter durations tending to be associated with better outcomes (Gantz et al. 1993). In contrast, aetiology of deafness has never been convincingly demonstrated to relate to performance with an implant. Various studies have identified other variables thought to be associated with better postoperative performance with an implant, including: lip-reading ability; performance on a visual monitoring task; motivation and involvement in healthcare; absence of depression. The study entitled 'Predicting outcomes of cochlear implantation in adults' (POCIA), begun in 1997 in some of the cochlear implant centres in the UK and set up and coordinated by the Institute for Hearing Research, should help to throw more light on which factors really are important.

The degree of hearing loss in adult patients considered for an implant has changed somewhat over recent years. The 'traditional' candidate for cochlear implantation had little or no usable residual hearing and gained no appreciable benefit from conventional amplification. In current practice, many patients with some limited useful hearing are now receiving implants with clear benefit. The National Institutes for Health (NIH) Consensus Conference (1995) recommended that postlingually deafened adults who scored up to 30% correct in an open-set (sound alone) speech-recognition test with appropriately fitted hearing aids should be considered as possible candidates for cochlear implantation, and this relaxation in criteria is widely accepted in the USA. The rationale behind this apparent 'softening' of the audiological criteria is that results with modern cochlear implants have improved greatly, so that implant surgery in patients with less than profound deafness can be justified. In the UK, a more conservative approach has been adopted and the results in adults with preoperative aided scores of up to 20% correct are currently being evaluated in some British implant centres participating in the POCIA study already mentioned.

In the paediatric population, a large number of congenitally deaf children around the world have now been given implants and data concerning the benefits for this group have grown enormously over the past five to ten years. Many implant teams and surgeons now accept that the best long-term outcomes in children are likely to be achieved if implantation occurs at a very young age. One would expect that a reduction in the period of auditory deprivation should lead to benefits to the child and this seems to be borne out in the outcomes seen.

Many children under the age of two have received implants and there is a view that implant surgery needs to take place before this age in order to achieve the best chances for spoken language acquisition. It is less clear whether implanting congenitally deaf children older than about six, i.e. the age by which most language acquisition is usually thought to be complete, can be completely justified, and many paediatric programmes operate an upper age limit of between five and seven years for this reason. Nonetheless, many children up to the age of ten or even older do receive implants with some apparent benefit. One might expect a big difference in the potential to benefit from an implant between a ten-year-old who has experienced a predominantly oral/aural education with emphasis on spoken language, and a child of the same age whose exposure to spoken language has been limited and where the main mode of communication is manual. Of course, children with postlingually acquired deafness are likely to be able to benefit greatly from an implant regardless of age and this subset of children tend to be the ones demonstrating the best outcomes in terms of speech recognition.

In young children, establishing their precise hearing levels can sometimes be difficult. In most cases, however, hearing aids should have been fitted and aided hearing thresholds should be obtainable by the usual behavioural methods. This has led McCormick, Cope and Robinson (1998) to propose an audiometric criterion based on aided hearing thresholds at 2 and 4 kHz of 55 dB(A). This figure is obtained from an analysis of speech recognition performance on the McCormick toy test in a large number of children with hearing aids and relating this to their aided levels. Adoption of this method allows the audiologist to identify from routinely available data those children who might be candidates for an implant (but does not determine which ones should be implanted).

In children and adults, many variables need to be carefully assessed and taken into consideration when deciding if an implant is the best treatment for each individual. This decision making in a paediatric programme can sometimes be very difficult indeed. Older children should be involved as far as possible in decisions about their own treatment, but ultimately the responsibility falls on parents and the implant team has a duty to explain all the reasons for and against an implant for the child. In all cases, establishing appropriate expectations is crucial and time spent devoted to this is unavoidable. Many teams use the Children's Implant Profile or 'ChIP,' which is a useful way to bring together the relevant information to help form a decision. An adult version known as the Adult Implant Profile or 'AIP' has been developed and is equally useful.

## Imaging

Imaging of the internal anatomy of the cochlea, middle ear and mastoid is an important part of the assessment process when considering a possible cochlear implant. The surgeon needs to assess whether it is surgically possible to insert an electrode array into the cochlea itself and also how easy the surgical approach through to the cochlea is likely to be. The information provided by radiological imaging frequently determines the choice of ear for surgery. In conditions known to increase the risk of ossification within the cochlea, such as meningitis, this is crucial, although as already mentioned it is increasingly rarer for surgeons to be unable to insert an electrode array at least partially.

Imaging techniques have been refined considerably in recent years and MRI scans are now frequently made use of in addition to (and sometimes in place of) CT scans. Three-dimensional computer reconstructions can provide an amazingly clear image of the internal anatomy of the cochlea and thereby give surgeons greater confidence in electrode insertion.

## Surgery

Cochlear implant surgery inevitably remains a fairly large and somewhat complex procedure but has become routine in the hands of experienced surgeons. The basic approach, involving a skin flap behind the ear and drilling through the mastoid, has undergone relatively minor variations only. Some surgeons have developed a smaller post-aural incision, which has the benefit of resulting in a smaller scar, and is especially suitable for children.

Cochleas obstructed by new bone growth, as is sometimes found in post-meningitic cases, do not present the problem they have done previously, as many surgeons have much greater confidence in drilling through ossification by various techniques. Multiple electrode arrays (see pp. 312–13) have also been successfully used in cases where full insertion of the normal intra-cochlear array is difficult or impossible.

The surgical complication rate has generally been acceptably low and major complications are generally rare. Minor post-surgical complications are slightly less rare but still uncommon compared with other forms of surgery. However, it would be wrong to underestimate the 'annoyance factor' to patients of apparently minor postoperative side effects, for example loss of taste, minor wound infections or slight pain around the implant package site, which occasionally occur.

## Programming

The dynamic range for electrical stimulation of the auditory nerve is much less than that obtained with auditory stimulation. It is therefore important to ensure that levels of electrical stimulation in cochlear implants do not exceed comfortable levels, and that any non-auditory sensations are avoided. All implant systems therefore require careful programming and this activity inevitably occupies much time for audiologists working with implanted patients.

Implant programming requires the audiologist to establish both the lowest level of electrical stimulation that produces an auditory sensation (threshold or T-level), and the highest comfortable level (C-level) for each of the stimulating electrodes. These values, often expressed in terms of stimulation-level units that relate to the current and pulse-width delivered, are stored as a 'map' in the speech processor.

Adults are usually able to describe the sounds they are perceiving and to report loudness growth, pitch changes, etc. In children, the programming is inevitably slower and more time-consuming. In the very young child, a conditioned response to sound may not be established and the audiologist must therefore rely on observation of involuntary responses to stimulation, such as stilling, blinking, head turns, etc. Modified Visual Reinforcement Audiometry can sometimes be used to obtain estimates of threshold levels, and some objective measures (see below) can provide estimated stimulation levels. Accurate estimation of the highest comfortable levels is frequently difficult in young children. Congenitally deaf children, even if the audiologist is able to communicate with them through sign, may not understand the concepts of 'louder' and 'softer', and establishing the true dynamic range is therefore much harder. Recent evidence that electrically elicited stapedius thresholds correlate closely to C-levels may point to a potentially new method (Cullington et al. 1998).

## Objective measures

Techniques for objectively measuring performance of cochlear implants and responses to them have been considerably refined in recent years. This approach is particularly valuable in assessment of young children, where behavioural responses and feedback from the child may not be relied on as it is with adults.

A number of responses can be recorded to provide information about the functioning of the implant and the effects of electrical stimulation on the auditory system. Many current implant designs are capable of reverse telemetry, whereby the implant itself feeds information back to the audiologist, confirming the function or otherwise of electrodes, their impedances and the integrity of the implanted receiver package itself. Electrically evoked auditory brainstem responses are also widely used to give estimated threshold levels and the electrically evoked stapedius reflex is frequently used intraoperatively to provide both evidence of functioning electrodes and estimated C-levels. Perhaps the most exciting development has been a technique known as Neural Response Telemetry, in which action potentials from the cochlea are elicited by stimulation through the implanted electrodes and also recorded by different electrodes in the array. It is hoped that this new method will provide direct evidence of the quality of neural tissue surrounding each stimulating electrode and so potentially help optimize performance by 'tailoring' electrical stimulation to match the neural conditions in the cochlea.

## Rehabilitation and results

Many adults receiving modern, 'third-generation' cochlear implants can obtain surprisingly good performance, including open-set speech discrimination, sometimes including telephone conversations, very quickly with relatively little rehabilitation support. However, even with the best devices available a small but significant subset of implant users still gain marginal benefit, which may amount only to awareness of sounds, enhanced lip-reading and reduced awareness of tinnitus, with no open-set speech recognition. These patients require ongoing encouragement, and both analytical and synthetic auditory training have an important role to play in enabling them to maximize their potential benefit and in monitoring their progress. Speech or hearing therapists are therefore an indispensible part of the implant team and although technically implants can be provided to most adults, without their input the outcomes are likely to be reduced.

In the paediatric programme, much of the responsibility for ensuring that children receive the most appropriate input and make the best use of their implant falls on their family, carers and the adults providing their education. It is widely accepted that it is important for exposure to spoken language to be available to the children with an implant, and considerable evidence that children in settings where this emphasis is made gain more from their implants than those in settings where manual communication predominates. The paediatric implant rehabilitation team comprising teachers of the deaf and speech and language therapists have a key role in monitoring progress, developing rehabilitation plans and advising those who are in daily contact with the children how to maximize their potential to benefit.

## The future

All aspects of cochlear implants have moved on so fast since they first came on the scene that it is sometimes difficult to anticipate what might happen next. As already mentioned, much work is being done on speech processing and much is yet to be learned about the possibilities for improving performance by manipulating parameters of stimulation, such as stimulation rate, channel selection, etc. There is certainly a feeling that performance of implants can be refined and improved in these ways but also a recognition that gains in performance may be asymptotic (see Wilson 1997 for a more detailed review of the future of cochlear implants). It is to be hoped that performance in background noise can be enhanced. Even the patients who perform well in quiet conditions are often badly affected by noise and this naturally limits the benefit they gain in real-life conditions. Small numbers of patients have now received bilateral implants and this should throw light on the question of whether binaural integration can occur with electrical stimulation.

The trend in relaxation of selection criteria is probably likely to continue though, as mentioned above, the practice in the UK lags behind that in the USA in terms of implantation of patients with significant levels of residual hearing. Also, the trend towards younger and younger children receiving implants seems to continue.

There is no doubt that most implant manufacturers have a strong commitment to technological refinement and development of the implant systems themselves. Most are likely to be able to offer patients a choice of ear-level or body-worn speech processors in the near future and this has already arrived for two devices. It is difficult to predict whether this represents a trend towards increasing miniaturization with the ultimate goal being a completely implantable device without external hardware, but this prospect seems likely and the next few years will show whether such a development is a realistic possibility. There is no doubt that cochlear implantation will remain a hugely exciting field for many years to come.

# Chapter 20
# Implantable hearing aids

ANDERS TJELLSTRÖM

During the past few decades interest in implantable hearing aids has increased. In this chapter, we discuss implants used to excite the otic capsule and cochlea, and those that are attached to the ossicular chain (cochlear implants are not discussed here as they are covered in Chapter 19). The important difference between these two types of aid are that the former need a functioning cochlea, whereas the latter are used when the hair cells of the cochlea have degenerated or do not function normally. The physiology of hearing is discussed in Chapter 3 and the focus here is on hearing by bone conduction.

## Bone conduction

Hearing through bone conduction has been investigated during the past 50 years by scientists such as Barany (1938), Kirikae (1958), von Békésy (1960) and Tonndorf (1966). According to Tonndorf, the cochlea is excited in three different ways: by compression, by sound radiation and by inertia.

In compression excitation of the cochlea, there are spatial changes of the bone enclosing the cochlea. Displacement of the basilar membrane with the hair cells is partly due to the fact that scala tympani and scala vestibuli have different volumes, and partly because of the different mechanical properties of the oval and round windows. The different mechanical load of the two windows is a third factor. The cochlea is also excited by sound radiation from the bony walls of the external ear canal and from the walls of the middle-ear cavity. This sound is then transmitted through the windows. The most important factor in excitation of the cochlea by bone conduction, however, is the inertia of the cochlear fluids, which is affected by inertia of the middle-ear ossicles and the eardrum.

Compressional excitation contributes to the total bone-conduction response mainly for the high frequencies, and sound radiation in the middle- and high-frequency range, but the most important factor in excitation of the cochlea is the inertia of the cochlear fluids.

In 1960, von Békésy published an experiment where he showed that sound of a specific frequency presented through the external ear canal was almost totally cancelled by a sound of the same frequency produced through a bone vibrator placed on the mastoid process. The levels of the sound were adjusted to equal loudness and by adjusting the relative phase angle von Békésy showed that a previously audible sound could be made to disappear. This elegant experiment indicates that airborne sound and sound produced through vibrating the skull excite the inner ear in the same way and give identical stimuli to the cochlear nerve. Hearing through bone conduction is thus no different from hearing through air conduction.

Brandt (1989) studied the characteristics of sound transmission through the human skull in vivo by using patients with bilateral skin penetrating implants in the skull. The transcranial attenuation of bone-conducted sound between the temporal bones was found to vary considerably with frequency and was in the range of –5 to 55 dB. The negative value indicates an amplification. Brandt also found that the sound transmission was linear.

## Transducers for bone-conduction hearing aids

Transducers for bone-conduction hearing aids are named bone conductors, vibrators or transducers. The most commonly used type of transducers in bone-conduction hearing aids are electromechanical transducers. These transducers are small in size, have a high output capability, wide frequency range, low level of distortion and low consumption of current. These properties are of great value for a hearing aid. Piezoelectric and magnetostrictive transducers on the other hand are less suitable in this field because a poor low-frequency response and, for the piezoelectric transducer, a high voltage are needed. Ordinary hearing aid batteries are not designed for such working conditions and a high current consumption could cause voltage variations, which might interfere with the internal electrical stability. The electroacoustic performance of an electrodynamic transducer of the variable reluctance type is thus a favourable transducer in hearing aids.

## 'Old-fashioned' bone-conduction hearing aids

In the traditional bone-conduction hearing aid the transducer is positioned over the mastoid process and the vibrations are transmitted through the skin to the skull. The transducer is continuously pressed against the skin over the mastoid process by a steel spring, a pair of glasses or a headband. The force that these arrangements produce is 3–4 N. This force causes an uncomfortable sensation of pressure and the skin often becomes irritated and tender. A long static force will also often affect the soft tissues and deep impressions in the skin at the site of the transducer are not uncommon. The skin is mobile and it is difficult to obtain consistent transmission conditions. The skin also acts as an attenuater of the vibration signal, which results in the need for a high vibratory output. This can lead to distortion and decreased clarity of the sound. High signal levels also means that the transducer and the microphone have to be kept apart to avoid acoustic feedback in the hearing aid.

## Bone-conduction implants

Two different devices have been available for clinical use. The bone-anchored hearing aid, BAHA, was developed in Sweden by the present author, Dr Per-Ingvar Brânemark and Dr Bo Hakansson, Göteborg, Sweden. It is manufactured by Nobel Biocare AB, Göteborg, Sweden.

The other, the Audiant, was developed in the USA by Dr Jack Hough and his co-workers in Oklahoma City, Oklahoma, and Dr Jack Vernon, Portland, Oregon, and is manufactured by Xomed Inc., Jacksonville, Florida, USA.

The BAHA, which was introduced in 1977, has a direct contact between a screw-shaped implant placed in the bone of the mastoid process and the transducer through a skin-penetrating coupling. The implant, made of commercially pure titanium, is allowed to osseointegrate, using a technique described by Tjellström in 1989. The design of the BAHA is illustrated in Figure 20.1. An important feature of the device is that the air gap between the two parts of the transducer is 0.05 mm and it has a well-defined suspension arrangement. The short gap is of great advantage for the function of the hearing instrument. Audiological data as well as statistics concerning the skin reactions have been published by Hakansson et al. (1990a,b), Mylanus (1994) and Proops (1996). The current BAHA, HC 300 Classic is shown in Figure 20.2.

The Audiant was introduced in 1984. This hearing aid consists of two parts, one internal and one external. The internal part consists of a strong rare earth magnet housed in a titanium disc and coated with medical-grade silicone. This is attached to the skull via a Herbert orthopaedic screw. The external device is the sound processor, including a second rare earth magnet and an induction coil. The distance between the internal and the external parts is 4–6 mm, with skin and subcutaneous tissue in between. The transmission is thus transcutaneous and there is no skin penetration. The design is shown in Figure 20.3. Clinical experience with this device has been published by Gates et al. (1989).

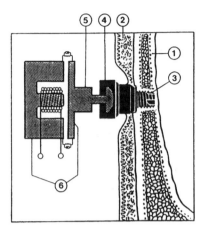

**Figure 20.1:** Percutaneous transducer used by BAHA. 1: Mastoid process; 2: soft tissue; 3: titanium screw (fixture); 4: skin-penetrating titanium coupling; 5: bayonet coupling; 6: external transducer unit.

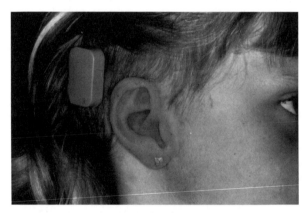

**Figure 20.2:** Current model of BAHA, HC 300 Classic fitted on an 8-year-old girl with bilateral artresia. Note: The external ear is a silicon prosthesis also retained on osseointegrated implants.

# Indications for bone-conduction hearing aids

For various reasons, some patients who need amplification cannot wear an air-conduction hearing aid with a mould in the external ear canal. The most obvious are patients who do not have any ear canals due to congenital malformation. Another indication is patients with chronic ear infection with constant or intermittent drainage from their ears despite attempts to eradicate the infection by medication and through surgical procedures. A third group of patients for whom a bone-conduction aid could be a good

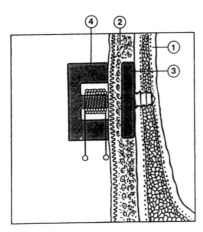

**Figure 20.3:** Transcutaneous transducer used by Audiant. 1: Mastoid bone; 2: soft tissue between the magnets; 3: implanted magnet with Herbert orthopaedic screw; 4: external part of the transducer.

alternative to a conventional hearing aid are those in whom the material of the earmould irritates the external ear canal. A maximum conductive hearing loss can sometimes be easier to overcome with a bone conductor than with an air-conduction aid.

One big advantage of implants in the cortical shell of the mastoid over tympanoplasty surgery is that there is no risk of inner-ear damage from surgical trauma. For the ear-level BAHA a bone-conduction threshold better than 45 dB for the speech frequencies is recommended. For patients with a sensorineural hearing loss greater than 45 dB, a stronger, body-worn aid, the Cordelle, is available from the same manufacturer. It should be noted that the size of the air–bone gap is of no significance, only the cochlear reserve. There are few contraindications to the device but patients with psychiatric disorders and those indulging in drug abuse should not be considered, as cooperation with the therapeutic team is essential. Children as young as two years of age have been treated with the BAHA and there seems to be no upper age limit.

The Audiant was initially tried by a large number of surgeons but as many patients did not experience the benefit of the device it has now been taken off the market. The reason the Audiant did not give the desirable loudness level for many patients was that the output from the Audiant 'saturated' at a level 20 dB lower than the BAHA. This meant that although tests showed that it performed well at threshold levels, it did not have enough gain at speech level, which is the level at which hearing aids are normally used.

As the Audiant is no longer available, the BAHA is, at present, the device of choice when a bone transducer is needed.

For patients with absence or malformation of the pinna (for example in congenital microtia) the osseointegrated percutaneous post allows attachment of a prosthesis.

## Middle-ear implants

Over the past decade there has been a growing interest in implants working on the ossicular chain. The ultimate goal is to have a totally implantable hearing aid with an implanted microphone and implanted rechargeable batteries. Such a device is not yet available, but several semi-implantable hearing aids in this category are under development.

In Japan, Suzuki and Yanagihara have been working on a semi-implantable as well as a totally implantable hearing aid (Suzuki et al. 1988). Both these have a framework attached to the wall of a mastoid cavity and a piezoelectric vibrator connected to an intact and mobile stapes (as illustrated in Figure 20.4). About 70 patients have had this device implanted. Few patients have been operated on outside Japan (Suzuki J-I, personal communication, 1998).

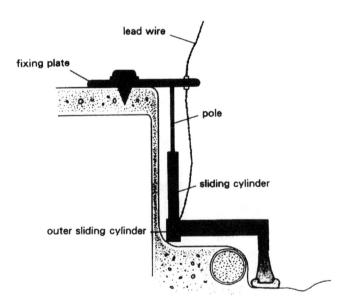

**Figure 20.4:** Schematic drawing of the Suzuki–Yanagihara vibrator fixed in the mastoid cortex and with the piezoelectric bimorph attached to the stapes. From Yanagihara, Gyo and Hinohira 1995.

A design reported by Fredricson and co-workers has a titanium shaft implanted into the incus (Fredrickson, Coticchia and Khosla 1996). This rod is driven by a transducer placed in the squamous portion of the temporal bone. Maniglia et al. (1997) use a very strong and biocompatible bone cement to fix a small but strong magnet to the incus as one part of a transducer; the other part is an electromagnet placed in the mastoid cavity, together with the internal wiring. Bench tests with both these devices are very promising and the fidelity of the sound is reported to be very good. However, none of these are at present available on the market for general use. Dr Hough, who was the original inventor of the Audiant, has a new device under development and there are plans to start clinical trials.

A new, strong vibrator called the Floating Mass Transducer (FMT) has been developed by Geoffrey Ball in California. This transducer is used in a new device called the VORP (vibrating ossicular prosthesis) or Sound Bridge, produced by the Symphonix company. The transducer itself is only 1.5 x 2 mm (Figure 20.5). It is attached to the long process of the incus, and the rest of the electronics are placed in the bony cortex of the mastoid (Figure 20.6). Short-term clinical results from a study with more than 100 patients in Europe are very promising, and the patients also report good fidelity of the sound with this device (Cooper, personal communication). A most interesting new refinement made by this company is an implantable microphone with good fidelity even when it is covered by 6 mm of skin and soft tissue. This, together with an implantable, rechargeable battery, is an important step in the development of a totally implanted hearing aid.

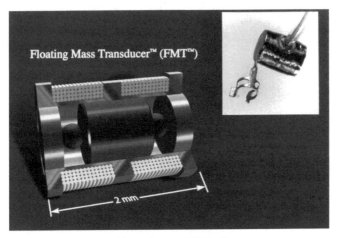

**Figure 20.5:** The Floating Mass Transducer (FMT). The permanent magnet inside is suspended by compressible plastic balls and surrounded by an external coil. The insert shows the transducer with the connecting wire and the attachment for the long process of incus. Provided by the Symphonix Devices AG.

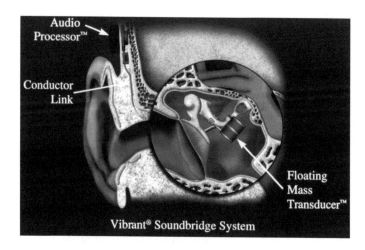

**Figure 20.6:** Schematic view of the arrangement with the FMT in place in the middle ear.

## Summary

Middle-ear implants have yet to establish a clear role for themselves in the rehabilitation of people with sensorineural hearing loss. In contrast, bone-anchored hearing aids have an important place in the management of some adults with conductive hearing loss and are considered by many to be the treatment of choice for children with bilateral congenital conductive deafness.

# References

Publication dates for the IEC and ISO standards listed below are not given, and readers are referred to the latest versions as listed on the IEC and ISO websites at www.iec.ch and www.iso.ch

Altshuler K (1971) Studies of the deaf: relevance to psychiatric theory. American Journal of Psychiatry 127.11, 1521–6.

Altshuler KZ (1986) Perceptual handicap and mental illness, with special reference to early profound deafness. American Journal of Social Psychiatry VI(2), 125–8.

Altshuler KZ, Deming WE, Vollenweider J, Rainer JD, Tendler R (1976) Impulsivity and early profound deafness: a cross-cultural inquiry. American Annals of the Deaf 121, 331–45.

American Psychiatric Association (1994) Diagnostic and Statistical Manual of Mental Disorders, 4th edn. Washington DC: American Psychiatric Association.

Andersson G, Melin L, Scott B, Lindberg P (1995) An evaluation of a behavioural approach to hearing impairment. Behaviour Research & Therapy 33, 283–92.

Baldwin M, Watkin P (1997) Diagnostic procedures. In: McCracken W, Laoide-Kemp S (eds), Audiology in Education. London: Whurr, pp 3–79.

Barany E (1938) A contribution to the physiology of bone conduction. Acta Otolaryngology (Stockholm) Suppl 26.

Barcham LJ, Stephens SDG (1980) The use of an open ended questionnaire in auditory rehabilitation. British Journal of Audiology 14, 49–54.

Basilier T (1964) Surdophrenia: the psychic consequences of congenital or early acquired deafness. Acta Psychiatrica Scandinavica 40.180, 362–72.

Beck J (1995) Cognitive Therapy: basics and beyond. Hove: Guilford Press.

Békésy von G (1960) Experiments in Hearing. New York: McGraw-Hill.

Békésy von G (1980) Experiments in Hearing. New York: Robert ER Krieger.

Brandt A (1989) On sound transmission characteristics of the human skull in vivo. Licentiate thesis No 61L, Chalmers University of Technology, Göteborg, Sweden.

British Society of Audiology (1988) British Society of Audiology recommendation –descriptors for pure-tone audiograms. British Journal of Audiology 22, 123.

British Society of Audiology (1998) Careers in audiology. Reading: BSA.

Chess S, Fernandez P (1981) Do deaf children have a typical personality? Annual Progress in Child Psychiatry & Child Development 19, 295–305.

Cody AR, Russell IJ (1987) The responses of hair cells in the basal turn of the guinea pig cochlea to tones. Journal of Physiology 383, 551–69.

Coles RRA, Davis AC, Smith P (1990) Tinnitus: its epidemiology and management. In Jensen JH (ed) Presbyacusis and other age related aspects. Conference 14th Danavox Jubilee Foundation, Copenhagen, pp 377–401.

Court SDM (ed) (1976) Fit for the Future. The report of the Committee on Child Health Services. London: HMSO.

Cullington H, Hodges AV, Butts SL, Dolan-Ash S, Balkany TJ (1998) The use of middle ear muscle reflexes in post-operative programming procedures. Presentation at the First International Symposium and Workshop on Objective Measures in Cochlear Implantation, Nottingham.

Davis AC (1989)The prevalence of hearing impairment and reported hearing disability among adults in Great Britain. International Journal of Epidemiology 18, 911–17.

Davis AC (1991) Epidemiological profile of hearing impairments: the scale and nature of the problem with special reference to the elderly. Acta Otolaryngologica (Stockholm) 23–31.

Davis AC (1995) Hearing in Adults. London: Whurr.

Davis A, Bamford J, Wilson I, Ramkalawan T, Forshaw M, Wright S (1997) Screening children's hearing: a critical review of the role of neonatal screening in the detection of congenital hearing impairment. Health Technology Assessment 1.

Davis A, Wood S (1992) The epidemiology of childhood hearing impairment: factors relevant to planning services. British Journal of Audiology 26, 77–90.

Denes PB, Pinson EN (1993) The Speech Chain: the physics and biology of spoken language. New York: WH Freeman.

Evans EK (1975) Cochlear nerve and cochlear nucleus. In: Keidel WD, Neff ED (eds) Handbook of Sensory Physiology, pp 1–108. Berlin: Springer.

Farrugia D (1992) Borderline personality disorder and deafness. Journal of the American Deafness & Rehabilitation Association 25.3, 8–15.

Field D, Haggard MP (1989) Knowledge of hearing tactics – assessment by questionnaire and inventory. British Journal of Audiology 23, 349–54.

Fortnum H, Davis A (1997)Epidemiology of permanent childhood hearing impairment in Trent region, 1985–1993. British Journal of Audiology 31, 409–46.

Fortnum HM, Haggard MP (1984) A population study of the use/non-use of hearing aids. Presented to a meeting of the British Society of Audiology, September.

Fredrickson JM, Coticchia JM Khosla S (1996) Current status in the development of implantable middle ear hearing aids. Advances in Otolaryngology 10, 189–204.

Fry S (1998) Moab is my Washpot. London: Random House, pp 100–1.

Gantz BJ, Woodworth GG, Abbas PJ, Knutson JF, Tyler RS (1993) Multivariate predictors of audiological success with multi-channel cochlear implants. Annals of Otology, Rhinology and Laryngology 102, 909–16.

Gatehouse S (1999) The Glasgow Hearing Aid Benefit Profile: derivation and validation of a client centred outcome measure for hearing aid services. Journal of the American Academy of Audiology 10, 80–103.

Gates GA, Hough JV, Gatti WM, Bradley WH (1989) The safety and effectiveness of an implanted electromagnetic hearing device. Archives of Otolaryngology Head and Neck Surgery 115, 924–30.

Gerber BM (1983) A communication minority: deaf people and mental health care. American Journal of Social Psychiatry III(2), 50–7.

Goldstein D, Stephens SDG (1981) Audiological rehabilitation: management model I. Audiology 20, 432–52.

Goodman R (1996) The Strengths and Difficulties questionnaire: a research note. Journal of Child Psychology and Psychiatry 38, 581–6.

Green R (1997) The uses and misuses of speech audiometry in rehabilitation. In: Martin M (ed), Speech Audiometry. London: Whurr.

Greenberg MT, Calderon R (1984) Early intervention for deaf children: outcomes and issues. Topics in Early Childhood Special Education 3, 1–9.

Greenberg MT, Kusche C (1993) Promoting Social and Emotional Development in Deaf Children: the PATHS curriculum. Seattle, WA: Washington University Press.

Gregory S, Bishop J, Sheldon L (1995) Deaf Young People and their Families. Cambridge: Cambridge University Press.

Grinker RR, Werble B, Dye R (1977) The Borderline Syndrome. New York: Basic Books.

Haggard MP, Hughes EA (1991) Screening children's hearing: a review of the literature and the implications of otitis media. London: HMSO.

Heller MF, Bergman M (1953) Tinnitus in normally hearing persons. Annals of Otology 62, 73–93.

Hákansson B, Lidén G, Tjellström A, Ringdahl A, Carlsson P, Erlandsson B-E (1990a) Ten years of experience with the Swedish bone-anchored hearing system. Annals of Otology Rhinology and Laryngology 99(10), 2 (Suppl 51).

Hákansson B, Tjellström A, Carlsson P (1990b) Percutaneous vs transcutaneous transducers for hearing by direct bone conduction. Otolaryngology Head and Neck Surgery 102(4), 339–44.

Hills CG, Rappold ES, Rendon ME (1991) Binge eating and body image in a sample of the deaf college population. Journal of the American Deafness & Rehabilitation Association 25.2, 20–8.

Hindley PA (1997) Psychiatric aspects of hearing impairment. Journal of Child Psychology and Psychiatry 34, 101–17.

Hindley PA, Brown R (1994) Psychiatric aspects of sensory impairment. In: Rutter M, Taylor E, Hersov L (eds) Modern Approaches to Child and Adolescent Psychiatry, pp 720–36. Oxford: Blackwell Scientific.

Hindley PA, Hill PD, McGuigan S, Kitson N (1994) Psychiatric disorder in deaf and hearing impaired children and young people: a prevalence study. Journal of Child Psychology and Psychiatry 55.5, 917–34.

Hood JD (1984) Speech discrimination in bilateral and unilateral hearing loss due to Ménière's disease. British Journal of Audiology 18, 173–7.

Hounsfield GN (1973) Computerised transverse axial scanning (tomography): part 1. Description of system. British Journal of Radiology 46, 1016–22.

IEC 60118-4 Hearing aids. Part 4: Magnetic field strength in audio-frequency induction loops for hearing aid purposes. Geneva: International Electrotechnical Commission.

IEC 60318-1 Simulators of human head and ear. Part 1: Ear simulator for the calibration of supra-aural earphones. Geneva: International Electrotechnical Commission.

IEC 60318-3 Simulators of human head and ear. Part 3: Acoustic coupler for the calibration of supra-aural earphones used in audiometry. Geneva: International Electrotechnical Commission.

IEC 60318-6 Simulators of human head and ear. Part 6: Mechanical coupler for measurements on bone vibrators. Geneva: International Electrotechnical Commission.

IEC 60645-1 Audiometers. Part 1: Pure tone audiometers. Geneva: International Electrotechnical Commission.

IEC 60645-2 Audiometers. Part 2: Equipment for speech audiometry. Geneva: International Electrotechnical Commission.

ISO 389-1 Reference zero for the calibration of audiometric equipment. Part 1: Reference equivalent threshold SPLs for pure tones and supra-aural earphones. Geneva: International Standards Organization.

ISO 389-3 Reference zero for the calibration of audiometric equipment. Part 1: Reference equivalent threshold force levels for pure tones and bone vibrators. Geneva: International Standards Organization.

ISO 389-4 Reference zero for the calibration of audiometric equipment. Part 4: Reference levels for narrow band masking. Geneva: International Standards Organization.

ISO 389-7 Reference zero for the calibration of audiometric equipment. Part 7: Reference threshold of hearing under free-field and diffuse-field listening conditions. Geneva: International Standards Organization.

ISO 6189 Acoustics – Pure tone air conduction audiometry for hearing conservation purposes. Geneva: International Standards Organization.

ISO 8253-1 Acoustics – Audiometric test methods. Part 1: Basic pure tone air and bone conduction audiometry. Geneva: International Standards Organization.

ISO 8253-2 Acoustics – Audiometric test methods. Part 2: Sound field audiometry with pure tone and narrow-band test signals. Geneva: International Standards Organization.

ISO 8253-3 Acoustics – Audiometric test methods. Part 3: Speech audiometry. Geneva: International Standards Organization.

Jastreboff PJ (1990) Phantom auditory perception (tinnitus): mechanisms of generation and perception. Neuroscience Research 8, 221–54.

Johnson M (1996) Models of disability. The Psychologist May, 205–10.

Jure R, Rapin I, Tuchman RF (1991) Hearing impaired autistic children. Developmental Medicine and Child Neurology 33, 1062–72.

Keller H (1910) Letter to Dr John Kerr Love, dated 31 March. Reprinted in Helen Keller in Scotland, a personal record written by herself (Kerr Love J, ed), p 68. London: Methuen (1933)

Kemp DT (1978) Stimulated acoustic emissions from within the human auditory system. Journal of the Acoustical Society of America 64, 1386–91.

Kennedy M (1992) The case for interpreters – exploring communication with children who are deaf. Child Abuse Review 1, 191–3.

Kerr P, Cowie R (1997) Acquired deafness: a multidimensional experience. British Journal of Audiology 31, 177–88.

Kiang NY-S, Moxon EC, Levine RA (1970) Auditory nerve activity in cats with normal and abnormal cochleas. In: Wolstenholms GEW, Knight J (eds), Sensorineural Hearing Loss, pp 241–68. Ciba Foundation Symposium. London: Churchill

Kirikae I (1959) An experimental study on the fundamental mechanism of bone conduction. Acta Otolaryngology (Stockholm) Suppl 145.

Kitson, N, Thacker A (1999) Adult psychiatry. In: Hindley PA, Kitson N (eds) Mental Health and Deafness: a multi-disciplinary handbook. London: Whurr.

Kyle JG, Woll B (1985) Sign language. Cambridge: Cambridge University Press.

Laszig R, Sollman WP, Marangos N, Charachon R, Ramsden R (1995) Nucleus 20-channel and 21-channel auditory brain stem implants: first European experiences. Annals of Otology, Rhinology and Laryngology 104(9), 28–31 (Supplement 166)

Luterman D (1987) Working with the deaf family. In: Luterman D, Deafness in the Family, pp 99–117). Boston, MA: College Hill.

Maniglia AJ, Wen HK, Garverick SL et al. (1997) Semi-implantable middle ear electromagnetic hearing device for sensorineural hearing loss. ENT Journal 76(5).

Martin JAM, Bentzen O, Colley JRT, Hennebert D, Holm C, Iurato S, Dejonge GA, McCullen O, Meyer ML, Moore WJ, Morgon A (1981) Childhood deafness in the European Community. Scandinavian Audiology 10, 165–74.

McCormick B, Cope Y, Robinson K (1998) An audiometric selection criterion for paediatric cochlear implantation. Presentation at the 4th European Symposium on Paediatric Cochlear Implantation, s-Hertogenbosch, The Netherlands.

McKenna L (1987) Goal planning in audiological rehabilitation. British Journal of Audiology 21, 5–11.

McKenna L, Andersson G (1998) Hearing disorders. In: Bellack A, Hersen M (eds) Comprehensive Clinical Psychology, Vol 9: Applications in Diverse Populations. Oxford: Elsevier.

McKenna L, Hallam R, Hinchcliffe R (1991) The prevalence of psychological disturbance in neuro-otology outpatients. Clinical Otolaryngology 16, 452–6.

Meadow-Orlans KP, Erting CE (1999) Deaf people in society. In: Hindley PA, Kitson N (eds) Mental Health and Deafness: a multi-disciplinary handbook. London: Whurr.

Misiaszek J, Dooling J, Gieseke A, Melman H, Misiaszek JG, Jorgensen K (1985) Diagnostic considerations in deaf patients. Comprehensive Psychiatry 26.6, 513–21.

Mylanus EAM (1994) The bone anchored hearing aid: clinical and audiological aspects. Thesis Proesfchrifa, Nijmegen, the Netherlands.

NIH Consensus Statement (1995) Cochlear Implants in Adults and Children. National Institutes of Health 13(2).

Proops D (1996) The Birmingham bone anchored hearing programme 1988–1995. Journal of Laryngology and Otology 110 (Suppl 21).

Quittner AL, Glueckauf RL, Jackson DN (1990).Chronic parenting stress: moderating versus mediating effects of social support. Journal of Personality and Social Psychology 59, 1266–78.

Reed H (1999) Deaf Children in Mind: personal and social initiative. Final report to the Department of Health. London: NDCS.

Richardson H, Clarke G, Hawthorne M (1998) A multi-array cochlear implant for the ossified cochlea: development and surgical technique. Presentation at the 4th European Symposium on Paediatric Cochlear Implantation, 's-Hertogenbosch, The Netherlands.

Sancho-Aldridge J, Davis A (1993) The impact of hearing impairment on television viewing in the UK. London: Independent Television Commission.

Sarlin MB, Altshuler KZ (1978) On the inter-relationship of cognition and affect: fantasies of deaf children. Child Psychiatry and Development 9.2, 95–103.

Schuknecht HF (1993) Pathology of the ear, 2nd edn. Lea & Febiger.

Sellick PM, Patuzzi R, Johnstone BM (1982) Measurement of basilar membrane motion in guinea pigs using the Mossbauer technique. Journal of the Acoustical Society of America 72, 131–41.

Sever JL, South MA, Shaver KA (1985) Delayed manifestations of congenital rubella. Reviews of Infectious Diseases 7, 164–9.

Sinkkonen J (1994) Hearing Impairment, Communication and Personality Development. Helsinki, Finland: Department of Child Psychiatry, University of Helsinki.

Stephens SDG, Hetu R (1991) Impairment, disability and handicap in audiology: towards a consensus. Audiology 30, 185–200.

Stephens SDG, Meredith R, Callaghan DE, Hogan S, Rayment A et al. (1991) Early intervention and rehabilitation – factors influencing outcome. Acta Oto-larygologica Suppl. 476, 221–5. From International Workshop on Hearing in the Aged, Elsingor, Denmark, November 1989.

Sullivan PM, Brookhouser PE, Scanlan JM (2000) Maltreatment of deaf and hard of hearing children. In Hindley PA, Kitson N (eds) Mental Health and Deafness: a multi-disciplinary handbook. London: Whurr.

Summerfield AQ, Marshall DH (1995) Cochlear Implantation in the UK 1990–1994. London: London.

Suzuki J-I, Yanagihara N, Toriyama M, Sakabe N (1988) Principle, construction and indication of middle ear implant. Advances in Audiology 4, 15–21.

Thomas A, Gilhome-Herbst K (1980) Social and psychological implications of acquired deafness for adults of employment age. British Journal of Audiology 14, 76–85.

Tjellström A (1989) Osseointegrated systems and their applications in the head and neck. Advances in Otolaryngology Head and Neck Surgery 3, 39–70.

Tonndorf J (1966) Bone conduction. Acta Otolaryngology (Stockholm), Suppl 213.

Tyler RS (1992) Audiological aspects of Cochlear Implants. London: Whurr.

Vaccari C, Marschark M (1997) Communication between parents and deaf children: implications for social-emotional development. Journal of Child Psychology and Psychiatry 38, 793–801.

Vernon McC, Andrews JF (1990) The Psychology of Deafness, chapter 8. New York & London: Longman.

Wilson BS (1997) The future of cochlear implants. British Journal of Audiology 31, 205–25.

Wilson BS, Finley CC, Lawson DT, Wolford RD, Eddington DK, Rabinowitz WM (1991) Better speech recognition with cochlear implants. Natyre 352, 236–8.

World Health Organization (1980) International Classification of Impairments and Disabilities and Handicaps. Geneva: WHO.

World Health Organization (1992) The ICD-10 Classification of Mental and Behavioural Disorders: clinical descriptions and diagnostic guidelines. Geneva: WHO.

World Health Organization (1997) International Classification of Impairments, Activities and Participation. Geneva: WHO (website: http://www.who.ch/icidh).

Yanagihara N, Gyo K, Hinohira Y (1995) Partially impalpable hearing aid using piezoelectric ceramic ossicular vibrator: results of the implant operation and assessment of the hearing afforded by the device. Otolaryngology Clinics of North America 28, 85–8.

# Index

balloning of, 156, 157
resonance, 29, 56
    resonant frequency, 56
    peak, 61
rhesus haemolytic disease, 181, 192
rheumatoid arthritis, 180
rigidity, 286
Rinne's test, 73–4
round window, 32, 41,42, 49
    membrane rupture, 173
    obstruction, 49
    stimulation test, 111
rubella, 18, 19, 181, 190, 283–4

salicylates, ototoxicity of, 163
scala media, 42
    contents of, 43–7
scala tympani, 41
    obliteration, 131
scala vestibuli, 41, 42
schizoid personality, 287
schizophrenia, 260, 282–3, 284–5
screening and surveillance, 194–9
    neonatal, 1, 115, 197–9
    programmes, 21
    satisfaction with, 21
    selective, 199
    tests, 89
    universal, 21, 199
sensorineural hearing loss
    acquired, chapter 10 passim
    causes, children, 182
    idiopathic, 178–9
    prevalence, 15
    sudden onset, 154
    and trauma, 154
    unilateral, 154
sensory nerves, 29
services for deafness, 20–4
    satisfaction with, 21–2
    prioritization of, 10
sigmoid sinus, 32, 37
sign language, signing, 5, 219, 272, 273–4
    and children, 275
    and infants, 277
silence, and hyperacusis, 251, 253
sinewave, 59, 60
social skills, 277

sound
    amplitude, 59
    enrichment, 253
    frequency, 49, 50, 58
    measurement, 59
    pressure, 49
    reinforcement, 253
    sound/electrical energy conversion,
        47–8, 102
    sound-field testing, 202
    source, 55–6
    waves, 58–64
source-filter model, 55
Spartan, 5
speech audiogram, 95–6
speech
    detection threshold level, 96
    development, 70–1
    discrimination, 153
        impaired, associated with hair cell
        loss, 154
        neonatal, 70
        and speech audiometry, 93
    perception, 6, 64–71, chapter 4 passim
        and noise-induced hearing loss,
        227–8
        paediatric tests, 204–6
    processing, processors, 313–15
    production, 5, 54–8
    quality, 56
    recognition, 290, 314
        curve, 98
        score, 96
        and speech audiometry, 93
        threshold level, 97
    sound, 55–6
        spectrographic representation,
        62–4
    synthetic, 65–6
    test material, 93–5
    variability, 64
Speech Chain, 1–2
speech-reading, 4, 67
stapedectomy, 146, 167–9
stapedial reflex, 106–7
    threshold, 106
stapedius muscle, 34, 106
stapes, 32, 33, 35, 49, 140